Library of
Davidson College

American medicine today is like a patient etherized upon a table, surrounded by a nation of diagnosticians wondering what to do. The question is, are Americans really getting the health care they are paying for? The answer is that they are not.

This book provides a searching and lucid diagnosis of what is wrong with the American system of medical care. It explains why so many Americans get more treatment than they need—unnecessary surgery is just one example—and why so many, prosperous as well as poor, get care that is second- or even third-rate. It explains why hospitals (whose charges have tripled in the last ten years) put money into new and enormously expensive facilities and equipment for which no real need exists. It explains why Medicaid has been such a disaster, and why the poor are made to pay so high a price in humiliation for those services that Medicaid was intended to secure for them.

Based on coast-to-coast investigation and research, this book is eloquently written in the one-man tradition of Lincoln Steffens and Rachel Carson. Here is the truth behind such things as crazy-quilt insurance coverage, the mad proliferation of hospitals, the indefensibly high price of prescription drugs, medical malpractice and greed, and the disappearance of the family physician, along with the invaluable personal services he performed. Here too are the facts about health maintenance organizations, and about how our fee-for-service medicine compares with medical care provided and paid for in different ways, as in Great Britain, Canada, and Europe.

Perhaps most important, *The Great American Medicine Show* offers cures as well as diagnoses. Mr. Klaw weighs the plusses and minuses of the various health-care programs now before Congress and proposes a number of very realistic reforms which, given a willingness to slaughter some sacred cows, could work for the benefit of us all.

THE GREAT AMERICAN MEDICINE SHOW

After graduating from Harvard in 1941, Spencer Klaw spent three years in the Army, mostly overseas in a liaison unit attached to a French armored division. After the war he covered the United Nations in New York for the United Press and worked as a "Talk of the Town" reporter at *The New Yorker* and on the staff of the *New York Herald Tribune*. From 1954 to 1960 he was an associate editor of *Fortune,* and for the last fifteen years he has been a freelance writer whose articles have appeared in many national magazines. His first book, *The New Brahmins: Scientific Life in America,* was published in 1968. Mr. Klaw currently teaches part-time at the Graduate School of Journalism at Columbia. His wife, the former Barbara Van Doren, is an editor and writer. They have four children and live in an old brick house in Greenwich Village.

"I think *The Great American Medicine Show* is very, very good—a fair, thorough, serious exposure of an American failure so extreme that it has taken on some aspects of a bitter joke, with intelligent and convincing suggestions for reform. Let me add that this book has, for me, the crucial additional virtue of being absorbing reading." —JOHN BROOKS

"For the layman contemplating the need to make intelligent choices about his own health care, and to weigh intelligently such complex issues as National Health Insurance, health maintenance organizations, peer review and malpractice, Klaw's book is the most readable, the most thoroughly researched, and the most fairly critical I have seen. The evidence he has compiled about the imperfections in our non-system of health care is overwhelming, and his sources are by and large impeccable. It's a responsible, dispassionate and thorough job of interpretive reporting."
—DAVID PERLMAN, Science Editor, *San Francisco Chronicle*

ALSO BY SPENCER KLAW

*The New Brahmins:
Scientific Life in America*

THE GREAT AMERICAN MEDICINE SHOW

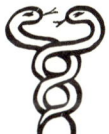 *The Unhealthy State of U.S. Medical Care, and What Can Be Done about It*

Spencer Klaw

**THE VIKING PRESS
NEW YORK**

Copyright © 1975 by Spencer Klaw

All rights reserved

First published in 1975 by The Viking Press, Inc.
625 Madison Avenue, New York, N.Y. 10022

Published simultaneously in Canada by
The Macmillan Company of Canada Limited

LIBRARY OF CONGRESS CATALOGING IN PUBLICATION DATA
Klaw, Spencer, 1920–
  The great American medicine show.
  Includes index.
    1. Medical economics—United States. 2. Medical care—United States. I. Title. [DNLM: 1. Delivery of health care—U.S. W84 AA1 K6g]
RA410.53.K58   362.1′0973   75-22040
ISBN 0-670-34836-8

Printed in U.S.A.

ACKNOWLEDGMENT is made to *Medical Economics* for material from articles by Arthur Owens, October 11, 1971, and April 15, 1974; and from Clifford R. Graves, March 18, 1974. Reprinted by permission.

*For Joanna,
Susan,
Rebecca,
and Margy*

I am more grateful than I can say to my wife, Barbara, for the skill and loving care with which she edited this book.

A Note to Doctors—
Especially Mine

Since there are passages in this book that may strike some doctors as unduly hard on them and their calling, let me say at once that I am not talking about the doctors who have taken care of me and my family. They have impressed me as intelligent and thoughtful people, and I know for a fact that they are conscientious. One, who was just starting out as a pediatrician when our first child was born twenty-eight years ago, is about as saintly a man as we are sometimes told that all doctors used to be. We do not, of course, insist on saintliness in our physicians. But I know there are tens of thousands of doctors like this fine pediatrician, and I ask readers to keep this in mind when I have critical things to say about American doctors in general—most of which, incidentally, are based on what doctors themselves have been saying about their profession. If that criticism seems harsh, it is because it makes me angry that so many Americans do not get the kind of care from doctors that my family and I have been lucky enough, so far, to take for granted.

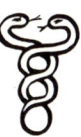

Contents

Introduction: What Crisis?   xi

1 Buying Health in a Sellers' Market   1

2 Buying Health in a Sellers' Market (Continued)   15

3 The Question of Quality   34

4 The Bitter Taste of Charity   49

5 The Price of Scientific Medicine   67

6 Some Notes on the Sociology of Healing   84

7 The Lingering Odor of Snake Oil   110

8 The Economics of Extravagance   132

9 The Business of Insurance   149

10 The Case for Health Maintenance Organizations   162

11 The Trouble with Medicare and Medicaid   181

12 Killing Rats in Mound Bayou: New Styles in Missionary Medicine   197

13 National Health Insurance: The Need for Heroic Therapy   209

14 Getting a Better Run for Our Money   231

15 How to Deal with the Doctor Shortage   252

16 Making Medicine More Human   262

Notes   277

Index   307

Introduction: What Crisis?

"America," Senator Edward M. Kennedy told an audience of doctors in New York City in 1971, "is beginning to realize that we have a health care crisis on our hands, and that the magnitude of the crisis is enormous." He added, "I have seen that crisis first hand, and I challenge even the most reactionary pillars of organized medicine, even the most affluent physicians in the most affluent suburbs of this rich city, to deny that a crisis exists, or that it exists for all Americans—not just the poor, not just the black, but each and every one of us."

Such a statement, by a leading political figure, would have been unthinkable a few generations ago. This is not because Americans were once better served by their doctors than they are today, which they were not. Until well into the twentieth century, medicine was assumed to lie outside the realm of politics, and medical care was regarded as a private matter between a doctor and his patients. When doctors and politicians did have business with one another it was generally transacted on the doctors' terms. Between 1910 and 1925, for instance, most states acted to raise the deplorably low standards of medical education in the United States by passing licensing laws that had the effect of closing down half of the country's medical schools. But these laws were adopted at the urging of the American Medical Association, and the politicians were called upon only to ratify what the doctors had decided must be done.

One reason why politicians were willing to leave medical care to the doctors was that it was still relatively cheap. Another reason was that it was looked on, with some justification, as a luxury rather than a necessity. In the last years of the nineteenth century, and the early years of the twentieth, doctors had learned a great deal about the nature of disease, but not much about its prevention or cure. In the presence of serious illness the doctor's characteristic role was still, as the poet Edwin Arlington Robinson wrote, "To flourish, to find words, and to attend: / Liar, physician, hypocrite and friend. . . ."

But over the past sixty years or so a striking change has taken place in the relationship between doctors and the rest of society. The power and complexity of modern medicine, along with its cobalt machines, artificial kidneys, and the rest of its elaborate technology, have turned medical care into a vast social enterprise, costing over $100 billion a year, and employing more than four million doctors, nurses, orderlies, x-ray technicians, drug-company detail men, inhalation therapists, processors of insurance claims, professors of hospital administration, medical records librarians, and makers of rubber gloves, incubators, and heart-lung machines. In the United States, it is true, most doctors still practice as independent entrepreneurs, and fiercely defend their professional and economic autonomy. But that autonomy is shrinking. In the future, the way that doctors are paid (and how much they are paid), the kind of quality controls to which their work will be subjected, and the nature of the settings in which they will work—hospital, clinic, private office, prepaid group practice—will increasingly be determined not by doctors, but by the rest of us. At the same time, American hospitals, most of which have traditionally been regarded as the private domain of the philanthropists who built and supported them, and of the doctors who used their facilities, are being subjected to stricter government regulation—regulation that is both inevitable and appropriate now that the government is paying a large and growing portion of the country's hospital bills. Medical care is now so indispensable and so expensive, and it has come to require so much planning and coordination, that it is unthinkable that politicians should *not* be concerned with its quality and cost, with where and how it is provided, and how it is to be paid for.

This concern has of course been heightened by a growing conviction that we are spending much too much money for medical care in America, and that much of what we get for our money is either inappropriate to our needs or of intolerably poor quality. This view is held not only by Senator Kennedy, but by the editors of *Fortune*. "American medicine, the pride of the nation for many years, stands now on the brink of chaos," the magazine warned in 1970, in an editorial titled "It's Time to Operate." *Fortune* went on to say that "most Americans are badly served by the obsolete, overstrained medical system that has grown up around them helter-skelter. . . ." The Panglossian complacency of the American Medical Association notwithstanding, there are even some doctors who would agree with this analysis. They include a New York internist, John W. V. Cordice, Jr., chairman of the 1970 Clinical Health Conference of the New York Academy of Medicine. In his address to the conference, Dr. Cordice tried to sum up in one long, angry sentence everything that he thought was wrong with health care in America. "I ask you," he said, "to picture our proud nation with its present technology and capabilities wallowing in its own garbage and excreta, breathing pollutants of all kinds, eating garbage, witnessing an increasing venereal disease rate, pandemic drug abuse, pandemic neuropsychiatric disease, pandemic alcoholism and malnutrition, pandemic home and automobile accidents, and an infant mortality rate about fifteenth among the nations of the world—a nation where the poor and the near-poor are being denied the possibility of having what those who have access to health care recognize as grossly inadequate, poorly coordinated, and blatantly expensive. . . ."

Most doctors are very irritated by this kind of talk. They point out, reasonably enough, that malnutrition, unsafe cars and highways, adulterated foods, and dirty air and water are not medical problems at all, and that doctors cannot fairly be blamed for the prevalence of alcoholism or drug abuse. It is true, also, as Dr. Cordice would concede, that lack of proper medical care is not the only reason why babies are stillborn or die in infancy (though, as we shall see, it is *one* of the causes of infant mortality, and one that we can clearly do something about by improving our arrangements for medical care). Doctors can also cite evidence that Americans are, in fact, reasonably satisfied with the kind of medical care they are getting. In late 1971 a Washington research group, Potomac Associates, put this question to a cross section of Americans: "All things considered, how much confidence do you have in being able to get good medical care for you and your family when you need it. . . ?" Only 14 per cent said they had "not so much" confidence, or none at all, while 84 per cent said they had at least "a fair amount" of confidence. On the basis of this and other similar findings, many doctors argue that if there is a crisis in American medicine it is one that has been invented by muddle-headed reformers, and seized on by politicians like Senator Edward Kennedy as a device for getting votes.

But this begs the question of why so many politicians of both parties have found the device so handy. The fact that five out of six Americans believe they can get good care when they need it does not mean that they are happy about what it will cost them, or about the way in which care is provided. Widespread dissatisfaction on these counts has been reported by, among others, the Citizens Board of Inquiry Into Health Services for Americans, whose members and staff traveled about the country in 1969 and 1970 asking people how they felt about the medical care they were getting—or, as it sometimes turned out, not getting. "We begin," the group noted in its final report, "by saying Americans are angry about health services. And indeed they are. Unless one has faced a room of angry consumers—whether on the edge of the Oakland ghetto, or in the plush living room of a Lake Shore home in a northern Chicago suburb—one cannot realize the extent or depth of that anger and frustration. Consumers feel that they are locked in a system of health care that exploits them financially and leaves them powerless and at the mercy of the health care providers."

The Citizens Board was made up largely of people, including a number of prominent public-health specialists, who had been working for years to change the medical-care system in America, and the board conceded that "We may have talked to a skewed sample of people; field representatives may have listened according to their own biases." But other observers have reported similar attitudes. "On the basis of my work," the well-known psychiatrist and author, Dr. Robert Coles, told a Senate committee in 1968, "I would say that no problem in American life so ironically unites all people in this country as the problem of medical care. Whether I am working with well-to-do suburban families or poor ghetto families, there is a strange similarity of dissatisfaction, confusion, and protest. Again and again people I work with fear financial disaster at the drop of any physical illness. Again and again I hear complaints about the coldness, the inhumanity, the mechanical quality of care that characterizes hospital wards, or even the outpatient clinics of these hospitals. Again and again I hear . . . complaints about regimentation, dehumanization, and, in general, a sense of fear and terror that pervades the minds of those who have been taken ill or anticipate being taken in the future. . . . And, in addition, there is almost universal resentment of the incredibly expensive costs of medical care, which threaten really almost everyone in the nation, except the very richest."

There is ambivalence, too, in the way people feel about doctors. While Americans continue to rate medicine as the most prestigious of the professions, they are not very happy about its practitioners. Joseph Lyford, writing about life in an Illinois town in the 1960s, noted that "Vandalia exhibits widespread resentment against doctors as a group. There is general irritation with rising medical costs and with the conspicuous affluence of most doctors in the area. There is also a frequently stated belief that some members of the medical profession do not have as much conscience as their fellow-citizens about paying their fair share of the income tax." Attitudes like these are not limited to residents of small towns. A national survey in 1962 indicated that while six out of ten Americans thought their own doctor was "sincerely devoted to his work," only one out of four was willing to say as much about the average doctor. Only two out of five persons described their own doctor as "completely ethical in his dealings"; fewer than half as many—only 18 per cent—said they thought this was true of the average doctor. Such skepticism was doubtless reinforced by the alacrity with which doctors raised their fees to take advantage of Medicare, and by reports, in the late 1960s, of widespread cheating by doctors collecting $100,000 a year and up from the government for the treatment of Medicare patients.

The main purpose of this book is not simply to describe, from the standpoint of a spectator, the forces that are transforming American medicine. It is, rather, to point out what exactly is wrong with medical care in the United States, and to suggest how we can best go about remedying its defects. This requires a certain amount of naiveté or faith, depending on one's point of view. The faults of American medicine are deeply rooted in the class structure of American society, and in an economic system that is powerfully resistant to change. Even after the passage of Medicare, for example, the humiliation and exploitation to which millions of elderly Americans are subject when they are sick is almost enough to convince the most stout-hearted reformer that the only way to get really good medical care in this country is to overturn the capitalist order. Nevertheless, I have managed to cling to the belief that we can change for the better the way we deal with illness in America without having a revolution. England, after all, is a country with economic and social arrangements that are much like ours. Yet everybody in England has a family doctor, nobody has to worry about the cost of illness, and there is virtually no discrimination against the poor. What England can do, we can do, though the means we choose to achieve these ends need not be the same.

If one wants to reform medical care in America, it is important to have a clear idea of exactly what needs reforming. It is not enough to know that medical care is terribly expensive; the question is whether, and in what ways, the cost is needlessly high. I shall begin, therefore, by examining in some detail the validity of what critics like Senator Kennedy have said about the shortcomings of American medicine. Next, I will undertake to trace the system's defects to their causes, looking, as it were, at the underlying pathology. I shall try to show, for example, why "the coldness, the inhumanity, the mechanical quality of care" to which Robert Coles refers are part of the price we pay for the enormous benefits of modern scientific medicine. I shall also go into such matters as the remarkable freedom and autonomy that American doctors enjoy, and what this means to their patients; the extravagance that is encouraged by the peculiar economics of the hospital business; and the stratagems by which drug companies induce doctors to prescribe high-priced drugs when cheaper ones (or none) would do as well or better.

Finally, I set forth a number of ideas for improving medical care in the United States. It is very likely that some form of national health insurance will be enacted soon. This will relieve Americans of the fear of being wiped out financially by a serious illness, and it will doubtless make it easier for the poor and the near-poor to get medical care. But other serious problems will remain. What is the best way to pay our doctors? How can we make sure of having the right kinds of doctors in the right places? How can we arrange things so that our hospitals, notably including the big teaching hospitals that are the temples of scientific medicine, will be run more for the benefit of the patients, and less for the benefit of the doctors? How can we reconcile the impersonality, and the division of labor, that medical technology fosters with our need, when we are sick, for sympathy and understanding? How can careless and incompetent medical care be discouraged without subjecting doctors to intolerable bureaucratic controls? What should consumers of medical care—that is to say, all of us—have to say about the running of hospitals, and what part should they play in monitoring the work of doctors? How can we avoid wasting billions of dollars a year on unnecessary operations, unused hospital beds, and seldom-used open-heart surgical units? How can we do away with poorhouse medicine, with the inconvenience and humiliation to which so many millions of Americans are routinely subjected when they try to see a doctor? These are questions we will be wrestling with in America for many years to come, and in my closing chapters I shall suggest how they might best be answered.

THE GREAT AMERICAN MEDICINE SHOW

Buying Health in a Sellers' Market

When Americans are asked what, if anything, they think is wrong with medical care in the United States they are as likely as not to begin by complaining about its fearful cost. Illness has never been particularly cheap, but in recent years its cost has soared spectacularly. Between 1964 and 1974 the daily cost of hospital care rose from an average of $38 to an average of $118, and in many hospitals a bed now costs its occupant (or his insurance company) well over $200 a day. Over the same ten years doctors raised their fees by more than 75 per cent, and medical care, taken as a whole, has gone up in price faster than just about anything else that Americans buy. As a nation, we are spending a larger and larger portion of our income on doctors, hospitals, and drugs. In the year ending June 30, 1974, the country's medical bill amounted to $485 per person, and the total of $104 billion that Americans spent on medical care came to nearly 8 per cent of the gross national product. This is proportionately a lot more money than is spent by most other industrial nations, including several—England, Norway, the Netherlands, for example—whose citizens, by and large, are at least as healthy as Americans.

Most Americans understandably worry less about such statistics than they do about how they are going to pay the bills in the event of serious illness. A study published in 1973 by the National Cancer Foundation suggests just how big these bills can be. The foundation collected information on expenses incurred by families in the New York area in which a family member had recently died of cancer. Of the 115 families surveyed, thirty-two, or 30 per cent, had expenses, including burial costs, of between $25,000 and $50,000. Three families had bills of more than $50,000. In most instances insurance covered only a small fraction of the families' medical expenses. Even a very brief illness can cost a staggering sum. "A ten-year-old boy was admitted to the hospital at 3:20 a.m.," John de Lury, President of New York's Uniformed Sanitationmen's Union, told a committee of the New York legislature not long ago. "The boy died at 10:34 the same night. The family of this child was charged $105.80 for drugs, $184.80 for x-rays, $220 for inhalation therapy, $655.50 for laboratory work. The total bill for the child was $1717.80." It is not only sanitationmen and other low-to-middle-income workers who worry about the costs of illness. David Halberstam, when asked recently by the magazine *Medical Economics* to give his views on American medicine, said, "The first rap is personal, and it terrifies me and all my friends—that is, the prospect that somebody in our families could get sick and the bills could total $30,000 or more. . . . I think I can deal with any bill that comes along except an enormous medical bill for myself or my wife. How does a man deal with that? No matter what kind of health insurance he has, that's a terrifying thing."

Even the angriest critics of American medicine do not contend, of course, that the steep rise in the cost of medical care is due entirely to extravagance, waste, and profiteering. One reason costs have gone up is that hospital workers are no longer willing to subsidize the care of the sick by working for sweatshop wages. In New York City, for example, orderlies, porters, laundry workers, and other unskilled employees who, fifteen years ago, were earning as little as $28 a week now earn a minimum of $181. Not all hospital workers have done this well, but wages everywhere have risen sharply, and since wages and salaries account for about 60 per cent of the total cost of running a hospital, this alone would have pushed hospital charges up.

More important, the cost of medical care has risen because of dramatic changes in medical technology. As Henry K. DeWitt, president of the American Hospital Supply Corporation, recently observed—happily, one assumes—"There was no thought ten or fifteen years ago of cobalt machines, heart pacemakers, cryosurgical instruments for cataract removal, artificial hearts, artificial heart valves, or microsurgical instruments for surgery performed under the microscope." Such devices necessarily cost a lot of money. Recently, for example, the Albert Einstein Medical Center in Philadelphia spent $300,000 for a linear accelerator capable of irradiating tumors at very high energies, and even a relatively low-powered cobalt machine can cost $100,000. To amortize, maintain, and operate the special equipment needed for x-raying the coronary arteries (a procedure that permits surgeons to perform certain kinds of heart operations they could not otherwise undertake) may cost $250,000 a year.

Even a medium-sized community hospital, one that does not offer angiography, as this technique is known, and that sends cancer patients who need irradiation to a nearby university hospital, is likely to have hundreds of thousands of dollars invested in diagnostic and therapeutic devices and machinery that either did not exist at all a few years ago, or else existed only in cruder and less effective forms. Recently, for instance, nearly half of all American hospitals have installed coronary-care units, in which patients are wired up, like astronauts, to instruments that record electronically how their hearts are functioning. The monitoring equipment for an eight-bed unit can cost $50,000. A single renal dialysis machine, or artificial kidney, may cost $10,000 or more, while the fluids and the disposable tubes and filters that are used up in the course of a year cost a minimum of $5,000 for each patient treated. "A fluoroscopic-radiographic room that could be fully equipped for $10,000 ten years ago now costs a minimum of $100,000," Edwin L. Crosby, chief executive officer of the American Hospital Association, pointed out in 1971. Since then the cost has risen even more.

The operation and maintenance of all this machinery obviously requires the services of many people—cardiopulmonary technicians, respiratory technologists, radiology aides, laboratory technicians, and others. Hospitals have also taken on the tasks of teaching amputees to walk again, and of helping stroke victims to regain their speech. These and similar developments have brought into being an army of specialized therapists. As a result, employees of the average community hospital now outnumber the patients by more than three to one; twenty years ago the ratio was less than two to one.

The need to pay hospital workers decently, and the growing complexity of medical technology, account for a large part, but by no means all, of the dizzying rise in the amount of money that Americans spend each year for medical care. It is true that such outlays have shot up even in countries that have much stricter governmental controls over costs. In England, for example, where many people think that too little money is spent on medical care rather than too much, hospital costs rose by 60 per cent between 1965 and 1971. The evidence is quite clear, however, that, in one way or another, Americans are being badly overcharged for medical care. This overcharge may amount to as much as $20 billion a year.

To begin with, evidence has been mounting that Americans are paying a great deal of money each year for surgery that benefits no one but the surgeon. More than sixty years ago, in his preface to *The Doctor's Dilemma*, George Bernard Shaw wrote, "That any sane nation, having observed that you could provide for the supply of bread by giving bakers a pecuniary interest in baking for you, should go on to give a surgeon a pecuniary interest in cutting off your leg, is enough to make one despair of political humanity. But that is precisely what we have done. And the more appalling the mutilation, the more the mutilator is paid. He who corrects the ingrowing toenail receives a few shillings: he who cuts your inside out receives hundreds of guineas, except when he does it to a poor person for practice." In a similar vein, a contemporary commentator, Dr. Charles E. Lewis, Professor of Preventive Medicine and Public Health at the University of California at Los Angeles, has observed that "medicine as currently structured is one of the few fields where if a wife really wants a new coat, all you have to do is maybe a couple more hysterectomies this week and you can buy it."

Venality is not the only reason why doctors operate unnecessarily. A surgeon who has done a particular operation hundreds of times may be unduly skeptical of an alternative, nonsurgical form of treatment even when its superiority has been clearly proven. Moreover, as Shaw suggests, some unnecessary operations are done for practice—most commonly by surgical residents who are getting their training in municipal hospitals, where the patients are almost all poor, and where there may be little supervision by senior staff physicians. Dr. Sidney Wolfe, an associate of Ralph Nader, recently described the results of an investigation of female surgery at Boston City Hospital. "A premium seemed to be placed on getting as many operations under the belt as possible for the residents," Wolfe testified at a public hearing in Philadelphia. "You hear residents who are trying to get one more, one more, one more hysterectomy to their credit. You hear remarks such as 'What is that woman doing with her uterus? She doesn't deserve to have a uterus; she's over forty'—things like that." Wolfe's report tends to bear out the contention of many women who are active in the women's movement, including some doctors, that there would be a lot fewer hysterectomies if all surgeons were women.

But the fact that most American surgeons are still paid on a fee-for-service, or piecework basis is almost certainly the main reason why they perform so many more operations than their English counterparts, who now work almost entirely on straight salaries. Writing in the *New England Journal of Medicine,* Dr. John P. Bunker, a professor of anesthesiology at the Stanford Medical School, has shown that, in the mid-1960s, nearly twice as many operations were performed in the United States, after allowing for the difference in the size of the two countries, as in England. Bunker cautioned that this "does not necessarily force the conclusion that we operate twice as often as the public health would justify. An alternative explanation might be that, as a wealthier country, the United States may simply be affording the luxury of surgical procedures that are desirable but not essential, and that the British public would be better served by more operations." It is true that nonurgent surgery has, in effect, been rationed under the British National Health service, so that people with hernias or varicose veins or hemorrhoids may have to wait as long as two years for surgical relief. But this does not explain, in Bunker's view, why tonsillectomies and hysterectomies, two operations that are particularly tempting to unscrupulous surgeons working on a fee-for-service basis, are so much more common in the United States than in England. Specifically, his figures showed that Americans were undergoing twice as many tonsillectomies as the English, and two and a half times as many hysterectomies. Noting that the United States has twice as many surgeons, proportionately, as England, Bunker concluded, "Until new evidence is available, it is reasonable to assume that there is a disproportionate number of surgeons in the United States . . . and it seems likely that some unnecessary surgery is being performed."

In the light of evidence already on hand, Bunker's tone of voice is remarkably bland. Again and again, when American surgical records have been reviewed by qualified specialists, the reviewers have found a dismayingly large number of cases in which there seemed to have been no need at all for surgery. This is particularly true of operations in which the surgeon has removed the patient's uterus, appendix, or tonsils. In 1961, for instance, two researchers at the School of Public Health of the University of California at Los Angeles, Paul A. Lembcke and Olive G. Johnson, studied the records of several hundred such operations carried out at a medium-sized suburban hospital. They concluded that 45 per cent of the hysterectomies and 38 per cent of the appendectomies were unjustified. The percentage of unjustified tonsillectomies was even higher. Authorities in the field of otolaryngology are in agreement, and have been for many years, that doctors should ordinarily leave tonsils alone unless a patient's hearing is impaired, or unless he has been suffering from recurrent abscesses or recurrent middle-ear infections. In only four of the 157 cases studied by Lembcke and Johnson did the records disclose any such justifications for taking out the patients' tonsils.

It is possible that doctors are performing fewer unnecessary operations than they were ten or fifteen years ago. At most hospitals a surgeon's work is now subject to audit by his colleagues, a process that can stay the hand of an over-eager operator. Lembcke and Johnson, in the course of their studies of unnecessary surgery, compared surgical records at a large community hospital before and after internal auditing was begun, and found an encouraging decline in the amount of unnecessary female surgery. But internal auditing is often ineffective, especially in smaller hospitals, and even in the hospital studied by Lembcke and Johnson 31 per cent of the hysterectomies performed after the new system had been put in operation were, so far as they could tell, medically unjustified. In any case, the effects of peer review in cutting down on needless surgery may have been offset, at least in part, by the passage of Medicaid and Medicare, and by the expansion of private health insurance, all of which have made it profitable for an unscrupulous surgeon to perform unnecessary operations on patients who could not afford to pay his fee out of their own pockets.

Perhaps the best way to get an idea of how much unnecessary surgery is done in American hospitals is to use, as a standard, the amount of surgery undergone by people who belong to prepaid group practice plans. Group Health Cooperative of Puget Sound, for example, furnishes virtually complete medical care, for a fixed annual sum, to some 200,000 people living in and around Seattle. Its doctors work on salary, and, unlike Shaw's surgeons, have nothing to gain by carving up patients unnecessarily. Furthermore, the plan, generally considered to be one of the best of its kind, is managed by elected representatives of the membership, who are charged with seeing to it that, among other things, their constituents get all the medical services they need. Yet in 1970 the plan's members underwent 20 per cent fewer operations than other residents of the Seattle area. Other comparisons have indicated that families of government workers covered by conventional health insurance undergo four times as many tonsillectomies and nearly twice as many appendectomies as families enrolled in prepaid plans such as Group Health of Puget Sound and the Kaiser-Permanente Health Plan.

The likelihood that at least one out of every five or six operations in the United States is medically unjustified is also suggested by the results of a program put into operation in the 1950s by the United Mine Workers. Worried about the large sums it was spending for surgery for its members, the union stipulated that in the future all operations would have to be approved in advance by a qualified surgical specialist if the union was to pay for them. Appendectomies fell off by 60 per cent, and hysterectomies by 75 per cent; surgical procedures of all kinds declined by 17 per cent. A similar requirement was put into effect in New York City, in 1972, by the United Store Workers Union, which retained as consultants a panel of specialists on the staff of the New York Hospital-Cornell Medical Center. In the first year, the required consultations brought about the cancellation or indefinite postponement of one out of five operations that had been recommended by the doctors whose advice had first been sought.

The figures I have just quoted would suggest that, of the roughly sixteen million operations that are performed in the United States each year, perhaps two to three million are unnecessary. Assuming that each such operation costs $1250—tonsillectomies cost less, but a complete hysterectomy is likely to run a lot higher—the total cost of all this needless surgery may amount to well over three billion dollars a year.

This is not the only price we pay for unnecessary surgery. All operations are risky, including so simple a procedure as a tonsillectomy. Of every thousand patients whose tonsils are removed, one dies as a result of the operation, and many more suffer harm. "Serious complications and sequelae occur in 15.6 per thousand cases each year," Robert P. Bolande, a professor at Case Western Reserve Medical School, has written. "These include deaths from anesthesia, postoperative hemorrhage and sudden postoperative deaths, and the morbidity associated with aspiration pneumonia, lung abscess or focal bronchiectasis." Bolande goes on to speak of other harmful effects. "Emotional changes lasting for more than two weeks are reported to occur in less than 10 per cent of the patients," he writes. "The symptoms are most often night terrors, increased dependence on parents, hostility to doctors and less frequently enuresis, asocial behavior, excessive appetite and aggressive behavior. . . . The psychiatric literature is replete with evidence that childhood tonsillectomy often has profound, life-long and irreversible repercussions."

On the basis of long-range statistical studies of the results of tonsillectomies it has been calculated that no more than 5 to 10 per cent of all children stand to benefit by having their tonsils out. Yet figures collected in 1969 by the Massachusetts Department of Public Health indicated that 30 per cent of the children in that state would sooner or later lose their tonsils. In many instances tonsils are taken out only because a surgeon needs the work to keep up his standard of living. A young pediatrician told me that after he had finished his training he had been at the point of joining a fee-for-service medical group in a midwestern city, but had changed his mind when he was told that he would be expected to produce an average of two tonsillectomies a week for the group's general surgeon.

Doctors are not exclusively to blame because so many children have their tonsils needlessly removed. There are communities where having a tonsillectomy is a sign of affluence, like taking ballet lessons. Often, too, parents who are having a hard time coping with a sick, irritable, and difficult child will become so frustrated that they will press hard for what amounts to a military solution—a solution which, in many cases, furnishes only temporary relief. But even in the face of such pressures, Bolande points out, "the tenet *'primum non nocere'* [first do no harm] exhorts the thoughtful and humane physician to attempt to eliminate cruel surgical ritual from our culture."

Bolande estimates that from one to three hundred deaths are caused each year by tonsillectomies, most of which are unnecessary. A Los Angeles surgeon, writing under the pseudonym Lawrence P. Williams, claims in a recent book called *How To Avoid Unnecessary Surgery* that at least 500 persons a year are killed by unnecessary hysterectomies, and 500 more by unnecessary appendectomies. Unnecessary surgery of all kinds, according to Williams's estimate, takes the lives of at least 10,000 Americans a year. This figure is only a guess. But even if the actual loss of life were only one tenth what Williams thinks it is, unnecessary operations would still be killing more Americans than infectious hepatitis, or complications of pregnancy and childbirth, or syphilis and its sequelae, each of which causes fewer than a thousand deaths each year.

America's yearly hospital bill is inflated not only by unnecessary surgery, but by the unnecessary hospitalization of people with nonsurgical ailments. This occurs for a variety of reasons that will be examined later, and that have mainly to do with the kind of health insurance that most Americans carry, and with the way doctors and hospitals are paid for their services. To be sure, doctors may reasonably disagree as to whether a particular patient should be admitted to a hospital, and they may disagree as to how long he should stay once he is there. Moreover, a decision to hospitalize, or not to hospitalize, a patient tends to reflect general notions about the appropriate use of hospitals that have no firm scientific basis, and that vary widely from country to country. In Russia, for example, half again as many people spend time in a hospital each year as in the United States; this is not because Russians are that much sicker than Americans, but because they are often admitted to hospitals for the treatment of quite minor disorders, or even as a preventive measure. If an epidemic of influenza breaks out in Russia, an elderly man with a chronic chest ailment or a bad heart, to whom the disease might prove fatal, may be advised by his doctor to go into a hospital to ride out the epidemic there.

But most investigators who have looked into the matter have concluded that, on any given day, tens—perhaps hundreds—of thousands of beds in American hospitals are occupied by people who could just as well, and much more cheaply, be cared for in nursing homes or as outpatients. Recently, for example, a team of Yale researchers examined the records of children being treated in three community hospitals in Connecticut. They reported that 38 per cent of the "patient days" covered by their survey seemed quite unnecessary. In other words, roughly one child in three would have been as well off, or better off, at home. Further evidence of how much unnecessary time Americans spend in hospitals is provided by the records of prepaid group practice plans. Operating on a fixed budget of so many dollars per year per patient, the plans and their doctors have every reason to keep patients out of the hospital unless they really need to be there. As a result, surveys of federal employees and their families who are enrolled in prepaid plans indicate that they spend only about half as much time in the hospital as employees who are covered by Blue Cross, or who have commercial hospital insurance. The prepaid plans that government workers have the option of joining have been thoroughly examined by public health specialists, and there is no evidence that they deny hospital care to anyone who needs it.

This is not to suggest, however, that American hospitals would lose half their patients if everybody in the country belonged to Kaiser-Permanente or a similar plan. The comparison I have just cited understates, probably by at least 10 per cent, the number of days that members of such plans actually spend in the hospital. This is because members occasionally go outside the plan for hospital care (a patient may want to be operated on by a particular surgeon who doesn't belong to the plan's medical group) even though they have to pay the bill themselves. A more realistic estimate is that the time Americans spend in hospitals could be cut by 20 to 25 per cent, without risk or serious inconvenience to patients, provided that patients needing convalescent or long-term nursing care could readily get it at home or in a so-called extended care facility. According to the General Accounting Office, this could reduce the country's medical bill by as much as $3 billion a year. The GAO's estimate was based on 1970 hospital costs; at present cost levels, the potential savings would be appreciably larger.

The economics of hospital care in America has also encouraged hospitals to compete with one another, at the expense of the taxpaying, insurance-buying public, in installing technologically glamorous machines and facilities even if no real need for them can be shown. One popular form of conspicuous consumption has been the purchase of expensive teletherapy units, used for treating certain kinds of cancer. Pierre de Vise, a former assistant director of the Hospital Planning Council for Metropolitan Chicago, has complained that teletherapy units concentrated on Chicago's near-South Side could, if properly dispersed, take care of the needs of the entire state of Illinois. Evoking the image of the woman in John Steinbeck's *Tortilla Flat*, who was persuaded to buy a vacuum cleaner even though she had no electricity—a lack she made up for by humming loudly as she pushed the machine around the room—de Vise adds, "There are teletherapy units in Chicago that have never been used because no one knows how to use this equipment." The Chicago Regional Hospital Study has estimated that a more rational distribution of teletherapy and coronary-care units might cut the operating costs of Chicago hospitals by as much as 10 per cent.

Facilities for open-heart surgery, in which a patient's blood is rerouted through a heart-lung machine while the surgeon repairs a hole in his heart, or replaces a valve or a section of the coronary artery, have also been much in vogue. Open-heart surgery is a very complex business, and the Inter-Society Commission for Heart Disease Resources, a government-supported body whose members include some one hundred experts in cardiovascular diseases, has taken the position that a center for such surgery can function efficiently only if it does an average of at least four to six operations a week, or a minimum of two hundred a year. Nevertheless, the Commission has reported that in 1969, when 360 American hospitals were equipped to do open-heart surgery, only fifteen actually performed 200 or more operations, while 220 hospitals averaged less than one operation per week.

This is not only extravagant—in 1971, Pennsylvania's Insurance Commissioner, Herbert S. Denenberg, estimated that the unnecessary proliferation of open-heart units was adding five to ten dollars a day to the average Philadelphian's hospital bill—but dangerous as well. In a report on other, less risky forms of heart surgery, the President's Commission on Heart Disease, Cancer and Strokes noted some years ago that mortality rates were higher in hospitals where such surgery was not regularly performed. This is likely to be true also of open-heart operations. When hospitals are called on only rarely for open-heart surgery, the Inter-Society Commission for Heart Disease Resources has pointed out diplomatically, "their professional staffs may find it difficult to maintain the special skills required in the cardiac surgical field."

Many American hospitals not only have expensive surgical and other facilities that are seldom used, but also many more beds than they can fill. In the hospital industry an average occupancy rate of 85 per cent is thought to be about right, allowing reasonably efficient operation while providing the flexibility that is needed to cope with emergencies, and to handle the rise in the demand for hospital beds that occurs each winter. Yet while many municipal hospitals, catering mainly to the poor, run at 90 to 95 per cent of capacity, there are thousands of other hospitals with one third to one half of their beds ordinarily unoccupied.

Low occupancy rates make hospital trustees and administrators unhappy, but such are the economics of running a hospital that they can usually compensate simply by boosting their charges. Indeed, there is so little risk in the hospital business that new hospitals are now going up all over the country in areas where hospital beds are already in more than ample supply. "I was in San Antonio recently and went through four hospitals without anyone knowing who I was," James Brusstar, an official of the Bay Area Health Planning Council in San Francisco, recalled not long ago. "In one hospital two floors had five patients between them—and six or seven nurses. They have a new state medical school there connected to the county general hospital. Right next door is Southwest Texas Methodist Hospital, and next door to the county hospital a 900-bed V.A. hospital is under construction. I don't know where they're going to get the bodies." The *Washington Post* has estimated that a "misguided boom" in hospital building will saddle the District of Columbia and its suburbs with 2300 unneeded hospital beds.

Already the average occupancy rate for all of the country's acute-care hospitals—hospitals other than psychiatric hospitals and hospitals for long-term care of patients with chronic diseases—has fallen to 75 per cent. The United States has, all told, about 900,000 acute-care beds, and some simple arithmetic suggests that, even if there were no reduction in unnecessary surgery or other unnecessary use of hospitals, more than 100,000 of these could be eliminated without pushing the average occupancy level above 85 per cent. Depending on what accounting formula one uses, the cost of maintaining these 100,000 surplus beds works out to between $1 billion and $2.5 billion a year.

The same economic arrangements that encourage extravagance in the building and equipping of American hospitals also encourage inefficiency. In the late 1950s Paul Lembcke of the University of California at Los Angeles took a close look at the operations of a medium-sized general hospital in the Swedish city of Karlskoga. He reported that the hospital was set in extensive grounds and was beautifully maintained; that the food was attractive and nourishing; and that there was no indication that the quality of care was being compromised in the interest of efficiency. Yet the staff was much smaller than in an American hospital of comparable size. Specifically, Lembcke added up the hours worked by the staff in the course of a year and divided the total by the number of patient days, giving him a figure of 6.27 staff hours per patient day. By contrast, the corresponding figures for some thirty hospitals in the United States, which Lembcke had chosen for comparison, ranged from 8.98 to 13.02 hours. The median was 10.72 hours, 66 per cent higher than at the Karlskoga hospital. In other words, it seemed to take five American hospital workers to do what three workers were able to do in Sweden.

Part of the explanation may be found in the fact that the average patient in a Swedish hospital stays several days longer than the average hospital patient in America. This means that on any given day many Swedish patients are up and around, making relatively few demands on the time of the hospital staff.

But this alone could not account for the figures reported by Lembcke, who suggested that one reason for the greater efficiency of the Swedish hospital was that, unlike its American counterparts, it seemed to run itself. "Nearly everyone is a productive worker," he noted. "Supervision is minimal and there is freedom to experiment."

One need not go to Sweden to find evidence that American hospitals are inefficient. In the late 1960s the American Hospital Association compared the costs of twelve hospitals, all "recognized as providing outstanding care, with the scope of service and teaching and the quality of staff considered to be essentially equivalent." Even after adjusting for differences in wage and salary levels, their costs ranged from $46 to $96 per patient day, with wide variations appearing "in every aspect of hospital operations—dietary, housekeeping, nursing, administration, etc." The conclusion to be drawn from these figures—and variations of this magnitude have shown up in survey after survey—is inescapable: if outstanding care can be provided for $46 a day, the $96-a-day hospital must be wasting an awful lot of money.

One authority on medical costs, Rashi Fein, Professor of the Economics of Medicine at the Harvard Medical School, has argued that hospital costs in the United States could be cut by 60 per cent without affecting the quality of care. His estimate would seem to assume an efficiency in the use of hospitals that is unattainable in the real world. But if we could eliminate most unnecessary surgery, limit the use of hospital beds more strictly to people who cannot safely be treated as outpatients, and close down a good proportion of the empty maternity wings, half-empty hospitals, and seldom-used open-heart surgical units, we should be able to shave our yearly hospital bill by half as much as Fein believes we could. In 1974 Americans spent around $44 billion on hospital care, and the possibility of making savings of even this magnitude would suggest that some $13 billion of this $44 billion was spent unnecessarily. This huge sum is only a part—though the largest part—of the total amount by which Americans, in one way or another, are being overcharged for medical care.

Buying Health in a Sellers' Market (Continued)

Dr. John H. Knowles, who for many years was director of the Massachusetts General Hospital in Boston, one of the world's leading medical institutions, recently outraged the touchier members of the medical profession by denouncing a great many of his fellow physicians as unconscionable profiteers. Not only are too many doctors getting rich by performing unnecessary operations, he told an interviewer, but 30 to 40 per cent of all American physicians are "making a killing" by charging too much. Knowles, who had just left his job in Boston to become President of the Rockefeller Foundation, was later censured by the Massachusetts Medical Society for declining to appear before it and explain where he got his facts. If he had done so, he would doubtless have had a hard time getting his hearers to agree with him on exactly what constitutes a killing in medical practice. But he would have had no difficulty in showing that the steep rise in the cost of medical care in recent years has been due, in part, to the uninhibited enthusiasm with which doctors have taken advantage of the sellers' market in which they have been operating.

Before 1966, when Medicare and Medicaid went into effect, doctors' fees had for many years been rising much faster than the overall cost of living. Now, with government payments adding billions of dollars a year to the effective demand for medical care, doctors boosted their fees by an additional 38 per cent in just five years. Medicare and Medicaid were also making it possible for them to charge (and collect) reasonable sums for taking care of people whom they had formerly treated free, or for less than their regular fees. As a result, between 1965 and 1970 doctors managed to increase their net incomes by more than one third. For a time during the early 1970s the rise in fees, and in doctors' earnings, was slowed by federal controls, and when these were lifted in the spring of 1974 the leadership of the AMA pleaded with the rank and file not to incur the wrath of Congress by hiking their fees too precipitously. The AMA's appeals may have had some effect: in the six months after controls were taken off, the rise in doctors' fees—up by 8 per cent—was only 25 per cent greater than the rise in the overall cost of living over the same period.

Even before they were freed from the yoke of federal price controls doctors were making out extremely well. Not long ago, for example, *Medical Economics* ran an illuminating sketch of a Florida physician named Jerry M. Robinson. *Medical Economics* is a plump and glossy fortnightly that regularly offers its readers, most of whom are doctors, tips on what to do with their money, printed under headings like "Try Texas for Little Stocks with BIG Potential," and "Commodity Trading? I've Had a Pork Bellyfull!" The article was one of a series on how doctors and their families spend their incomes. "Neither inflation nor the energy crisis has had much impact on the lifestyle or spending habits of the Jerry M. Robinsons in Deltona, Fla.," it began. "A 35-year-old G.P., Robinson still orders chateaubriand for two and eats all of it himself. He still buys up to a dozen custom-tailored suits a year. . . . He and his wife both drive late model Lincoln Continentals, while his oldest daughter tools around in a 1974 Pontiac Firebird. The doctor's house has a pool that costs $100 a month to heat, two fireplaces, and eight TV sets—four color and four black-and-white. Two of the color sets, purchased last year, stand side by side in the family room; the doctor likes to watch two sports events at once."

Robinson's tastes are obviously not typical of all doctors, and neither is his income, which amounts to $70,000 a year before taxes. In 1971, according to *Medical Economics*, which periodically surveys the earnings of physicians in private practice, only one self-employed doctor in eight made $70,000 or more, and the median income of all self-employed physicians, after deduction of professional expenses was only $42,500. But these figures do not accurately reflect the earnings of doctors who, like Robinson, are taking advantage of the tax savings available to any doctor who forms a so-called professional corporation and puts himself and his office help on its payroll. (A doctor practicing by himself who establishes such a corporation is normally its only stockholder as well as its highest-paid employee.) Incorporated physicians now constitute over a third of all practicing physicians, and *Medical Economics* reported that *their* median earnings—salary plus bonus plus retirement-plan contributions—came to $62,500. Doctors' incomes have, of course, gone up since 1971 (in 1973 an AMA survey indicated that the average physician in private practice was netting close to $50,000) and it is clear that doctors make a lot more money than any other sizable occupational group in America, with the exception of executives of large corporations. In 1968, for instance, the Internal Revenue Service analyzed the income of professionals practicing in partnerships, and reported that doctors earned half again as much as lawyers, nearly twice as much as dentists, and well over twice as much as architects.

Whether doctors as a class deserve to make as much money as they do is not an easy question to answer. Some doctors are, by any reckoning, grossly overpaid. Knowles has explained (though not to the Massachusetts Medical Society) that when he complained of doctors making a killing he had particularly in mind those who earn salaries well above $50,000 "by virtue of excessive charges for use of technology such as laboratory, x-ray, and surgical equipment that the hospital generally buys for specialists." Knowles could have been thinking of physicians such as Dr. Vernon E. Martens, a pathologist in charge of laboratory work at the Washington Hospital Center in Washington, D.C. The *Washington Post* disclosed in 1972 that Dr. Martens was netting $200,000 a year from this job, even though he worked only part-time at the Hospital Center, having a similar position at another Washington hospital, Hadley Memorial. At the Hospital Center Dr. Martens was receiving a percentage of the net profits realized by the hospital on its laboratory operations; at Hadley Memorial he was getting a percentage of the gross income. Such arrangements are quite common. A hospital can pass muster with the Joint Commission on Hospital Accreditation only if its laboratories are run by a certified pathologist—that is, by a specialist in the processes of disease—and few pathologists will consent to take on the job at a community hospital except on a share-the-profits basis. Chief pathologists at large hospitals not infrequently clear $300,000 a year, and the

Post reported that one pathologist in the Washington area was clearing $500,000.

Other specialists who have exclusive contracts with hospitals also make far more money than they are worth. Knowles has pointed out that anesthesiologists and radiologists at the Massachusetts General Hospital start at around $25,000 a year and can earn up to $60,000 near retirement. But, he adds, "we constantly lost such people after five years to community hospitals where they were paid twice that amount." A West Coast radiologist, writing in *Medical Economics,* recently cited the case of a chief of radiology "netting nearly $150,000 before taxes under the lucrative percentage contract he had with the hospital. For this rich reward, he put in a bare six hours a day, never saw a patient, and rarely consulted with an attending physician."

Pathologists, anesthesiologists, radiologists, and over-eager surgeons are not the only doctors who make too much money—or who, at any rate, make it the wrong way. There are a fair number of doctors in private practice who squeeze every dollar they can out of patients who have little power to resist their demands.

Doctors who treat old people often refuse to settle for what the Medicare administrators consider to be a reasonable fee—one that is in line with what other doctors in the community charge—and bill their patients for large extra amounts. "Many of the doctors around here automatically assume that every old lady has five or ten thousand dollars squirreled away in a bank somewhere," I was told by a social worker whose clients are old people living on the upper east side of Manhattan. "They see no reason why they shouldn't get a little of this money." There are also doctors who pad their bills. A California surgeon, Clifford L. Graves, who spends one day a month reviewing disputed claims for a nonprofit insurance plan called the San Diego Foundation for Medical Care, reports that 10 to 15 per cent of all surgical claims processed by the foundation are singled out for review. "Of these approximately half show minor padding," Dr. Graves writes. "The others prove to be grossly inflated. How else would you describe a $400 charge by a plastic surgeon for suturing a lacerated chin? . . . Or two separate and full billings by a neurosurgeon and an orthopedist who had teamed to do a disk-and-fusion procedure—and then an additional bill from each doctor for assisting the other?" Dr. Graves notes that a surgeon's fee for an operation used to cover the preoperative examination. "Today," he points out, "it regularly appears as a separate item. That may be defensible, but it sure looks chintzy on a bill for $2000. . . . I have seen a $32 charge for preoperative examination of a patient with a cut finger!" Some surgeons, Graves adds, have begun charging large extra amounts for any incidental tinkering (his word) that they may have to do in the course of an operation. "The real moneymaker in this scheme is the spleen," he writes. "Every surgeon occasionally has to remove it for no other reason than to gain access to his primary target. Yet I find that in such situations, some surgeons bill for an extra $300. . . . In a few cases where spleen excision truly complicates an operation, this extra charge is permissible. But more often than not, I discover that the splenectomy couldn't possibly have added more than ten minutes to the operating time."

The question remains whether the average American doctor, who neither pads his bills nor blatantly exploits his market power, makes more money than he should. In defense of their high earnings, doctors point out that their work is very demanding, and that they put in very long hours. In 1971, for instance, a survey of physicians in and around Hartford, Connecticut, disclosed that one out of four was, by his own estimate, working sixty-one hours or more a week, and that only one out of five was working less than fifty hours. Doctors also argue that because it takes them so long to learn their trade—four years in medical school, plus three to five years of postgraduate training as interns and residents—they are entitled to extra income to make up for lost time, and to pay off the heavy debts they are likely to have incurred.

But these arguments are not completely convincing. Many people, including shopkeepers, moonlighting factory workers, small farmers, and housewives with small children, also put in very long hours without expecting to be paid $40,000 a year or more. Moreover, even when interns made only $50 a month plus board, and residents not much more, an analysis of 1960 census data indicated that doctors were making a lot more money in the course of their lives than people in other professions, and thus were being more than compensated for the lean years of their apprenticeship. Today, interns and residents earn

$10,000 to $18,000 a year, and the earnings of doctors in practice, even after allowing for inflation, are a lot higher than they were in 1960.

Instead of asking whether doctors deserve to make forty or fifty thousand dollars a year, which is an unanswerable question, it may be more useful to ask whether we need to pay them quite so handsomely. If we paid them less, could we still persuade competent young men and women to go into medicine in large enough numbers to meet the country's needs? The answer is almost surely that we could. Each year since World War II, American medical schools have had a great many more applicants, most of them well qualified, than they could accept. In 1965, when the real earnings of doctors averaged several thousands of dollars a year less than they do today, there were more than twice as many applicants as the schools had places for. Obviously one of medicine's appeals is that doctors make a lot of money. But the college students who are beating on the doors of medical schools in record numbers—there were 42,500 applicants in 1974, more than twice as many as there had been ten years before—seem to be more attracted by other advantages of a medical career. Chief among these, apart from the interest of the work itself, is the security it offers. In recent years students have been uneasily aware of unemployed engineers, unemployed physicists, and unemployed teachers, but it has been a long time since a physician has had to worry about how he was going to earn his living.

It has not always been that way. In the early years of this century, American medical schools were turning out more doctors than the country could absorb, and young graduates often grew so discouraged about their prospects that they turned to other lines of work. This changed, however, after 1910, when the Carnegie Foundation published a stinging critique of medical education in the United States. Its author, Abraham Flexner, was merciless in characterizing many of the country's medical schools as "very weak," "wholly inadequate," "miserable," "dirty," and "utterly wretched." He urged that such schools should be put out of business, and medical education concentrated in fewer and larger schools, closely tied to universities, in which the students would get more basic science, more laboratory work, and more work with patients than most American schools of the time were capable of providing.

The reforms that Flexner proposed had the enthusiastic backing of the American Medical Association, and were quickly put into effect. By 1926 more than half of the schools that had been in existence when Flexner began his investigations had shut their doors, and all but two of the forty-eight states were refusing to license, as medical practitioners, graduates of those remaining schools that did not measure up to the standards set by Flexner. In time this greatly improved the quality of medical practice in America, but it had other consequences as well. Under the new arrangements it was not the state licensing boards that sat in judgment on the medical schools, but the AMA's Council on Education, whose ratings were accepted as final by the boards. The AMA thus had the power to restrict the yearly production of new doctors to a level that would insure plenty of work for everyone. In fact, between 1904 and 1927 the number of students in medical schools fell from 28,000 to 20,000, even though the population of the United States grew by 34,000,000 over this same period. In the depression of the 1930s, and again after World War II, the AMA forced the medical schools to reduce their enrollments, and in 1949 the schools actually graduated fewer students than they had in 1930.

While this was undoubtedly good for doctors, it was not, in the end, so good for their patients. By 1960 the evidence was piling up that the United States was not producing enough doctors—not enough of the right kind, at any rate—to meet the mounting demand for their services. The signs were unmistakable: hospitals staffed with house officers trained (not always adequately) in foreign medical schools; emergency rooms overrun by patients with nonemergency problems, but with no family doctor to take them to; general practitioners too busy to give most of their patients more than perfunctory care. Even so, it was not until 1968 that the AMA at length conceded there was an "urgent and critical need for more physicians." The prosperity of American doctors, and the magnitude of their fees, thus reflect, in part, the AMA's success in limiting the supply of doctors and thereby driving up the price of their services.

Since 1968, twenty-five new medical schools have opened their doors, and the number of first-year medical students rose from 9500 in 1967 to 14,700 in 1974. If enough new doctors elect to go into family practice, and to set up shop in city slums and rural areas where doctors are hardest to come by—and neither of these things will happen automatically—the shortage should ease in five to ten years.

But the recent history of surgical fees offers little hope that more doctors will necessarily mean lower charges. Although the United States has too few family physicians, it has many too many surgeons, most of whom are only partially employed at their trade. In 1972 a survey by *Medical Economics* indicated that one third of the country's 23,000 general surgeons were performing, on the average, fewer than four operations per week. A spot check two years later showed no change. "I could easily do five times as many operations as I'm doing," one surgeon reported. "Of the 200 surgeons in my town, I estimate that only six are working at more than 80 per cent of capacity." Given the circumstances, one might suppose that it would be poor business for surgeons to hike their fees. But in fact, surgeons' fees have risen almost as steeply as those of doctors in other specialties. Between 1970 and 1973, *Medical Economics* reported, the median fee for an appendectomy rose by 25 per cent. "You don't have to do much if you charge enough," a West Coast surgeon told the magazine. "If a young surgeon comes to town, hangs around the emergency room, and takes out three or four appendixes a month, he can make a living." Surgeons have also been sweetening the pot, as we have seen, by charging extra for preoperative and postoperative examinations. Partly for these reasons, *Medical Economics* pointed out, surgery "is prospering as never before." In 1972, according to the magazine, one out of four self-employed general surgeons netted at least $60,000, and general surgeons who had incorporated their practices apparently did even better. "Nor has [the surgeon's] traditional edge over other doctors narrowed," the magazine added. "[Our] survey shows self-employed general surgeons netting a median of 11 per cent more than all self-employed M.D.s combined—about the same spread as in 1964."

Surgeons seem to be particularly favored by the economics of medical practice, and doctors in other specialties, finding themselves with too little work to go around, might not be able quite so easily to defy the laws of supply and demand. But obviously competition in the marketplace cannot be relied on to prevent the overpricing of doctors' services. How the price of a doctor's care can be kept in line is necessarily bound up with the question of how doctors should be paid, a question that will be considered in a later chapter.

Besides wasting billions of dollars a year on unnecessary operations, Americans annually consume, and pay for, billions of capsules and pills, prescribed by their doctors, from which there is no reason to think they will benefit in any way. The waiting room of the average family doctor is perpetually crowded, and writing a prescription is often a convenient way to bring a visit to a close so that the doctor can get on with the next patient. The patient, for his part, feels that the doctor is concerned about his condition, and is doing something about it. Most Americans tend to think there is a pill for everything, and to feel cheated if all they get from a visit to the doctor is his assurance that they will probably feel better soon, or a lecture on the virtues of eating less and exercising more.

But this does not entirely explain why American doctors are so quick with their prescription pads. Despite years of outraged protests by senators, journalists, and academic experts on pharmacology, overprescribing is unrelentingly fostered by the drug manufacturers. Merck, Lilly, Squibb, Hoffmann-La Roche, and the other fifteen or so companies that dominate the prescription-drug business in the United States spend a bigger proportion of their sales revenue to advertise and promote their wares than any other American manufacturers except, perhaps, those that sell cigarettes, soap, and cosmetics. The target of these promotional efforts, which cost the industry at least a billion dollars in 1974, are the country's 275,000 practicing—and prescribing—physicians. As Pierre Garai, an advertising man with years of experience in the merchandising of prescription drugs, has pointed out, "perhaps no other group in the country is so insistently sought after, chased, wooed, pressured, and downright importuned as this small group of doctors who are *de facto* wholesalers of the drug business."

Drug-company wooers, including the fifteen thousand or so detail men who regularly call on doctors in their offices, are at least partly responsible, for example, for the fact that Americans take a great many more antibiotics than they need or than is good for them. It is the firm conviction of virtually all experts on infectious diseases that antibiotics are called for only when it is quite certain that the patient has a bacterial infection. They should not be prescribed for ordinary colds, for which they are totally ineffective. Nor, for reasons I shall come to presently, should they be given as a means of warding off possible infections to patients awaiting surgery.

Yet a great many doctors regularly ignore these precepts. Market surveys made by or for drug manufacturers have shown that at least half of all cold victims who consult a doctor leave his office with a prescription for an antibiotic. A survey of 86,000 hospital patients, made in the early 1960s, disclosed that nearly half of the patients to whom an antibiotic had been given had nothing on their charts to indicate there had been any need for it. These patients, the survey reported, "were given antibiotics to prevent infections which did not exist, should not occur, and in all probability will never happen. Such prophylactic use has been denounced for years as a dangerous, unnecessary, and expensive practice." The denunciations have continued, but with little effect. Not long ago Dr. Harry Dowling, a well-known authority on drugs, told a Senate committee that, in the 1972 fiscal year, the Food and Drug Administration had cleared for marketing more than five million pounds of the eight most commonly prescribed antibiotics. This was enough, he calculated, to treat two illnesses of average duration for every man, woman, and child in the United States. The average person, he went on to say, has an illness requiring antibiotic treatment no more often than once in every five to ten years.

Antibiotics are not the only drugs that doctors commonly administer or prescribe even when there is little or no chance of their helping the patient. Vitamin B_{12}, for instance, while it is indispensable and highly effective in the treatment of pernicious anemia, is of no known use in treating anything else. Yet two medical researchers, Paul D. Stolley and Louis Lasagna, note that "millions of injections of Vitamin B_{12} . . . are given yearly for a remarkably wide spectrum of diagnostic conditions with the desired pharmacologic action often listed as 'placebo,' 'stimulant,' 'sedative,' or 'hematinic [blood-improving] properties.'" Vitamin B_{12}, they point out, is neither a stimulant nor a sedative, and it has no effect on the blood of anyone except victims of pernicious anemia. (However, as another commentator on B_{12}'s popularity has observed, its "red color, nontoxicity, and injectability make it an excellent placebo.") In another article, Stolley, who is a professor at Johns Hopkins' School of Hygiene and Public Health, has called attention to market research data indicating that most persons who don't get an antibiotic when they see a doctor about a cold get an antihistamine instead. "According to well controlled trials," Stolley writes, "neither of these medications are effective against the viruses that cause colds, nor do they relieve cold symptoms." Medical journals carry ads for dozens and dozens of drugs, some of them best sellers, that have been found by the FDA, on the basis of a two-year study by a group of experts assembled by the National Academy of Sciences, to be no more than "possibly effective" in treating the condition doctors are being urged to prescribe them for. This rating signifies that while there is no proof that a drug *doesn't* work, neither is there any convincing evidence that it does.

Usually when a doctor writes an unnecessary prescription the only harm is to the patient's pocketbook. But on occasion there are other and much more serious consequences. One out of every twenty hospital patients who gets an antibiotic reacts badly to it, and one out of seven of these reactions is serious enough to threaten the patient's life. Moreover, the enormous benefits of antibiotics have been partly offset by the change their widespread use has brought about in the bacterial ecology of hospitals. More and more patients are contracting infections caused by so-called Gram-negative bacteria; these are not affected by the most commonly used antibiotics, and flourish in hospitals where competing bacteria, like the familiar staphylococcus, which used to be responsible for most hospital infections, now have a hard time surviving.* Surveys have shown that about 1 per cent of all patients admitted to certain large teaching hospitals now contract Gram-negative infections, and that one third to one half of these patients die as a result. Extrapolating these figures to all United States hospitals, three specialists in infectious diseases, writing in *Annals of Internal Medicine,* recently warned that Gram-negative bacteria may be killing as many as 100,000 persons a year. Whatever the actual total may be, most experts believe it could be greatly reduced if doctors

---

* The term "Gram-negative" does not imply weightlessness. Rather, it refers to a standard technique for classifying bacteria—the Gram strain—named for its Danish inventor, Dr. Hans Gram.

were to stop promiscuously dosing their hospital patients with antibiotics.

Other drugs besides antibiotics are also widely prescribed in the face of evidence that the risk of unpleasant or dangerous side effects may well outweigh any probable benefit to the patient. Speaking of his own practice in Silver Spring, Maryland, Dr. Martin Shargel recently told Senator Kennedy's Subcommittee on Health, "We are seeing more and more patients with complaints consequent to their medicine taking and have hospitalized a significant number of them." He added, "It is becoming an impossibility to keep track of what all of these drugs do to human bodies. . . . Often the hazards of prescription medication are discovered only through widespread public use after the usual drug company promotion." On the basis of studies carried out in a large university hospital, Colonel Robert H. Moser, chief of medical services at the Army's Walter Reed Hospital, and an expert on drug-induced diseases, has testified before another Senate committee that perhaps as many as 1,500,000 persons are admitted to United States hospitals each year because they have reacted badly to a drug. There is reason to think that Moser's estimate is on the high side, but there is no question that the number of such admissions runs into the hundreds of thousands. In most cases the drug that has caused the trouble has doubtless been properly prescribed, in the sense that the patient stood to gain far more than he stood to lose. But the evidence is strong that tens of thousands of people, at the least, are being hospitalized each year because they have reacted badly to a drug they should not have been given in the first place.

In 1959, when the late Senator Estes Kefauver of Tennessee undertook to educate Americans about the remarkable pricing practices of the drug industry, the subject of one of his first lessons was estrodiol progynon, a drug used for the treatment of menopausal disorders. At the time, estrodiol was sold exclusively in the United States by the Schering Corporation. Investigation by the staff of the Senate Subcommittee on Antitrust and Monopoly, which Kefauver then headed, turned up the fact that Schering was buying the drug in bulk, for $3.50 a gram, from a French firm, and putting it up in bottles holding sixty tablets each. Each bottle contained 3/100ths of a gram of estrodiol, and the staff had calculated that the total cost to Schering of buying, processing, and bottling the drug came to no more than 11.7 cents per bottle. Yet Schering was charging druggists $8.40 a bottle for estrodiol, a price that, as Kefauver pointed out, represented a markup of 7079 per cent.

While conceding that this was pretty steep even by drug-company standards, Kefauver was able to show that markups ranging up to 1000 per cent or more were not unusual in the industry. They are still not unusual today. According to testimony at a patent-licensing hearing in Canada, the cost of manufacturing Valium, a tranquilizer that is more frequently prescribed than any other drug on the American market, comes to $487 a kilogram, including the cost of making it up into pills, putting it in bottles, and distributing it to the drugstores. This translates into just over 24 cents for a bottle containing 100 five-milligram tablets. At the time of the hearing, the manufacturer, Hoffmann-La Roche, was charging American druggists $6.95 a bottle, which works out to a markup of just under 2800 per cent. Assuming that the druggist tacked on a 67 per cent markup of his own, the customer who walked in with a prescription for Valium ended up paying 48 times what it cost the manufacturer to make, package, and ship the drug.

The big drug companies are understandably reluctant to say how much money they make on individual products. But a comparison between prices charged in the United States and the prices charged for the identical products in other countries—countries in which drugs are not patentable, or where drug prices are controlled by the government—suggests that gross profit margins of several hundred per cent are common in the American market. "The price of 100 tablets of propoxyphene, Darvon, sold by the Lilly Co. to the druggist in the United States is $7.02," Senator Gaylord Nelson of Wisconsin said in a Senate speech not long ago, "but the price charged by the same company for the same product in Ireland is $1.66, and in the United Kingdom is $1.92. Bristol charges $21.84 for 100 tablets of ampicillin in the United States, but $9.31 in Ireland . . . ; the Pfizer Company charges $20.48 in the United States for oxytetracycline, Terramycin, but $4.63 in Brazil and $3.68 in New Zealand." There may be an even greater difference between the price that a druggist has to pay for a drug, and the much lower price at which its manufacturer is willing to offer it to a city hospital system or to a federal agency. In 1967, for instance, the Department of Defense asked for bids on reserpine, a drug used in the treatment of high blood pressure. CIBA offered to sell the department its own brand of reserpine, Serpasil, for $3.95 a bottle, or exactly one tenth what drugstores were paying for it. Even so, CIBA lost the business to other firms that were able to supply the identical drug for about 90 cents a bottle.

By means of a number of ingenious stratagems, which will be examined in a later chapter, the big drug companies can often command an enormous price for a product even after its patent has run out. In 1973 this was true in the case of no fewer than thirteen of the fifty most frequently prescribed drugs, even though in every instance the same drug, subject to the same government tests for potency and purity, could be bought much more cheaply from one of the smaller drug firms specializing in the sale of generic—that is, unpatented and unbranded—products. The difference in price between a branded drug and its generic twin can be at least as big as the difference between the price of a Rolls-Royce and a Volkswagen. Consider, for example, the price of Butisol, a best-selling sedative, manufactured by McNeil Laboratories, that just missed the top-fifty list in 1973. (It ranked sixty-seventh.) In *The New Handbook of Prescription Drugs,* a widely read and admirably astringent guide both for laymen and for doctors who are unwilling to accept drug-company detail men as their only tutors, Butisol is rated as completely dispensable. "With a handsome purple or green or orange dye added to the tablet, and called by an easy-to-remember name," the author, Dr. Richard Burack, writes, "Butisol is nothing more than an old-fashioned sedative. Its official name is butabarbital, and by that name it can be very inexpensive." In 1974, butabarbital was being offered by some small houses for as little as $2.50 for a thousand pills, while McNeil's price for the same quantity of Butisol was $15.30. Similarly, Schering was charging druggists $18.41 per thousand tablets for Chlor-Trimeton, an antihistamine often prescribed for hay fever; the same drug could be bought under its generic name, chlorpheniramine maleate, for $1.24 per thousand.

As Richard Harris has written in *The Real Voice,* his absorbing account of Kefauver's dogged (though largely unavailing) efforts to reform the drug business in America, "If one were to awaken any one of a thousand drug executives in the dead of night and ask him where all those profits went, the answer would undoubtedly be 'Research.' " Spokesmen for the drug industry also argue, along similar lines, that drug prices have to be high because the drug business is such a risky one. "Only one out of about 6000 compounds tested by drug companies turns out to be a marketable product, and even then it can reach the market only after years of animal and clinical testing," C. Joseph Stetler, President of the Pharmaceutical Manufacturers Association, has explained. "In addition, a competitor's new or improved product for treatment of the same disease can appear at any moment to overshadow or make obsolete a profitable product perfected at great cost."

But critics from Kefauver on have, with reason, found these arguments singularly unconvincing. While it is true that the big drug companies do put a good deal of money into research, even after they have paid off all their scientists and technicians they still have a lot of money left over. In 1973, the earnings of the fifteen drug companies on *Fortune*'s list of the 500 largest manufacturing corporations amounted, after taxes, to 18 per cent of the stockholders' equity. This was more than was earned by any other industry group, and half again as much as the average earnings of all the companies listed by *Fortune*. Moreover, 1973 was a fairly typical year for the drug industry. Although drug companies on occasion may invest hundreds of thousands of dollars on products that don't pan out, they never seem to lose more than they can comfortably afford. "Losses, or even low profits, are practically unheard of among large drug companies," a witness told the Senate Subcommittee on Monopoly not long ago. "In this respect the drug industry is practically unique among important American industries." The witness, Dr. Willard Mueller, who was then chief economist of the Federal Trade Commission, went on to say that, over a long period of years, large drug companies "not only earned a higher return than any other of the major manufacturing industries . . . but none of the drug companies ever experienced losses during the period, nor did any companies experience profit rates below 5 per cent. . . . No other industry matched drugs in the frequency with which companies had profit rates exceeding 15 per cent."

The drug companies' high profits are less costly to the consumer, however, than the promotional activities by which these profits are created and sustained. Working from subpoenaed records, the Kefauver committee calculated that in the late 1950s the big drug companies were spending 25 cents out of every dollar they were taking in on advertising and sales. This was slightly more than four times as much as they were spending on research. A government study published in 1968 indicated that the big companies were still spending one dollar out of four to promote their products, and there is no reason to believe that the proportion is much different today. The public, of course, pays for this huge promotional enterprise, and thereby subsidizes the drug companies in their successful efforts to sell Americans more drugs than they need, at prices a great deal higher than they should be paying. As a witness testified some years ago at a Canadian inquiry into drug prices, "for every dollar the drug industry spends on research, they spend four dollars telling you about it, and charge you ten dollars more for listening."

In the eyes of many Europeans, accustomed to the notion that taking care of sick people is properly a communal responsibility, like cleaning the streets or teaching children to read, one of the more barbaric aspects of life in America is the extent to which the costs of illness are expected to be borne by the ill themselves. The American insurance industry often congratulates itself on the rapid growth of the private health insurance business over the past thirty-five years. Yet the Social Security Administration has estimated, on the basis of house-to-house surveys, that, at the end of 1973, some forty-one million Americans who had not yet reached the age of sixty-five—that is, who were too young to be eligible for Medicare—had no health insurance of any kind. Many of these people are self-employed (as handymen, for instance), or work as casual or seasonal laborers, or as domestics, or are employed by small, marginal enterprises whose owners do not offer such fringe benefits as health insurance. A man or woman in such circumstances can, in theory, buy an individual insurance policy. But it may not be easy to get one. Some companies refuse to insure people in certain occupations, no matter how healthy they look. Metropolitan Life, for example, in a manual issued to its agents in 1972, listed as "unacceptable for any form of Personal Health Coverage" people holding many kinds of unskilled jobs. The list included dishwashers, carwashers, hod carriers, kitchen helpers, scrubwomen, bootblacks, farmhands, porters, and pinboys. Even if he does find an agent willing to sell him a policy, a carwasher or a farmhand may decide, on discovering that reasonably good coverage for himself and his family is going to cost him, say, seventy dollars a month, that he can't afford insurance.

A serious illness not covered by insurance can, of course, be financially disastrous. "A 62-year-old man, Paul R., developed heart trouble and had to retire," a union-sponsored publication reported recently. "He drew $81 a month in Social Security and could not afford medical insurance. When he had to enter the hospital, $400 was required as a deposit. His daughter and her husband paid it from the $700 they had saved over 14 years. His son paid the rest of the $2000 bill. Now Mr. R. has lung cancer. His son-in-law writes, 'We have been to Social Security and they say they can do nothing. We went to Welfare. They said that Medicaid does not cover him. We pay taxes and we stand for Medicaid and then it doesn't cover anything. . . . The children have spent all their money. The old man has spent all his money. What are we going to do now? We can't just let him die!'"

Besides those Americans who have no health insurance at all, there are millions of others who are only skimpily covered. Among them are many who cannot get in on a group plan, and have to settle for an individually-written policy. Such policies are very expensive, and are likely, at best, to cover only a fraction of the expenses of a long illness. Moreover, the circumstances in which benefits will be paid are often defined so as to exclude the most likely cause of illness.

"The waiver is one of the best and most useful tools of the health insurance business," Leonard Woodcock, President of the United Auto Workers, and a vigorous supporter of national health insurance, has observed. "By this method the company sells policies with hay fever or heart trouble or lumbago or sinusitis or any of dozens of other conditions written out, so that the illness the consumer is most susceptible to is what he is not covered for. If he is a farmer, he may find himself with coverage for accidental injury except when it is caused by operating, repairing, or otherwise coming into contact with farm machines."

Group insurance policies, too, may leave a lot to be desired. Some plans have serious gaps in their coverage. Often they exclude surgery or medical treatment required by an infant during its first fifteen days of life. The policyholder is happily unaware of such gaps until he is stuck with a $5000 hospital bill. Tens of millions of Americans have policies that will pay all or part of their hospital bills, and at least a part of all doctors' bills for treatment in the hospital. But often the patient is left to pay for drugs, nursing-home care, home nursing, physical therapy, and visits to the doctor's office. Holders of so-called major medical expense policies, which now cover more than 110 million persons, are much better off. In the event of a serious illness they can count on the insurance company to reimburse them for, say, 80 per cent of all expenses, both in and out of the hospital, over and above a specified deductible of $500 or so, and up to a total of twenty or thirty thousand dollars or even more. Yet for all their advantages, policies of this kind often have serious shortcomings, quite apart from the fact that they do not usually cover check-ups, measles shots, Pap tests, or other forms of preventive care. Between deductibles and co-insurance—the portion of the bills the patient is expected to pay himself—the out-of-pocket cost of a three-week hospital stay, followed by a long convalescence, can easily amount to a couple of thousand dollars. Even more serious is the ceiling on total liability. Twenty thousand dollars may sound like a lot of money, but tens of thousands of people every year run up hospital and medical bills that far exceed this amount.

The plight that millions of families have found themselves in, even when they thought they were reasonably well insured against the costs of illness, may be illustrated by the case of Mrs. Patrick Smythe, who testified before Senator Kennedy's Health Subcommittee at a hearing in Denver in 1971. Mrs. Smythe explained that her husband had undergone open-heart surgery two years before, and had had to return to the hospital a few months later for a second operation. In response to questioning by Kennedy, she said that she and her husband earned, between them, $620 a month after taxes, out of which they were paying $150 a month on one hospital bill, $30 a month on another, and $50 a month to each of two doctors.

SENATOR KENNEDY: Now you had medical insurance which paid $15,000 of the approximately $30,000 bill, is that right?

MRS. SMYTHE: That's right. . . .

SENATOR KENNEDY: How do you live?

MRS. SMYTHE: It's pretty slim. As a matter of fact, I was kind of reluctant to use the gas to come over here today. I have that gauged down as to how I can get to work with X number of gallons, and this has to come out each month.

SENATOR KENNEDY: What about your house?

MRS. SMYTHE: We lost our house. We sold it. We took what we could out of it to pay some other bills. . . .

SENATOR KENNEDY: How long do you think you will be paying off medical bills?

MRS. SMYTHE: For the rest of my life.

SENATOR KENNEDY: What do you think now of the insurance policy you had?

MRS. SMYTHE: I think our insurance policy wasn't big enough, as I think most American insurance policies aren't big enough, but can most Americans afford a bigger policy?

3

The Question of Quality

It is often said, with some justification, that American medicine is the best in the world. As generators of new knowledge about human biology, American medical schools, and their affiliated teaching hospitals, have few if any equals. Nourished on a rich diet of federal money, biomedical researchers in the United States have not only been enormously successful in penetrating the mysteries of heredity and other fundamental life processes, but they have probably done more than scientists in any other country to apply such knowledge to the control of disease. The medical centers associated with Harvard, Yale, Stanford, Johns Hopkins, Columbia, Chicago, and other leading universities have attracted gifted scientific pilgrims from all over the world, and in the past twenty-five years more Nobel Prizes for physiology or medicine have been awarded to American scientists, most of them on the faculties of medical schools, than to scientists of any other country.

American medicine is distinguished not only by the preeminence of its researchers, but also by the sophisticated training its practitioners are given in the diagnosis and management of disease. From a technical standpoint, the care that a patient gets at a teaching hospital such as Massachusetts General, especially if his disease is organic (not rooted in emotional disturbance) and if it is also intellectually challenging, is at least as skillful and imaginative as is to be had anywhere in the world. Moreover, an American does not have to be seriously ill to get better care than is generally available in most other countries. "The [American] general practitioner is . . . more likely to be 'on his toes' than his counterpart in Europe," Dr. Milton I.

Roemer, professor of public health at the University of California at Los Angeles, and a longtime student of the ways in which doctors practice their trade, has written. "The community general practitioner in Great Britain or on the Continent tends to practice a relatively superficial 'symptom-relieving' brand of medicine. His office is meagerly equipped and he rarely has technical aides at hand. . . . He rarely has his horizon widened by postgraduate education, and he is very likely to cling to methods of treatment he learned years before." Dr. Roemer's observations were made some ten years ago, and since then the quality of European general practice has improved; certainly this is true in England. But, by and large, family doctors in the United States still know their business better, and are prepared to do more for their patients, than the average family doctor in most European countries.

Yet the evidence is overwhelming that, for all the dazzling triumphs of American medicine, tens of millions of Americans get medical care that must be rated, considering how rich this country is, and how much we know about the prevention and treatment of disease, as scandalously poor in quality. The fault lies not only with the inadequacy of our arrangements for medical care—too few family physicians, for example—but also, to an extent seldom realized by their patients, with the carelessness, incompetence, and venality of many American doctors.

To begin with, there is the evidence provided by the statistics on the number of babies born in the United States who die before their first birthday. Infant mortality is sometimes used as a rough gauge of the state of a nation's health, and of the quality of its health services, and by this test, as everybody knows, the United States does not come off very well. In 1972, the latest year for which the United Nations has published complete statistics, seventeen countries—Australia, Canada, Denmark, East Germany, Finland, France, Hong Kong, Iceland, Ireland, Luxembourg, Malta, Japan, the Netherlands, Norway, Sweden, Switzerland, and the United Kingdom—all had lower rates than the United States. Infant mortality has dropped off steeply in most countries during this century (in 1900, one out of six babies born in America failed to survive their first year) and the death rate in the United States, in 1974, was down to 16.5 deaths for every thousand births. Even so, if the rate in this country from 1969 through 1973 had been as low as the rate in the Netherlands over the same five-year period, 120,000 fewer American babies would have died.

When American doctors are confronted with such statistics, as they have been more and more often in recent years, they are likely to protest angrily that they are being pinned with a bad rap. The way to reduce infant mortality, they argue, is not to tamper with the country's system of medical care, but to clean up the slums and to teach their residents to take better care of themselves and their children. As the AMA has put it, "Infant mortality is not a good measure of the health status of a population or the performance of the health delivery system in a country. If it is to be used at all, it should be used for discussion of a nation's social problems."

There is some basis for this lofty assertion. Babies do die because their mothers are poor and uneducated and do not eat properly while they are pregnant or care for their babies properly after they are born. Babies also die because their mothers do not really want them. Sweden's infant mortality rate, which for many years has been the lowest in the world (in 1973, it was less than ten deaths for every thousand births), can be accounted for in part by the fact that abortions, as well as birth-control information and devices, have long been widely available and widely accepted, and by the fact that Sweden has no counterparts of Watts or Bedford-Stuyvesant or rural Mississippi.

But the figures on infant deaths in the United States, and what they might seem to imply about the quality of medical care in America, cannot so easily be brushed aside. Infant-mortality rates in many other countries are not only lower than in the United States, but have been falling much more rapidly, and in some of these countries it seems quite clear that improved health services have had a good deal to do with this. In 1945, for example, the infant mortality rate was 20 per cent higher in Britain than in the United States. Today it is a few percentage points lower. Since Britain has been in economic difficulties almost steadily since the end of World War II, and since its government has not been notably more successful than the government of the United States in doing away with poverty, the shift in the two countries' positions can doubtless be credited, in part, to the beneficial effects of Britain's National Health Service, which was established in 1946.

In other countries, too, low infant death rates seem to be a result, again in part, of better medical care. "In Sweden," Dr. David D. Rutstein, Professor of Preventive Medicine at the Harvard Medical School, has written, "if a woman is found to be normal on her first medical examination, she is referred to a nurse-midwife who follows her closely throughout her pregnancy. The midwife must report any serious event in the pregnancy to the patient's physician—otherwise, she may lose her license. The nurse-midwife works closely with the patient throughout her pregnancy, visits her home, and keeps a close watch for warning signals." Dr. Rutstein notes that the nurse-midwife, working under a physician's supervision, "is in attendance on the patient from the moment she arrives in labor until after she is delivered. . . . The ability of the nurse-midwife to perform normal deliveries makes it unnecessary to schedule deliveries in Sweden as busy American physicians are often forced to do. As a result, in normal deliveries in Sweden, membranes are rarely ruptured, drugs to induce labor are infrequently prescribed, instruments are less commonly used, and there are fewer surgical interventions. The Swedish physicians then conclude, in the light of these facts, that it is not surprising for Sweden to have a lower infant mortality rate than the United States."

It is not necessary to look to other countries for evidence that high infant death rates in the United States are associated not just with poverty, but with poor medical care. Pierre de Vise of the Chicago Hospital Planning Council, in an essay titled "Slum Medicine: Chicago Style," writes: "At the age of six weeks, Miss J.'s baby was taken to St. Barnaby's emergency room with an acute case of diarrhea. The examining doctor recommended admission for the dehydrated infant, but the hospital refused. Instead the mother and child were sent to Cook County Hospital on the El on a cold winter day. After waiting several hours at the County emergency room, the baby was again seen by a doctor, who prescribed a white powder. Mother and child returned home on the El. During the night, the baby expired. The autopsy reportedly showed death due to dehydration and exposure." De Vise notes that deaths of this sort are fairly common in Chicago. It can be argued, of course, that they are a consequence of poverty, not of poor medical care. But this amounts to saying that a rich mother, unlike Miss

J., would have had a doctor of her own to go to, and would have taken her baby to his office in a taxi. Deaths like those of Miss J.'s baby must be charged to the faults of a system whose defenders often claim that no one in America has to go without good medical care simply because his pockets are empty.

In any case, it has been shown repeatedly that infant deaths fall off sharply in poor communities when there is a real improvement in arrangements for the care of expectant mothers and their babies. In 1965 the Denver Department of Health and Hospitals, with financial help from Washington, established a network of health centers and satellite stations to provide "team" care for more than 100,000 low-income residents of the city, among whom are included a large part of Denver's nonwhite population. Before the new program was set in motion, the infant-mortality rate for nonwhites—42 deaths per 1000 births—was higher in Denver than in any of the seventeen other American cities of approximately its size (that is, with populations of 400,000 to 1,000,000) except Kansas City. In three years, while the infant mortality rate for nonwhites fell by 18 per cent in the United States as a whole, it fell by 40 per cent in Denver. By 1968 only two other cities of its size, San Diego and San Francisco, had lower rates. A program like Denver's but on a smaller scale was started in 1969 in Holmes County, Mississippi. Among other things, it offered the county's residents, most of them black, and most of them very poor, the services of hospital-trained nurse-midwives. In two years, while the infant mortality rate across the country was falling by 7 per cent, the rate in Holmes County fell by 45 per cent.

Over the past twenty years researchers at a number of medical schools and schools of public health have tried to get a line on the quality of medical care in America by examining, case by case, the medical records of hundreds of thousands of hospital patients. In rating the skill and judgment of the attending physicians, the investigators have commonly used as their standard the kind of care that leading specialists in the relevant branch of medicine or surgery would consider appropriate under the circumstances. This method has obvious weaknesses. Doctors may reasonably differ both about the general value of a particular line of treatment, and about the advisability of following it in the case of a particular patient. Moreover, even in an age of scientific medicine, medical decisions are often based largely on faith and guesswork, and doctors may enthusiastically embrace forms of treatment that later turn out to be of far less value than they had assumed.* It was only a few years ago, for instance, that leading ear-nose-and-throat specialists were all in favor of removing tonsils, not because they were eager to drum up surgical business, but because they genuinely (though wrongly) believed that most people are really better off without them.

But while all this makes it hard to establish standards by which a doctor's performance can fairly be judged, there are areas in which the experts' views do rest on a fairly solid scientific basis, and when they do it is reasonable to expect the ordinary practicing physician to go along with the experts. Yet study after study has indicated that all too often American doctors operate when they shouldn't, give their patients the wrong drug, or the right drug in the wrong dosage, make incorrect diagnoses, ignore obvious symptoms that should be followed up, and generally make a botch of their work. In 1962, for example, leading New York specialists reviewed the hospital records of several hundred Teamsters' Union members and their families, all living in the New York City area. Summarizing their findings, Frank Fitzsimmons of the Teamsters' Union told a Senate committee, "Just look at the results of our study: One in five of the hospital admissions was actually unnecessary. Twenty of the sixty hysterectomies performed were unnecessary, and another six were highly questionable. One out of five of the hospitalized patients received poor care, and another one in five received only fair care. . . . More than half of the thirteen Caesarean sections were questionable. One in five general surgical cases appeared to have been the victims of unjustifiable delays in performing the surgery." Fitzsimmons went on to give some examples of what the reviewers regarded as poor care: "In one instance of an unnecessary hysterectomy, the pa-

* In the opinion of one respected authority, Dr. Kerr White, who is chairman of the Department of Medical Care and Hospitals at Johns Hopkins, *most* medicine is unscientific. At any rate, that would seem to be the burden of a syntactically graceless but widely quoted pronouncement he made in 1969 before an audience of public-health experts assembled at Yale. "I know of no evidence," he said, "to suggest that more than 10 to 20 per cent of all that doctors and nurses do for or to patients are based on objective evidence that . . . [the treatments] are likely to be more beneficial and useful than they are harmful and useless."

tient developed a blood clot six days following discharge, necessitating a second eight-day hospital stay. The surveyor noted that if an operation had not been performed in the first place, a second admission would not have been required." Fitzsimmons also cited the case of a man who had complained of stomach pains off and on for four months. "A great deal of laboratory work was done," he told the committee, "but, the surveyor commented, 'the massive investigation was on a schoolboy level. It covered the waterfront and never followed through on the intestinal complaints that were the major cause of admission.'" A second Teamsters' Union study, which was carried out two years later, and which differed from the earlier one mainly in that each case was reviewed by two surveyors instead of one, was equally critical. In four out of ten cases, the quality of hospital care received by the teamsters and their families was rated as only fair or poor.

As Fitzsimmons' remarks suggest, the specialists who carried out these investigations were not asking for the impossible. Their standards were, in fact, met in nine out of ten cases in which the patient was treated in a hospital run by, or closely connected with, a medical school. Similar findings were reported by the Yale investigators who examined the records of some 400 children treated in four Connecticut hospitals. Eighty-seven per cent of the children in one of the four, a large university hospital, were judged to have received "optimal care"; in the other three, all of them smaller community hospitals, the figure was only 57 per cent. Doctors were faulted for, among other things, subjecting children to the discomfort and risk of unnecessary laboratory tests, dosing them unnecessarily with antibiotics, and failing to deal appropriately with psychosomatic disorders. "For example," they noted, "a child was hospitalized for school phobia and chronic abdominal pain, the cause for which was not found. At discharge, the physician recorded his advice to keep the child in bed for one week without toys, books, friends, or television. He explained this might teach the child to appreciate school."

The average community hospital, to be sure, cannot be expected to cope with rare or complicated disorders as effectively as a university medical center. But the records of the Chestnut Hill Hospital in Philadelphia suggest that there is no reason why a community hospital cannot do just as well in handling the common run of medical and surgical conditions. In 1966, nearly half of all appendixes removed by doctors on Chestnut Hill's staff turned out, on examination by the hospital's pathologist, to be perfectly normal. The next year the hospital began reviewing critically the work of its attending physicians, and in 1968 and 1969 the number of normal appendixes taken out amounted to only 19 per cent of the total. (This is considered a pretty good batting average; the only sure way of telling whether an appendix is acutely infected—and is therefore likely to burst—is to take it out and look at it, and even the most skillful and least venal of surgeons remove a certain number of normal appendixes.) In the same two years, according to Dr. Clement Brown, Chestnut Hill's director of medical education, "we had fewer complications, fewer ruptured appendixes—and we did thirty fewer appendectomies." There were also fewer hysterectomies, and fewer complications resulting from hysterectomies, while inappropriate use of antibiotics was reduced, over a three-year period, from 70 per cent of all cases in which patients were given an antibiotic to 25 per cent. Unfortunately, few community hospitals have been as determined to upgrade the work of their medical staffs, and even fewer have been as successful. At proprietary hospitals, those which, unlike most community hospitals, are run as profit-making ventures, there are often no real checks at all on the quality of a doctor's performance.

Most investigators who have looked into the quality of hospital care have been concerned only with bed patients. But more and more Americans are showing up in hospital emergency rooms for the treatment of ailments that do not require hospitalization, and that would in the past have been taken care of in a doctor's office. A study recently reported in the *New England Journal of Medicine* suggests that, quite apart from the impersonality, long waits, and other disagreeable aspects of emergency-room care, there is a very good chance that the patient will not get the relief he is looking for. The authors of the study, Robert H. Brook and Robert L. Stevenson, Jr., undertook to find out what happened to 141 men and women who came to the emergency room of the Baltimore City Hospital in the spring of 1969 complaining of stomach pains, and who were examined and then referred to the hospital's x-ray department.

After interviewing each of the patients, and going over their hospital records, Brook and Stevenson concluded that only 38 of the 141 had gotten effective care.

In a number of cases where the x-ray photographs were unsatisfactory no one told the patient to come back for another try. Sixty of the patients were found to have been given inadequate diagnostic work-ups—that is, proper steps had not been taken to find out what was wrong with them. Of those patients whose x-rays revealed gallstones, hernias, ulcers, or other abnormalities, only about a third received appropriate treatment. "By every criterion included in this study," Brook and Stevenson reported, "the medical care was both inefficient and inadequate. The house staff performed incomplete physical examinations and too few routine laboratory tests. . . . A rewarding physician-patient relation was lacking, as indicated by the few patients who knew why they were scheduled for diagnostic x-ray studies or who learned the results. . . ." For these and other reasons, about a third of the patients experienced "prolonged symptomatology and loss of work," and eventually went elsewhere for help. Brook's and Stevenson's report indicates that it is not only the very poor who use hospital emergency rooms as their family doctors, and who must put up with treatment of this kind. Many of the men who came to the Baltimore City Hospital held skilled or semiskilled factory jobs, and the women were typically employed as secretaries, waitresses, and hospital workers. It cannot be assumed, moreover, that emergency rooms deal with genuine emergencies any more effectively than with ulcers. Investigators at Johns Hopkins reported not long ago that more than half of a group of automobile accident victims who had died from abdominal injuries "should have had a reasonable chance of survival" if mistakes in diagnosis and treatment had not been made in the emergency rooms to which they had been taken.

The haphazard character of medical care in a large American city that is suggested by Brook's and Stevenson's report has also been documented by a different kind of investigation recently carried out in Washington, D.C., by the Institute of Medicine, a branch of the National Academy of Sciences. Physicians examined a sample of 2150 children from both poor and middle-class Washington families, with the aim of determining how well certain common health problems of childhood—poor vision, ear infections, and anemia—were being cared for. The results were, to say the least, disturbing. One out of four four- and five-year-olds had ear infections serious enough to impair their hearing. Seventy per cent of the children wearing eyeglasses saw at least as well without them, and 5 per cent saw *better* when they took their glasses off. Only one third of the children whose blood tests showed them to be anemic had previously been diagnosed as such and were being treated for the disorder.

Most Americans, when they see a doctor, see him in the privacy of his office, and much less is known about what goes on in such encounters than is known about hospital medicine. Back in the 1950s, however, a team of internists, headed by Dr. Osler Peterson of the University of North Carolina, arranged to observe the work of eighty-eight North Carolina doctors, chosen at random from a roster of all physicians in general practice in the state. Peterson and his colleagues spent three or four days with each of the doctors, observing him as he dealt with patients in his office or visited them at their homes or in the hospital. Each doctor was then given a rating. In the end, only seven of the eighty-eight were rated as excellent clinicians; thirty-nine were found to have serious deficiencies.

Nearly half of the doctors in the sample used unsterilized syringes, forgot to wipe the patient's skin before a shot, forgot to wash their own hands after contamination, or were otherwise careless about sterile techniques. Only twelve of the doctors routinely examined the breasts of female patients during general check-ups. When treating patients suffering from hypertension, more than half of the doctors did not try to find out what might be causing the condition, but simply prescribed a drug without advising the patient to lose weight, stop using salt, get more sleep, or make other indicated changes in his or her way of living. About half of the doctors failed to take proper precautions when prescribing potentially dangerous drugs: that is, they failed to ask about previous reactions to penicillin shots, and failed to advise patients about the possibility of their reacting badly to such drugs as cortisone and the hormone ACTH. Twenty-nine per cent of the doctors consistently failed (or refused) to recognize obvious emotional problems. Most doctors kept only the skimpiest of clinical records; eleven doctors recorded only the patient's name and the fee.

There is no reason to suppose that the general practitioners in Peterson's sample were atypically careless or inept. In the late 1950s, a similar investigation of general practitioners in Canada, where medical training and practice are pretty much the same as in the United States, yielded equally discouraging results. The investigators reported that two out of five of the doctors whose work they observed were doing such a poor job as to arouse "grave misgivings." They added, "We must emphasize that the deficiencies to which we refer were *not* lack of knowledge of the details of recently discovered drugs or lack of familiarity with the abstruse complexities of rare diseases. The deficiencies were in the fundamentals of clinical medicine—failure to take an adequate history . . . failure to perform an adequate examination, and, in some cases, inability to distinguish between normal and abnormal physical findings. . . ."

There have, of course, been changes in American medical practice in the nearly twenty years since Peterson and his associates were frequenting doctors' offices in North Carolina. It is now almost unheard of for a young doctor, upon graduation from medical school, to take a one-year internship and then set up shop as a general practitioner, as most young doctors did fifty years ago. More and more Americans are regularly cared for by internists or pediatricians or gynecologists—that is, by specialists who have had two to three more years of postgraduate training than the doctors in Peterson's sample, and who, by and large, probably offer their patients a more sophisticated brand of care. But perhaps as many as 140 million Americans, when they have colds or chest pains or sprained ankles, or when they feel they need a check-up, go to a general practitioner, of whom there are still some 55,000 in the United States. Most of these GPs were in practice at the time Peterson's study was made, and there is no reason to suppose that their performance has improved very much over the years.

One test of the quality of medical care is whether people can get it when they need it. In America, a patient who is lucky enough to have a family doctor may have to wait many days for an appointment, and often the only way to get prompt medical attention is to go to the nearest hospital with an emergency room. The trouble is not that there are too few doctors to go around. The United States has more doctors in proportion to its population than a number of other countries—including Britain, Japan, Sweden, and the Netherlands—where people get just as good medical care as they do here. The difficulty, as I have pointed out, is that we have too many surgeons and too few family doctors, and that too few of the family doctors that we do have want to practice in the places where they are most needed.

In the suburbs, and in prosperous residential areas of the cities, doctors are fairly easy to get hold of. "There's no shortage around here," I was told not long ago by a New York City internist whose office is just off Park Avenue. "If I were to vanish tomorrow it wouldn't make any serious difference to anyone. Well, I suppose one or two of my older patients, who have gotten rather dependent on me, might be upset. But no one would have any trouble finding another doctor right away, and a good one."

Things are quite different, however, in a town I shall call Slaterville, in the mined-out coal fields of north-central Pennsylvania. Not many years ago, Slaterville had four general practitioners, but when I visited there, in 1971, there was only one, Harold Conroy, as I shall call him. Conroy is a thin, energetic man in his late thirties who, like many of his fellow townsmen, was growing a beard to mark the observance of Slaterville's bicentennial. Conroy's work schedule is something like this: Each morning at eight he goes to Slaterville's small community hospital, where, on an average day, he sees fifteen to twenty bed patients, takes care of anyone who comes to the emergency room, and puts in an hour or two in the operating room, assisting the town's only other doctor, who is a surgeon. From one-thirty until five Conroy sees patients in his office—twenty-five to thirty-five on a typical afternoon—and then leaves to make house calls. Two nights a week he is back in his office by seven, and by ten o'clock he will have seen an additional twenty to twenty-five patients. He also delivers two to three babies a week.

Because Conroy has, on the average, only seven or eight minutes to spend with each patient, there are many things he has no time to do. By his own account, he keeps inadequate records, often neglects to give Pap tests (to detect incipient cancer of the cervix or uterus), and doesn't give his older patients the thorough check-ups he thinks they ought to have. He tries to keep up with the medical journals, but he has to do his reading at night when he is apt to be dead tired. "I know we should have group sessions on obesity and on psychiatric problems," he told me gloomily. "I don't have time even to *think* about that." Slaterville badly needs at least one more doctor, and when I was there Conroy and a group of the town's leading citizens were trying hard to find one. But even though the town was offering free office space and a guarantee of $30,000 a year to start with, there had been no takers. Not many American doctors, who can earn a good living almost anywhere, are eager to settle in northern Appalachia.

As it is—or as it was in 1971—Slaterville is better off than many communities. Weldon Barton, a lobbyist for the National Farmers Union, told a Senate committee in 1972 that in the states of Montana, Minnesota, North Dakota, and South Dakota there are more than 800 small towns where there is no doctor. Barton pointed out that fifty years ago four out of five of these towns had doctors of their own. The shortage of doctors is not limited to Appalachia or to thinly settled areas of the Great Plains or the rural South. In 1970, the Illinois Medical Society's placement service listed a town of 22,000 that had only one doctor. In that same year Chelsea, Massachusetts, just outside Boston, had only six doctors, four of whom were over sixty, to take care of 28,000 persons. (This works out to one doctor for every 4666 persons. In England, general practitioners ordinarily have no more than 2500 patients on their lists.) In big-city slums the shortage is often even more acute. "Chicago's Negro west and south sides have been particularly hard hit by the exodus of physicians who have moved office and home to suburbs ten to twenty miles away," Pierre de Vise reported in 1969. "To cite but two examples, the west side community of East Garfield Park had 212 physicians back in 1930, when the population was all white. Today, there are only 13 physicians serving 63,000 Negro residents. The near south side community of Oakland-Kenwood had 110 physicians serving a population of 28,000 whites back in 1930. Today there are but 5 physicians serving a population of 45,000 Negroes."

The shortage of doctors that exists in many places would be much worse if it were not for the wholesale importation of doctors from abroad. In recent years nearly half of all doctors newly licensed to practice in the United States have been alumni of foreign medical schools, most of whom have come to this country right after graduation for advanced training in an American hospital, and many of whom have settled here permanently. By and large, doctors from abroad who come here for training get low marks from their American teachers and colleagues. When physicians at one hundred and fifty hospitals were asked to evaluate interns and residents with whose work they were familiar, the consensus was that the foreign graduates "as a group have a limited capacity for independent learning, require (but do not receive) close supervision, and are predictably less suitable than [American graduates] to become members of the local medical community."

Two out of three of the foreigners who arrive each year to take up internships and residencies in the United States are from India, Korea, the Philippines, Thailand, or other Asian countries, and the poor opinion that many American doctors have of their abilities may well be tinged with chauvinism and racial prejudice. There is no solid basis for questioning the competence of most of the foreign-born doctors who have finished their training and are practicing in the United States. But it is also true that when they arrive in this country a great many graduates of foreign medical schools do not know as much about medicine as their American counterparts. The main reason is that many medical schools in Asia—and in some non-Asian countries as well—do not give students the same chance to work with patients under close faculty supervision that they would have at an American school. Moreover, graduates of such schools are likely to get very little help in making up for their deficiencies after they get to this country. Typically they find themselves at hospitals that have no connection with a university medical center, and that are less concerned with the systematic training of the doctors on their house staffs than with getting the most possible work out of them. Partly as a result, some of these young foreigners fail again and again to pass the examination that must be taken by anyone who wants an unrestricted license to practice medicine in the United States. Often they stay on here anyway, obtaining limited, or temporary, licenses that permit them to practice under the supervision of a fully licensed physician. Other foreign graduates, perhaps as many as several thousand in all, have failed to qualify even for a limited license, but are nevertheless performing operations, giving anesthesia, interpreting x-rays, and generally doing a doctor's work. As a rule, they are employed by a hospital, and are carried on its payroll, usually at a fraction of the salary a licensed physician would command, as ward attendants, x-ray technicians, or medical assistants. No doubt many of these unlicensed and partially licensed doctors are doing a good job. But it seems like a poor idea to ease the doctor shortage in this country by importing men and women whose education has not been up to American standards and exploiting them as cheap medical labor.

Medical care in America has other weaknesses than those so far described. For one, there is the preoccupation of so many doctors with the heroic aspects of their trade, with battling death in fierce hand-to-hand encounters—a preoccupation that often leads to a disdain for the more mundane job of improving the quality of life in the communities where they practice. For another, there is the irritation and bafflement with which so many doctors react to patients who are so inconsiderate as to present them not with nice, clear-cut problems, like lumpy breasts or arthritic hands, but with symptoms of emotional and psychological distress. Four out of five of the North Carolina doctors observed by Peterson and his collaborators seemed indifferent or uneasy when confronted with psychological problems, and they spoke frequently of "malingering," "hypochondriacs," "problem patients," and "getting them out of the office quickly." There is also the tendency of doctors to resist with priestly arrogance the idea that patients, individually or collectively, have anything to say about the kind of treatment they get, or the terms on which they get it.

But before turning to these weaknesses, and their causes, it will be well to take a close look at perhaps the worst deficiency of American medicine, namely, the slovenliness, the chilly disdain, the condescension, and the exploitation that the poor have to put up with when they are sick.

The Bitter Taste of Charity

The hospital's physical plant is a hopelessly obsolete labyrinth of 22 buildings connected by unwashed tunnels. It is a nightmarish caricature of a community hospital 10 times too large. There is no parking within half a mile. There is an average waiting time of two hours to be seen; even 11 per cent of the ambulance cases are made to wait two hours. About 2 per cent of the patients are never seen; they give up, recover or die while waiting. Once admitted, the patient is crowded into a 50 year old ward which he shares with 60 other patients. Twentieth-century innovations like telephones, nurse-patient call systems, doctor paging system, and bathtubs are lacking.
  —*Pierre de Vise, Principal Investigator, Chicago Regional Hospital Study, describing Chicago's Cook County Hospital in 1970*

The family does not like the [hospital] clinics. They are dingy and poorly maintained. Mrs. Santos feels the clerks ask too many questions and sometimes talk so loudly that everyone can hear. She complains about the crowding, the yelling out of names and numbers. And then there is the waiting: waiting for charts, for the x-rays, for the doctors, for the medicine. Waiting half-dressed, with no privacy. Waiting, often for half a day.
  —*Harold B. Wise, former project director, The Dr. Martin Luther King, Jr., Health Center, the Bronx*

I thought I was expecting a baby once. I went into the hospital, and they had me undress in a little room. The nurse took my pressure and said she'd get a doctor. Then she left me. I was there six hours. Finally, I just got up and left—no one was there—nobody noticed me leaving.
  —*Anonymous*

There are doctors' offices in America, it must be said at once, where the poor are welcome, and where the care they get is as sympathetic and thorough as if they had money in the bank. There are city hospitals that are trying to reduce the waiting time in their clinics and emergency rooms, and to make sure that patients are dealt with courteously even if they are on welfare and don't speak fluent English. There are more than a hundred neighborhood health centers, relics of President Johnson's Great Society, where perhaps a million and a half poor people are ministered to by teams of doctors, nurses, and family health workers recruited from the communities that the centers serve, and where they are getting a brand of medical care that is generally a good deal better than the standard poorhouse medicine of which Mrs. Santos complains.

But even though Congress has formally declared that every American has a right to decent medical care, some thirty to forty million people find it hard or impossible to claim that right. While some Americans are having operations they don't need, many more are going without the routine care, both preventive and curative, that most families take for granted. In the late 1960s a team of physicians who investigated the health of black children in six Mississippi counties found, for example, that most of them were getting no medical care of any kind. "In child after child," the doctors reported, "we saw: evidence of vitamin and mineral deficiencies; serious, untreated skin infections and ulcerations; eye and ear diseases, also unattended bone diseases secondary to poor food intake; the prevalence of bacterial and parasitic disease, as well as severe anemia . . . diseases of the heart and the lungs—requiring surgery—which have gone undiagnosed and untreated; epileptic and other neurological disorders; severe kidney ailments, that in other children would warrant hospitalization. . . ." The horrified physicians also noted the prevalence of diseases and conditions "that we know once were easily correctable, but now are hopelessly consolidated: bones, eyes, vital organs that should long ago have been evaluated and treated are now beyond medical assistance, if it were available."

Obviously not all poor people are as badly off as blacks who live in rural Mississippi. Yet in 1966, when children in Head Start programs in some two thousand communities were medically examined, more than 20 per cent were found to have iron deficiency anemia. Seven per cent had visual defects, nearly half had not been immunized against diphtheria, smallpox, polio, tetanus, or whooping cough, and one third had not been seen by a physician for any reason over the two preceding years. A similar survey today might show some change for the better as a result of government health programs set in motion in the 1960s under the banner of the War on Poverty. But the Institute of Medicine's recent investigation of children's health in Washington, D.C., suggests that the improvement may not have been very great. While a disturbingly large fraction of children of all classes were found to have impaired hearing, the proportion was much the highest—23 per cent—among children from the poorest families. Doctors sometimes argue that it is up to parents to make sure that their children get their measles shots and are checked over periodically, and that in a city like Washington—if not in rural Mississippi—a mother who persists in demanding proper medical attention for her children will get it. But the obstacles, as we shall see, may be formidable. In any case, it is hard to take pride in a system of medical care that penalizes children (for example, by allowing them to attend school month after month, year after year, when they can't see the blackboard properly) just because their parents are too poor, too timid, or too uninformed to fight their children's battles with sufficient vigor and intelligence.

The Institute of Medicine's Washington survey was made six years after the enactment of Medicaid, which was intended to make it easier for the poor to get medical care without having to beg for it. But any way one looks at it, Medicaid, for reasons that will be explored in Chapter Eleven, has been a wretched failure. To begin with, unlike Medicare, which was enacted in the same year, and under which every American sixty-five years old or over, whether rich or poor, is entitled to have his hospital bills paid for by the federal government, Medicaid is a welfare program. Anyone who wants to take advantage of its provisions must take a pauper's oath. And many people who set out to establish their eligibility for Medicaid are so daunted by the bureaucratic minefields through which they must pass that they give up. In one state visited in 1970 by the Citizens Board of Inquiry Into Health Services for Americans, Medicaid recipients were entitled to one free outpatient visit per month. "To claim the right," the Board reported, "a recipient must first make an appointment with a doctor, then go with proof of the appointment to the county welfare department for a medical reimbursement form, then back to the doctor, form in hand." (The purpose, it was explained, was to keep doctors from cheating the welfare department by billing it for patients they hadn't seen.) In California, the Board learned, a farm worker's family might have little prospect of making more than, say, $3000 in the course of a year, but nevertheless stood to lose its Medicaid coverage if it happened to earn $500 of this amount in a single month. An informant familiar with the system explained, "Family planning in Tulare County . . . means getting pregnant during July so that the baby will be due when there are no cherries to pick and thus no income to endanger Medicaid eligibility."

More importantly, the original income ceilings for Medicaid recipients were drastically lowered during the late nineteen sixties. The law's benefits are now limited almost entirely to families on welfare, leaving tens of millions of "medically indigent" persons, such as the families of the working poor, whom the act was intended to cover, to shift for themselves. In many states, too, Medicaid does not pay for dental work, eyeglasses, hearing aids, and a number of other rather essential goods and services. In Vermont, for example, an angry Medicaid recipient told state officials, "Your program isn't much good if you can't help me when my eyes get so bad I can't see and my teeth get so bad I can't chew." Three years after Medicaid went into effect, a Blue Cross survey indicated that six out of ten poor people in America were afraid that free medical care might not be available to them in an emergency. Their fears on this score were (and are) not unjustified. A federal task force found in 1970 that only about one third of the people whom Medicaid was intended to protect were getting any of its benefits. The group concluded sadly, "The promise of Medicaid, that some care at least would be available to all who needed it, has vanished into the obscurity of state determinations of eligibility and the limitations of state resources and priorities."

When the poor do get medical care in America it is often in Dickensian settings and on Dickensian terms. "Once I called 20 different doctors asking for an appointment," a woman told the Citizens Board of Inquiry. "Each time the receptionist gave me an appointment. Then I would tell them I was on welfare—I think it's only fair to tell them—and suddenly they couldn't take any patients." This report may be exaggerated, but it is a fact that most doctors won't see people on Medicaid if they can help it. In Portland, Oregon, for example, a survey by the county medical society indicated that only a few more than a third of the city's doctors were willing to treat Medicaid patients, and some of these were limiting the number they would see. Many doctors who signed up with Medicaid in its early days have become convinced, in view of the low fees that Medicaid pays, and the long delays that doctors often have to put up with in collecting their money, that Medicaid is neither good business nor good charity. Some of them look back nostalgically (or say they do) to the days when they treated their poorer patients free, and when the patients comported themselves accordingly. "I joined Medicaid because I thought it was the right thing to do," a Washington, D.C. physician wrote recently on a questionnaire circulated by the District of Columbia Medical Society. "Patients I used to treat free now want more frequent visits which they don't need and [they] bug me on the phone."

By contrast, there are doctors who have chosen to practice in neighborhoods like East Harlem and Chicago's south side, and who specialize in treating the poor. In 1968 representatives of the New York City Health Department visited the offices of more than a hundred such doctors, and their findings were later reported in the *American Journal of Public Health* by the chief of the department's Medicaid office, Dr. Florence Kavaler. Dr. Kavaler wrote that most of the doctors had well-equipped offices and seemed to be working conscientiously to take care of a population which, she noted bitterly, other doctors had abandoned. But little attention was being paid to preventive measures, she pointed out, and most of the doctors were seeing so many patients that they had time only to give symptomatic relief in the form of shots and prescriptions.

Some doctors have been attracted to the slums purely because it is possible to make a lot of money there if one is not too finicky. Leon A. Katz, a member of the New York City Council who conducted an investigation of doctors with large Medicaid practices, reported that some of them were seeing two to three hundred patients a day. In one six-month period, he told the Council, an internist working part-time in a Harlem clinic had billed Medicaid for $106,000. An investigation in Chicago in the late 1960s, when doctors' earnings were a lot lower than they are now, turned up a number of doctors specializing in the treatment of welfare clients who were clearing between $50,000 and $100,000 a year. One of the biggest earners was a physician identified by the pseudonym of Dooley. "[His] patients arrive without appointment and wait one to three hours before being sent to one of six under-equipped examining rooms," an investigator reported. "Dr. Dooley sees 100 patients each day, which means cursory examination, unconcerned technique and inadequate explanation. This doctor doesn't even gown patients or wash his hands between examinations." Some welfare physicians in Chicago were regularly adding to their earnings by billing the Department of Aid for two visits if, say, a mother with a sick child happened, while in the doctor's office, to ask a question about another child whom she had not brought with her. ("Patient C.R., left at home, had symptoms of chapped lips according to the mother's report," an investigator wrote. "Dr. R.P. wrote four prescriptions for him and charged the agency for a diagnostic visit and a shot.") Another common practice was to make patients come back at frequent intervals: "Each week Dr. Dooley may see a patient with arthritis, spraying the back with ethyl chloride and renewing prescriptions of analgesic and muscle relaxant. This means he can bill the welfare department six dollars a week, twenty-four dollars a month for saying hello to the patient and signing a pre-typed prescription."

Some doctors were handing out two or three prescriptions to each patient, specifying that they be filled at a particular pharmacy of which the doctor happened to be a part owner. A year or so after this investigation, two doctors practicing in one of the poorest sections of Chicago were cited by the Chicago Board of Health for operating an unsanitary medical facility with broken stairs, peeling plaster, refuse in the hallways, and without sterilizing equipment or functioning toilets. In the preceding year, one of these physicians had been paid $95,729 for treating recipients of public assistance, and the other $87,643.

In New York City, hospital emergency rooms are furnishing primary medical care, the kind of care people have traditionally expected from their family doctor, to at least half a million persons, and perhaps to many more. Considering how hard it is for poor people to get a doctor to see them, and given the sketchiness of the care they are likely to get in those doctors' offices where they are welcome, the figures are not surprising. A mother who takes her sick child to an emergency room can at least be sure that the child will be examined by a doctor—provided, that is, she goes to a county or city hospital that is required to treat people free if they can't pay; or, if she goes to a private hospital, provided she can convince the clerk that she can pay for the visit, or that Medicaid will foot the bill.

But unless the visitor to an emergency room is bleeding heavily, or seems to be in danger of dying if he doesn't get immediate attention, he may be in for a long wait. The *New York Post* recently reported, for example, the case of a postal clerk who had to wait more than six hours in the emergency room of Harlem Hospital to get some advice on what to do about minor pains in his neck and shoulder. The *Post* also reported that the staff of the pediatric emergency room at Lincoln Hospital in the Bronx was so overworked "that sick children squirm for four hours in a jammed waiting room, swapping respiratory infections." Even people who are seriously ill may be ignored for hours. The bureaucratic indifference that is often to blame for such delays has been portrayed by a Columbia student, Barry Siegel, who spent some time in 1972 as an observer in the emergency room of a small hospital on the edge of Harlem. "It's 12:30 p.m.," his account begins, "and four patients have been lined up at the window of the waiting room for almost 45 minutes, since I've been here, trying to register to see a doctor. I'm getting nervous about the first patient in line, Jim, a big muscular black man about 40. He's sitting in a chair, his head buried in his arms, which rest on the counter before the window, and he's moaning . . . he seems to lapse into semi-consciousness every few minutes. A friend, Ralph, stands next to him, patting his shoulder." Three quarters of an hour later, even though two nurses were on emergency-room duty, Jim was still sitting there. "I can hear the two nurses arguing in the back room about a paperwork procedure," Siegel's account continues. "They can't decide which supervisor's directions they should follow. One of them comes out and walks down the hallway. I walk up to her and ask her why no one is at the window. 'There's usually someone there,' she says vaguely. . . . 'We can't handle them until they're processed. That's the clerk's job. . . .' She walks over to the door leading into the waiting room and calls in a patient, a Mr. Simon, who had registered before the clerk left the window. But Mr. Simon isn't there; he left a half-hour ago. The nurse doesn't call another patient."

A visit to an emergency room, even if it is well organized and well staffed, is likely to be a humiliating ordeal if one is poor, and more particularly if one is also black or Puerto Rican or Mexican-American. The patient who shows up with a cough or a fever or a stomachache not only has to sit for hours, straining to hear if it is his name that is being called out over the low-fidelity public-address system, but he must also be prepared to be treated like a recruit at a Marine boot camp. The attitudes he is likely to encounter have been described by Julius Roth, a sociologist who has made a special study of what goes on in emergency rooms. "The workers on emergency wards with large slum-area clienteles develop a negative conception of their patients," he writes. "They seek to establish a defensive position against the lower depths of our society. They often exchange stories demonstrating how unintelligent, untrustworthy, and immoral the patients are. New clerks, aides, nurses, and doctors are instructed by the older hands not to tolerate any abuse or disobedience from the clientele, not to accede to their demands, or do burdensome favors for them." Roth points out that some of this is just talk, and that the clerk who speaks of patients as "garbage" may, in fact, treat most of them quite politely. Nevertheless, he continues, the patient "will often wait until employees get around to him, be made to stand while questioned even if ill or aged, be notified peremptorily about the rules and procedures ('Sit down over there'; 'Put out the cigarette'; 'You can't go back there') and be subjected to questioning that would be considered impertinent by middle-class people ('Are you on welfare?'; 'Is there a father in the home?'; 'Are you able to pay for this visit?')"

An emergency-room staff may perform brilliantly when confronted with third-degree burns, multiple fractures, bullet wounds, and other life-threatening emergencies, but it does not follow that the patient with ordinary aches and pains will get equally good care. He may be seen by an inexperienced intern, working under inadequate supervision. In any case, the doctor who sees him will have time to hear only about the particular symptom that brought him to the emergency room. If the patient's problem is a swollen and possibly broken ankle, or something in his eye, that is all the doctor really has to know. But more and more people who come to emergency rooms these days have ailments that are complicated, or poorly defined, or of social or psychological origin. Their sufferings can only depress and frustrate the compassionate physician who knows that in his brief, impersonal encounter with such patients he has no hope of discovering what is really wrong, let alone of doing or saying anything really helpful. And even when a patient's complaint is relatively simple—a sore throat, an earache, a bad case of poison ivy—the staff is likely to feel that it is being imposed on by being asked to deal with such trivia. It is, of course, the poor who suffer most in these circumstances. "Welfare cases are more likely to be denigrated than patients of private physicians," Roth observes, since doctors and nurses tend to resent having their valuable time taken up by freeloaders. "Thus if the patient has no problem which is a 'real emergency' by the definition of the staff," Roth adds, "he is more likely to be given short shrift, superficial diagnosis and careless treatment."

Many poor people go regularly for medical care not to the emergency rooms of hospitals but to their outpatient clinics. These differ from emergency rooms in several ways. They are open only at specified hours, and patients are seen only by appointment. They often undertake to give continuing care to people with diabetes, high blood pressure, and other chronic diseases. They are primarily for people who can't find or can't afford private doctors. And they commonly serve to provide medical students, interns, and residents with patients whom they can thump, poke, question, draw blood from, bandage, tranquilize, cut open, sew up, and generally practice on.

Patrons often prefer hospital clinics to private physicians. This was true, for example, of more than half of a group of welfare clients questioned recently in New York City. "A hospital is better equipped," one woman said. "There's more exchange of ideas." A number of people said hospital examinations were more thorough than the examinations they would be likely to get from a private doctor. A middle-aged Irish-American woman said, "The doctors in the clinic are registered, not just picked up. The clinic knows how to pick good doctors better than someone like me." Much the same point was made by a black woman in her fifties with whom I spoke in the pediatric clinic of New York's Columbia Presbyterian Medical Center, where she had taken her two granddaughters for check-ups. I asked her whether, assuming she had won a million dollars in the New York State lottery, she would take them to a private pediatrician instead. Her reaction was indignant. "Why should I?" she asked. "Where in the world would I find better doctors than right here?"

Such confidence is to a degree justified. The care to be had from doctors working in the clinics of university hospitals like Columbia Presbyterian is likely to be thorough and technically expert. And a few hospitals are trying to reorganize their clinics so as to offer patients the equivalent, if not of a family doctor, at least of a good group practice. In general, however, the care that poor people get at hospital clinics is very far from ideal.

To begin with, when a patient's condition has been tentatively diagnosed, and he has been referred to the appropriate clinic, he may have to wait months for an appointment. Brook and Stevenson, in their report on the Baltimore City Hospital, noted that patients referred to the hospital's gastrointestinal clinic for treatment were given appointments two and a half months in the future. When the appointed day does come around, the patient may have to wait for hours to see a doctor. (At many clinics it is customary for the doctors not to show up until an hour or two after the first batch of patients has been instructed to appear.) Occasionally a patient will go to an emergency room and, after examination by a doctor, be referred to one of the hospital's specialty clinics—only to discover, when he arrives to keep his appointment weeks or months later, that he has been sent to the wrong clinic. A resident in urology at a leading New York hospital told me that many of the patients he sees in the hospital's urology clinic have to be told, sometimes after having waited for up to five hours to see a doctor, that what they have is a slipped disk, not an infected kidney, and that what they need is an appointment at the orthopedic clinic. Clinic patients also waste a lot of time, and undergo a lot of unnecessary anxiety, because it is usually impossible to consult the clinic doctors by telephone. During a morning that I spent in Columbia Presbyterian's pediatric clinic I estimated that about half of the parents who came in with their children had problems that more fortunate mothers are able to resolve by phoning their pediatrician.

Another thing wrong with outpatient care at big teaching hospitals is that it is provided by as many as forty or fifty separate clinics. This suits the convenience of the residents in training, and of the senior cardiologists, orthopedic surgeons, neurologists, and other specialists and subspecialists who want, both for teaching purposes and for their research, a steady flow of patients with the particular diseases in which they are interested. But it means not only that every member of a family must ordinarily go to a different clinic, but that a patient who has two or three different things wrong with him may have to attend two or three different clinics. No one is responsible for considering whether and how his seemingly separate ailments may be related. In these circumstances, a patient with an injured knee or an infected ear may get excellent treatment, but the system has little to offer to the patient who has recently lost his job, who has intermittent pains, and who suffers from insomnia and impotence.

From a human, if not from a strictly technical standpoint, clinic medicine has another serious drawback: its brusque impersonality, which is particularly disagreeable when, as often happens, the clinic doctors seem to think of their patients simply as teaching material. A young San Francisco woman recently tried to make clear to Senator Kennedy's Subcommittee on Health just how unpleasant this can be. Explaining that she had gone to a large San Francisco hospital for prenatal care because she and her husband could not afford a private obstetrician, she said, "[We] would all be given an appointment at nine o'clock in the morning and if you were lucky and happened to get there early you might be able to see a doctor by ten-thirty—or sometimes you had to wait until eleven-thirty or so. After this you see the doctor for five minutes. I never saw the same doctor twice . . . it was always a different person and there was never any kind of attempt made to treat anybody who is there like they were a person or like they deserved any kind of attention as being a person—it was just a pregnant 'being' who had to get this baby delivered." Toward the end of her pregnancy, she testified, "one of the interns or doctors examining me decided there was something slightly irregular about the position of the baby; and so he went out, without saying anything to me, and called in five or six other people, who all proceeded to poke and stick their fingers in me. I was only nineteen years old, and it was my first pregnancy."

Finally, the care that poor people get in emergency rooms

and clinics inevitably suffers because the poor tend to be disliked, as patients, by the doctors who treat them there. Partly this is because of the nature of clinic practice, which too seldom permits a doctor the gratification of getting to know a patient and watching the patient respond to treatment. But beyond this, the young, mainly middle-class medical students and interns and residents who staff the clinics of big urban hospitals quickly become angered and depressed by the overwhelming problems of their patients, and by their own inability to do much about solving those problems. "I sincerely doubt," a Harvard medical student told Daniel Funkenstein, a psychiatrist who has made a specialty of studying medical-student attitudes, "that the majority of recent graduates have the 'nobility of soul' required to endure the self-sacrifice and lack of patient gratitude inherent in urban ghetto practice. Two years ago, I thought I had it; I have found that I do not."

As this comment suggests, one reason why doctors don't want to spend too much of their time treating poor people is that, as they look at it, the poor are bad patients. A good patient is one who is well-educated and articulate, who shares many of the doctor's interests and values, who does exactly what the doctor tells him to do, and who is grateful to the doctor when this makes him feel better. Poor people, by contrast, often seem to take the doctor's services for granted. The clinic doctor may find this all the more annoying if he suspects that the patient with whom he is dealing is largely to blame for his own troubles. As recently as 1968, a national survey showed four out of ten American physicians to be in agreement with the statement, "A dissolute way of life is the cause of many diseases among the poor." And while the proportion of recent medical-school graduates who feel this way is probably not so high, even idealistic young doctors are resentful and impatient when the patients whom they see in hospital clinics don't follow instructions and won't give clear, straightforward answers to the questions that are put to them.

The clinic doctor could, in principle adapt his questioning and his explanations—and even his expectations as to gratitude—to the language and attitudes of his patients. He could learn some Spanish, and read up on the theories of folk medicine to which many Puerto Ricans subscribe. But doctors usually feel that they have been trained, at great effort and expense, to diagnose and treat the patient's ills, and that it is up to someone else to see to it that the patient plays his part successfully. This attitude emerged quite clearly in a talk I had with a young, politically liberal, and unusually candid young physician, a cardiologist, who is on the staff of a large New York hospital. Speaking of why doctors seem to be reluctant to practice in the ghetto even when the pay is good, he said, "I think one of the reasons is that the doctors haven't liked their experience with ghetto patients. I know that the patients whom I see at the clinic that I can talk to, I enjoy. And they probably get better care. The patients who come in who are hostile, who are not particularly interesting, who are Spanish-speaking—well, for instance, you tell a woman, 'Now don't dress up like you're going off to a ball; you know I want to listen to your heart.' And then they come in all dressed up, you know, and corseted, and it's impossible to get at them. There's just no way that I can imagine myself or anyone else giving these people the same kind of concern and sympathetic attention I would give to a patient whom I liked."

It is often said that if one is seriously ill in America the next best thing to being very rich is being very poor. The main basis for this belief is the fact that each year hundreds of thousands of poor people are cared for, often at little or no expense even if they are ineligible for Medicaid, as teaching patients in university hospitals like Columbia Presbyterian in New York City, Massachusetts General in Boston, or Johns Hopkins in Baltimore. Although such patients are under the direct care of interns and residents, each stage in their diagnosis and treatment is ordinarily reviewed by specialists who teach at the hospital and its affiliated medical school. The result, as we have seen, is that the patient stands to get better care from a technical point of view (he is less likely to have his condition misdiagnosed, or to be operated on unnecessarily, or to be dosed with the wrong drugs) than the average private patient gets at many community and proprietary hospitals.

But the poor pay heavily for this. As in the clinics, they have to submit to being worked over and talked about by relays of medical students and house officers. This may entail having samples of their blood drawn repeatedly for tests whose main purpose is not to help the patient but to satisfy the curiosity and further the education of the house staff. Even when tests or other procedures are clearly in the patient's interest, the young house officers who order them may not bother to explain what is being done, and why. Too often the patient is seen as having obligations, but no rights, his main obligation being to make things as easy as possible for the hard-pressed staff. Rose Lamb Coser, a sociologist who has studied life in the ward of a university hospital, found that most of the doctors and nurses were convinced that the patients were antagonistic ("they won't give you a decent history"); that patients should be "good" (nurses disciplined "bad" patients by not answering their calls right away); and that the patients were children ("we don't tell them anything"). Most people who have spent time in a hospital have no doubt encountered such attitudes. But they are particularly common on the wards of university and municipal hospitals, where the patients have no doctors of their own and, being objects of charity, are in no position to fight back.

The advantages of being treated in a university hospital, such as they are, are available to only a minority of the poor. There are not nearly enough teaching beds to accommodate all of them, and the physician whose job it is to assign patients to such beds knows that his colleagues will be angry with him if he fails to reserve them, by and large, for patients whose ailments are mysterious, rare, or complicated, or who are suffering from a common disease that happens to be of current interest to a hospital research group. Poor people who need to have their hernias repaired, or their gall bladders removed, stand little chance of admission to a university hospital if the residents in surgery have already tried their hands at a sufficient number of such operations, and are looking for more challenging problems. This is also true, to give one more example, of men suffering from a form of inflammation of the penis, not dangerous, but often uncomfortable, that can be relieved only by circumcision. "If a guy comes to the clinic and needs a circumcision, I tell him we'll put him on the waiting list," I was told by the same young urologist who sees so many patients with slipped disks. "But there are five hundred people on the list, and in my year working in the clinic I have never heard of anyone being called. The chief resident doesn't want to use up precious operating room time on circs." In theory, a man who needs a circumcision can, if he is on Medicaid, get admitted to a university hospital as a private patient—that is, under the care of a surgeon in private practice who does some teaching at the hospital and who is entitled, as a quid pro quo, to treat his own patients there. But surgeons who qualify for such appointments usually have plenty of business without taking on work for which they will be paid only the relatively low fees that Medicaid ordinarily allows.

Voluntary hospitals that are not closely affiliated with medical schools also may admit charity patients from time to time. But a great many hospitals, even though their exemption from taxes is granted to them because they are supposedly charitable as well as nonprofit enterprises, customarily demand proof that their bills will be paid, or insist on sizeable cash deposits, before they will admit a patient."In Prestonburg, Kentucky," *Health Law Newsletter* has reported, "a 21-year-old woman died soon after the birth, at home, of her third child. The child was born at home because the Prestonburg General Hospital refused to admit the mother without a $250 deposit and refused to accept a check for that deposit. The same hospital refused to treat a 5-year-old boy's broken leg because the parents had no money." Some hospitals refuse to honor a Medicaid card unless the holder has been accepted as a private patient by a doctor on the hospital's staff. By enforcing this rule, and by granting staff privileges only to doctors practicing in other (and richer) neighborhoods, a hospital can largely avoid treating Medicaid patients even if it is located in the middle of a slum. In 1970, according to Pierre de Vise of the Chicago Hospital Planning Commission, some 18,000 emergency patients, many of whom were presumably on Medicaid, were refused admission to private hospitals in Chicago, and were taken instead to Cook County Hospital, whose amenities are catalogued at the head of this chapter. "Hundreds of these transfers were unsafe and resulted in about fifty deaths," de Vise has written.

Thus more often than not the poor end up in public hospitals, whose wards and corridors are seldom seen by middle-class Americans. Few cities and counties have been willing to spend enough money on their hospitals to maintain and run them properly, and they tend to be overcrowded, obsolete, inadequately staffed, and chaotic. In 1970, for example, staff physicians at the District of Columbia General Hospital, one of the largest in the country, complained to the Joint Commission on

Accreditation of Hospitals that certain commonly used drugs were often out of stock for a week or more at a time; that it took as long as two weeks to get a routine x-ray taken, and that pictures were lost with astounding regularity ("One physician recently reported the loss of three repeated x-ray studies on one patient within a 24-hour period. . . ."); and that records were so poorly handled that "in a recent sampling of 55 requests for patient records . . . only one out of six could be retrieved." A resident physician at San Francisco General Hospital, told a Senate committee, in 1972, that accident victims brought there "frequently had to wait for extended periods of time. In other areas of the hospital exposed wiring was evident. Skylights were cracked and leaked when it rained. Stench emanated from dirty utility rooms, in some cases a mixture of raw urine and stale dirty water. Toilets were filthy and rarely supplied with soap and towels. . . ."

In 1970 the Society of Urban Physicians, whose members are all chiefs of service at one or another of New York City's municipal hospitals, published an angry report on the inadequacy of nursing care in their institutions. The report noted that "three thousand patients on general medical wards of thirteen municipal hospitals were cared for by thirty-five registered nurses during a recent night . . . and one third of the nurses on duty were at a single hospital." Hundreds of patients were dying in the municipal hospitals every year, the Society charged, because of inadequate nursing. Some patients were said to be dying because they were not turned over often enough to keep them from developing bedsores. "At least fifteen cases of the following," a doctor noted in a report on Coney Island Hospital. "Bedsores develop, eroding skin, causing infection. Patient's blood is poisoned, he goes into shock, and dies, of septicemia." A year later, Edmund O. Rothschild, a physician serving on the board of the New York City Health and Hospitals Corporation, which runs the city's hospitals, complained bitterly that nothing much had changed. "Mr. Shapiro (or Rivera, Spinelli, Wilkins, Wong, or Ryan) is about to die," he wrote in *The New York Times.* "His tracheotomy tube, the metal one temporarily placed in his windpipe to help him breathe, is becoming clogged with mucus. He needs to have it suctioned clean, but there is no nurse around right now. He will die tonight because of inadequate nursing care. Mr. Shapiro could have avoided this fate in another hospital, but he is in a New York City municipal hospital. He will die because he is poor or because he is old or because he does not have a private physician. He is a victim of the two-class system of medical care in this nation."

Many doctors who work in public hospitals are compassionate and dedicated. But others grow cynical and callous, readily finding excuses for withholding their sympathy from patients whose troubles can be blamed on their own moral deficiencies. Thus David Sudnow, a sociologist who spent many months studying attitudes toward death in a large county hospital, observed that the young interns and residents who staffed the hospital, working almost entirely without supervision from older physicians, were quick to give up on certain kinds of patients. "Not only were gravely ill alcoholic patients more readily assessed as terminal," Sudnow writes, "but so were other classes of patients whose character and social background were regarded as less than desirable. Victims of violence from lower-class settings, prostitutes, suicidal cases, vagrants, narcotic addicts, and the like, when encountered in grave borderline illnesses, were normally accorded a more rapidly fatal fate." Sometimes, Sudnow suggests, the belief that a patient is "undeserving" becomes a license for treating him as nonhuman. "A woman was brought into the emergency unit with a self-inflicted gunshot wound which ran from the sternum downward and backward, passing out through the kidney," he writes. He continues:

> She had apparently bent over a rifle and pulled the trigger . . . she was quite alive and talkative, and though in great pain and very fearful, was able to conduct something of a conversation. She was told that she would need immediate surgery and was taken off to the operating room; following her were a group of physicians, all of whom were interested in seeing the damage done in the path of the bullet. (One doctor said aloud, quite near her stretcher, "I can't get my heart into saving her, so we might as well have some fun out of it.") During the operation the doctors regarded her body much as they do one during an autopsy. After the critical damage was repaired and they had reason to feel the woman would survive, they engaged in numerous surgical side ventures, exploring muscular tissue in areas of the back through which the bullet had passed but where no damage had been done that required repair other than the tying off of bleeders

and suturing. One of the operating surgeons performed a side operation, incising an area of skin surrounding the entry wound on the chest, to examine, he announced to his colleagues, the structure of the tissue through which the bullet had passed. He explicitly announced the project to be motivated by curiosity; one of the physicians spoke of the procedure as an "autopsy on a live patient," about which there was a little laughter.

There is no way of knowing how much of this sort of thing goes on in public hospitals. But the openness of the proceedings (they were carried out, after all, in the presence of an outside observer) suggests that at this particular hospital, at any rate, young doctors in training saw nothing wrong at all with casual human vivisection.

It would be naive to suppose that we will ever have one-class medical care in America in the sense that all sick people will be treated in identical settings, with identical dispatch, sympathy, and technical skill. There are few places in the world—and none in Europe—where generals, politicians, managers of big industrial enterprises, and other rich and powerful persons do not contrive to get extra care and attention when they are sick. But in Norway and Sweden, in Britain and Canada, in Hungary and Czechoslovakia, the poor have access to the same hospitals and clinics and doctors' offices, and are treated on the same terms, as the vast majority of their more prosperous countrymen. It should be a matter of national shame that this cannot be said of the United States.

5

The Price of Scientific Medicine

Much that is wrong with medical care in America can be blamed, paradoxically, on the power that doctors have acquired to prevent and cure a wide variety of human diseases. As L. J. Henderson, a widely respected physiologist and medical sociologist, pointed out some forty years ago, doctors have not had this power very long. "I think it was about 1910 or 1912," Henderson observed, "when it became possible to say of the United States that a random patient with a random disease consulting a doctor chosen at random stood better than a fifty-fifty chance of benefiting from the encounter."

The potency that medicine has achieved in this century was made possible by the discoveries of Pasteur, Koch, and other nineteenth-century pioneers in the new field of bacteriology, who formulated the germ theory of disease and demonstrated its validity. Among the first to benefit by their work were surgical patients. The wearing of sterile gowns, and the use of sterile instruments, one historian has written, "rejuvenated surgery entirely and transformed surgical wards, after centuries of hospital gangrene, into places which one could enter with the hope of leaving alive." At the same time, by showing that certain diseases were invariably associated with the presence of certain specific microorganisms, the bacteriologists gave physicians some understanding of a whole group of diseases, including tuberculosis, pneumonia, diphtheria, and malaria, whose causes were as dimly perceived before the turn of the century as the causes of cancer and schizophrenia are today. This understanding led in time to prevention and cure. Thus diphtheria and paralytic polio have all but vanished in the United States, while measles, whooping cough, and scarlet fever are disappearing. Pneumonia and influenza, which were the two principal causes of death in the United States in 1900, are seldom fatal now if properly treated with antibiotics. And while medicine's most striking victories have been won over infectious diseases, physicians have also learned to bring under some degree of control certain chronic and noninfectious disorders, such as diabetes and pernicious anemia.

All this has inevitably, and rightly, enhanced the respect that physicians command. But their new therapeutic prowess, and the basis on which it rests—that is, an understanding of human physiology, and of how it is affected by disease, at a cellular and molecular level—has just as inevitably changed in complicated ways the nature of the physician's calling.

To begin with, the traditional general practitioner is almost certainly headed for extinction in the United States. There is so much to know about disease and its treatment, and that knowledge is being so rapidly augmented, that young doctors understandably despair of being able to deal competently with the wide variety of conditions, from broken ankles and chicken pox to tubal pregnancies and leukemia, that they will be called on to cope with if they elect to go into general practice. And so, whereas more than half of all medical-school graduates in the 1920s ended their formal training after a year's internship and became general practitioners, today more than nine out of ten young doctors choose to take advanced training in surgery, internal medicine, or other specialties in which they can enjoy the comfortable feeling of knowing a little better what they are doing.

There are other reasons, of course, why most doctors now become specialists. For one thing, a neurosurgeon or urologist is not so constantly at the beck and call of his patients as is the family doctor. For another, specialization pays off in both money and prestige. Because Americans can afford to spend so much more money than they used to for medical care, and, more importantly, because there is so much more that doctors can do for them, the demand for doctors' services has soared. The average American sees a doctor twice as often as he did forty years ago, and in a given year he is more than twice as likely to be admitted to a hospital. Yet until recently the output of American medical schools has been held, as we have seen, to a relatively low level, and for the past thirty years a young doctor has been able to choose just about any branch of medicine that appealed to him without having to worry where his patients would come from. Moreover, quite apart from any real benefits a patient may stand to gain by consulting a specialist, the consultation itself tends to enhance his status. "My cardiologist," or "Grace's obstetrician" falls more pleasantly from the tongue than "our local M.D." Thus while Americans may complain about the growing scarcity of general practitioners, they have been unwilling to pay the GP as well as his more highly trained competitors. Even in pediatrics, the worst-paid of the major specialties, earnings average several thousand dollars a year higher than in general practice.

The exodus from general practice has been further speeded by the contempt in which the GP is held by members of medical-school faculties. The best that most academic physicians can find to say about him is that he is the victim of circumstances that force him to be an incompetent bungler. This point of view has been expressed by, among others, Dana W. Atchley, an authority on psychosomatic illness and for many years a prominent member of the faculty of Columbia University's College of Physicians and Surgeons. At a time, several years ago, when the American Academy of General Practice was urging medical schools to train more GPs, Atchley characterized the Academy's leaders as "nostalgic artisans struggling counter current to survive." He went on to say, "One motive of some members of this group is the urge to turn back the clock to the time when the goal of medicine was to graduate an artisan rather than a scientist. The student is [to be] moved out of the academic environment in order to become familiar with home conditions, family life, economic facts, and the practical problems of general practice. . . . What could an apprenticeship to a general practitioner contribute to our goal? What could a department of general practice teach at the undergraduate level except artisanship of a disillusioning nature . . . ?"

The prevalence of this attitude in academic medicine, and the extent to which it rubs off on students, are suggested by a poll taken a few years back at the medical school of the State University of New York's Downstate Medical Center in Brooklyn. Seniors at Downstate were asked how they thought various kinds of doctors were regarded within their profession. Not one student said he thought general practitioners were "very highly admired," and only 4 per cent thought they were "quite respected." By contrast, 94 per cent said it was their impression that internists—specialists, that is, in the nonsurgical treatment of adult diseases—were either highly admired or quite respected, and 64 per cent placed surgeons in one or the other of these categories. Not surprisingly, in the year the poll was taken only seven out of 170 members of the junior and senior classes at Downstate said they themselves planned to go into general practice.

The general practitioner's low standing reflects in part the ignorance and snobbery of his detractors. "The intern does not see all the fine preventive work done outside the hospital," Robert J. Haggerty, an expert on child care, and himself a professor at a medical school, has observed, "but the fact of the family doctor missing the diagnosis of a rare disease like Moschkowitz's syndrome is bantered about the house staff lounge as an indication of the poor level of most family doctors." Still, a strong argument can be made that the average general practitioner, after four years of medical school and a year or two as an intern, simply can't know enough to do a good job, and that people are better off under the regular care of specialists. Many pediatricians and internists do act as general medical advisers, seeing their patients again and again over a period of years, and diagnosing and treating a wide variety of ailments. In addition, more than 200 hospitals are now offering three-year residencies leading to certification in a new specialty called family practice. The family practitioner will not be expected to spread himself as thin as the usual GP—he may deal with simple fractures and, on occasion, deliver babies, but he will not ordinarily take out anybody's appendix—and sponsors of the new programs hope that graduates will command the earnings and respect that other specialists enjoy. In any case, the idea is to attract students who want close, continuing relations with patients, and who rather like the idea of having to cope mainly with fairly commonplace disorders, but who want to be able to deal with them in a more informed and sophisticated fashion than the limited training of a general practitioner would permit.

In 1973, 770 young doctors began residencies in family practice; in 1974, the number rose to 1200. The total is still small, however, compared with the more than 16,000 men and women who begin residencies each year in general surgery, internal medicine, psychiatry, pediatrics, obstetrics and gynecology, pathology, and other traditional specialties. To be sure, some young physicians trained as internists and pediatricians will elect to spend much of their time doing work that has traditionally been done by GPs. Together with the new family practitioners they will replace most of the 1500 GPs who retire or die in harness each year. But young doctors by and large remain highly skeptical about the rewards of family medicine. In 1972, when *Medical Economics* questioned graduating medical students about their plans, only one out of eight expressed an interest in full-time family practice. (This compares with one out of four doctors now practicing in the United States who is either a GP, or else is an internist who conducts a limited general practice—i.e., no surgery—for adults, or a pediatrician who does the same for children.) One third of the students who were polled said they had no interest at all in family medicine, and recent history suggests that, as time passes, more and more of them will come to feel this way. Many of the students rejecting family medicine gave reasons such as "long, irregular hours," "underpaid," "monotonous and noncreative." Others shared the view of a student who wrote: "Family medicine is a specialty doomed to die because of the explosion of scientific knowledge and the desire of patients to get the best care possible." All that is certain is that scientific medicine has deprived a great many Americans of the services once provided by general practitioners; that these services—some of them, at any rate—are badly missed; and that nobody knows how they will be provided in the future, and by whom.

As medicine has become more scientific, and more effective, there has been a striking change in the way doctors view their job as healers. Seventy-five years ago a physician typically was less concerned with curing his patients, which in most cases was out of the question, than with relieving their anxiety and pain. The poet Mark Van Doren, whose father was a country doctor who practiced in Illinois around the turn of the century, recalls in his autobiography that his father's "controlling desire as a doctor was that his patients be comfortable.... He wanted them to feel better, and the thing I have heard most often from those he visited is that they did so as soon as he entered the house. His theory, he once told me, was to 'treat the symptoms' and trust the disease to become discouraged and go away, having no longer any power to express itself." Once, while attending an old man who was burning with fever, and who seemed unlikely to live through the night, the elder Van Doren granted his patient's wish to be dunked in the cold water of the rain barrel that stood at the corner of his house. The doctor saw no reason not to treat the symptoms, and by doing so to ease the last hours of a dying man. As it turned out, the patient recovered. But that was an act of Providence and, in a way, quite beside the point.

The style of medical practice is altogether different today, and the difference is not just that doctors no longer have time to sit up all night with dying patients. Today the physician's attention is focused not so much on the patient as on the nature of the disease that has invaded his body, disease being viewed primarily as a disturbance of the body's physiological processes that can be dealt with most effectively by studying it and treating it at the cellular or subcellular level. This way of going about their work is precisely what has conferred on doctors their new power to prevent illness and restore health. But it has had serious side effects as well.

One of these side effects is that doctors too often think of patients not as fellow humans to be listened to and comforted, but as temporary and dimly seen hosts to a disease that it is the doctor's job to identify and subdue. The coldness and inhumanity to which this can lead have been depressingly portrayed by Raymond S. Duff and August B. Hollingshead in a book called *Sickness and Society*. The authors, who are professors at Yale (Duff is a physician and Hollingshead a sociologist) closely observed, over a period of several months, how patients were treated in a large teaching hospital, affiliated with a leading American medical school, to which they give the name Yankee Hospital. Most of the patients whom they interviewed were frightened, they write, yet for the most part their fears "were outside the interests of the physicians and nurses. No ward patient thought there was a physician to whom he could talk about his fears of hospitalization, illness, or treatment. . . . Visitors and [researchers] who watched the desperate behavior of the patients and listened to their conversations were swept along in the current of intense, sincere, emotionally painful yet awe-inspiring, and tragic efforts of the sick to cope with their fears. These efforts were almost entirely ignored by the physicians, nurses, and other members of the hospital staff."

The same sort of insensitivity to patients also made a powerful impression on Emily Mumford, a sociologist who recently did a study of interns in training at a university hospital. She notes that an intern making rounds with other house officers and medical students "might hesitate to extend a gesture of acknowledgement or reassurance as a physician lest it look foolish to the doctors around him." She adds, "It sometimes happens that when an intern says much to his patient while the group stands at the bedside, some two exchange knowing glances, smile, or quip about the neophyte's fumbling efforts. Besides, in his concern over how the patient is receiving rounds, the intern could miss something that a professor is saying about a case." What the professor says may frighten or depress the patient if it is overheard by him, Dr. Mumford adds, and it is the nurse who is left to repair the damage. "House-staff members, absorbed in discussion as they walk away from a bedside, may seldom note the emotional debris they have left in their wake."

The concentration on the processes of disease that has so greatly enhanced the physician's ability to prolong life has also tended to change his attitude toward death. Commonly he sees it not as the inevitable end of life, but as an adversary whom he is bound to attack with every weapon at his command. In the duel between physician and death the patient is cast in the role of bystander. Death, when it comes, is felt by the doctor as a humiliating defeat.

One serious consequence is that doctors too often are unwilling to let their patients die in peace. Recently, for example, a Mrs. Deborah Josephs, writing in the *New York Times*, described the suffering that had been inflicted, in her view, unnecessarily, on her young brother-in-law after he had been found to have an incurable cancer. Doctors at the hospital where he spent most of the last eleven months of his life had assured the patient and his relatives that his pain could be controlled. Yet during those eleven months, Mrs. Josephs wrote, he "had not a day without pain and most of his pain was created by doctors continuing in their efforts to help him. . . . There must be a point where a patient is left alone and permitted to die. People with terminal illnesses should not be seen as threats to hospitals and doctors. There should be a time when operations, when radiation, when everything is stopped so that patients can die in relative comfort."

Sometimes dying patients are made to suffer, not for their own good, but for the benefit of others. David Sudnow, in his account of death in a county hospital, reports that many dying patients "were subjected to treatments that had, as their essential aim . . . the satisfaction of professional curiosity." He continues, "Relatively radical procedures were undertaken as experiments or to gain experience. These included massive doses of antibiotics in excess of prescribed limits, massive surgical maneuvers, and the use of potent drugs in even more potent combinations. These were described as 'last resort measures,' but the fact that the patient was 'terminal' was frankly regarded as providing the opportunity for scientific or educational experience." Experimenting on dying patients is not uncommon in public and university hospitals, and was strongly defended by a young house officer interviewed by Duff and Hollingshead, who argued that "in keeping some patients alive only to suffer and die in pain we learn something more about keeping patients alive to live."

To experiment on a dying patient without his consent, when the patient himself does not stand to benefit, is plainly indefensible. There are many who feel it is indefensible even if the patient agrees. A dying man, the argument runs, is in no position to make a rational cost-benefit analysis of the doctor's proposal to inject him with untried drugs. Usually, however, as seems to have been the case with Mrs. Josephs' brother-in-law, experiments on the dying are justified on the ground that there is some chance they may prolong the patient's life. This may encourage the doctor to go ahead even without explaining to the patient exactly what he is up to, an omission that, in turn, is justified by the time-honored principle that, where the patient's health is concerned, the doctor knows best.

Even when doctors scrupulously refrain from pressuring dying patients into subjecting themselves to painful experiments, they may cause a great deal of unnecessary suffering simply by insisting on fighting death to the bitter end, without considering the odds, and without regard for what the patient wants and how he feels. "It has always bothered me that our job as doctors is not to alleviate suffering but to prolong life," one doctor at Yankee Hospital told Duff and Hollingshead. "We're doing it in the hope that maybe something will happen, maybe a miracle will occur. We throw people into oxygen tents; we do all sorts of heroic things. We even rip open chests and squeeze hearts of patients who have massive myocardial infarctions or cancer involving their hearts. Everything is justified to save the life of a salvageable patient. But where death is inevitable I wonder if it isn't the best thing to make them comfortable and leave them alone. Usually, we don't. . . ."

People like to do what they do best, and doctors today are happiest when they are confronted with organic disease—with disorders, that is, whose symptoms can be accounted for by specific physical and chemical disturbances of normal physiological processes. These are the disorders that scientific medicine can deal with most successfully, and for which there may be tidy explanations even when there are no cures. But doctors are often irritated by patients whose headaches, ulcers, nausea, fatigue, or dizziness are symptoms of emotional disturbances. They resent wasting time on vague and formless ailments that can not be traced to genetic defects, or to the ravages of an invading microorganism, but that reflect the patient's inability, as the doctor sees it, to cope with the mess that he and other people have made of his life. This attitude is not limited to cardiologists, urologists, and other specialists who might argue that emotional disorders are clearly not in their line. E. Jack Geiger, a physician who took part a few years ago in a study of general practitioners, recalled recently that "for all that vaunted crap about family practice, tender loving care, and the guy that knows the patient, and so on, it was demonstrable that on the whole the general practitioners were the least adept of anybody at psychosocial aspects of medicine, at psychosomatic medicine, who were the most uncomfortable with it and disliked it the most."

It is at medical school, or as interns and residents, that doctors learn to refer to certain patients as "crocks," a crock being defined as someone whose sickness is all in his mind, and who therefore doesn't really have anything wrong with him. These are the years, too, when doctors are taught that, when confronted with a patient whose illness is real—that is, organic—it is not their business to consider whether, and how, social or emotional difficulties may have contributed to the patient's condition, or may be hampering his recovery. It is true that students are periodically reminded that there is more to medicine than treating blocked arteries or infected kidneys, and that they must not neglect the "whole patient." But a student or house officer who takes such exhortations to heart, and concerns himself with the family life and emotional frustrations of his patients, is likely to be pulled up short by his teachers. The physician and novelist Michael Crichton, who interned at the Massachusetts General Hospital, asks, rhetorically, what a house officer at such a hospital is being trained to become. "The answer," he writes, "is an academic physician specializing in acute, curative, hospital-based medicine. This is heavily scientific and not very behavioral; it must be so. (As the [visiting instructor] said: 'Tell me about his kidneys, not his marital troubles.' And he was right: the hospital is geared to treat his kidneys, and not his arguments with his wife.)"

The trouble with this hard-boiled, no-nonsense approach is that it is not very helpful in treating the large number of patients whose disorders are both organic and emotional in origin. Severe stomach pains may be caused by a gastric ulcer, but the ulcer may be caused in turn by the patient's repressed anger at his boss, and the doctor who fails to take this into account is unlikely to work a lasting cure. Indeed, the physician who ignores the emotional determinants of illness may do his patient more harm than good. On this score, too, Duff and Hollingshead found much to criticize at Yankee Hospital. They describe, for example, the case of a Mrs. Helms, a fifty-two-year-old woman who had been admitted to the hospital complaining of viselike headaches and fainting spells. Her difficulties, Duff and Hollingshead concluded after studying her medical chart and talking with her at length, were almost certainly emotional in origin. The headaches had begun shortly after her daughter had left home, against her mother's wishes, to join the WAVES; and they had grown worse after the daughter had married a sailor and become pregnant. Mrs. Helms told her interviewers that she was afraid she might be mentally ill. But she did not tell this to her doctors, and they, not wishing to offend a private patient by suggesting that her illness was imaginary and that she should see a psychiatrist, fell back on a diagnosis of cerebrovascular insufficiency—that is, an inadequate supply of blood to her brain. On her chart, this diagnosis was preceded by the word "probable," but the patient was not told of this qualification. Instead, Duff and Hollingshead report, she was told that her trouble might be caused by a defective heart valve or "the narrowing of a blood vessel at the base of her brain." Her doctor indicated there was not really much to be done about this, and sent her home. "Frightened by this diagnosis," the authors write, "Mrs. Helms left the hospital troubled not only by her personal and family problems but also about the possibility of heart or brain disease. Her fears mounted enormously." Her doctors, they add, "felt they had done their job and wanted Mrs. Helms to stop pestering them like a dissatisfied customer."

Duff and Hollingshead report that at Yankee Hospital there were many patients like Mrs. Helms, and that their illness was often wrongly diagnosed and inappropriately treated. There was "no tangible effort to diagnose mental illness even though it was evident and frequently contributed to the patient's symptoms," they write. "Physicians had a prime concern with sick organs; when sick organs were found, symptoms of the patient were attributed to them; if sick organs could not be found the symptoms remained unexplained or were attributed in some instances to functional [nonphysical] disorders. Even then, a psychiatric diagnosis was not applied."

It is obviously not very helpful to tell a sick person that there is nothing wrong with him, or to provide him with a dubious physical explanation for his symptoms that may make him acutely anxious and, further, reduce the likelihood of his taking steps to cope with his emotional difficulties. Although the internist or the surgeon may feel that emotions are not really his business, the patient doesn't know whether it is a virus or his wretched marriage that is making him feel bad. He turns to the doctor because he would like to feel better, and Duff and Hollingshead argue persuasively that the doctor's job is to try to help him understand the sources of his distress, whatever they may be. The physician, they write, "should function as a kindly and cautious Socratic teacher who uses what the patient is, knows, and desires in making his choices of advice, information, diagnosis, and treatment." This view is incompatible, of course, with the notion that the only real disease is the kind that can be studied with a microscope.

Many doctors, like many television viewers, are bemused by the hospital drama that begins with the arrival of a desperately ill patient whose symptoms are contradictory and baffling, and ends, after suitable diagnostic and therapeutic maneuvers, with his swift and total recovery. But the main causes of death and disability in the United States are the chronic and incurable diseases that come with advancing age, and that now afflict roughly half of all Americans. And while surgeons can dramatically intervene to help people suffering from some kinds of cancer and heart disease, the physician who undertakes the care of a diabetic, or a victim of arthritis or hypertension or arteriosclerosis, must be content to be a counselor rather than a miracle worker. However, this is not a role that most doctors have much desire to play. At Yankee Hospital, for instance, the authors of *Sickness and Society* report that the young interns and residents in training there "found it unpleasant to associate with patients facing progressive and irreversible disease. Thus, the house staff looked down upon the admission of [such] uninteresting patients (turkeys), endured them when they could not avoid them, and 'shipped' (discharged) them as soon as possible."

Preoccupation with the heroic aspects of modern medicine has not only caused doctors to resent the patient who is chronically and incurably ill. It has also tended to divert attention from other ways of saving lives and improving people's health. On the whole, doctors have shown little interest in the prevention of disease, either in their own practices or as a community enterprise. In their defense it must be said that doctors can do less to keep their patients healthy than is popularly supposed. There is good reason for thinking, for instance, that for the average person who feels perfectly well it is a waste of time and money to have an annual checkup. And it is true that doctors don't know how to prevent cancer or diabetes or heart disease, or how to keep people from becoming alcoholics or from eating too much. But it is also true that even when it is quite feasible to prevent disease by vaccination, or to lessen its impact by catching it early, the necessary measures are not always taken.

One reason is that arranging for children to get their whooping cough or measles shots has traditionally been regarded as the job of public health officers, and most physicians regard public health as a field for people who lack the courage to be real doctors—that is, to accept responsibility for the life and health of individual patients. Most physicians do not consider taking social action to prevent disease to be the real business of medicine.

The peculiar sense of values to which this can lead has been deplored by, among others, John Knowles. Recalling an occasion on which he had been making rounds at Massachusetts General with a group of medical students and house officers, he notes that "the first five patients presented to me all happened, by a curious coincidence, to have the same problem. And it serves to point up the incongruity of what we're doing here. All five were elderly, chronic alcoholics with massive GI bleeding and end-stage liver disease. All five were in a coma and we were treating them vigorously, with everything medicine has to offer. They had intravenous lines, and central venous pressure catheters, and tracheotomies, and positive pressure respirators, and all the rest. They had house staff and students and nurses working on them around the clock. They had consultants of every shape and sort. They were running up bills of five hundred dollars a day, week after week." Knowles concedes that they deserved such treatment, and that Massachusetts General was the kind of hospital that should be providing it. "But you can't help reflecting," he added, "as you look at all this stainless steel and tubing and sophisticated equipment, that right outside your door there are people with TB who aren't getting antibiotics, and kids who aren't getting vaccinations, and women who aren't getting prenatal care."

It would be unfair to judge the quality of medical care in America entirely by institutions like Massachusetts General or Yankee Hospital. Most encounters between doctors and patients take place in doctors' offices, not in hospitals. And most people who need hospital care get it in a community hospital, where the technical quality of the care may be lower than in a university hospital, but where at least they stand a better chance of being treated as humans, and not as challenging (or, worse yet, boring) problems in medical technology. One reason is that, in the community hospital, the patient is likely to be under the care of his family doctor. The family doctor who has hospitalized a patient following a heart attack may share responsibility for his care with a surgeon or cardiologist, but he is impelled by self-interest, if nothing else, to act as a sympathetic counselor to the patient who is paying his bill. More importantly, perhaps, the prospect that he will be seeing the patient regularly for years to come gives him a perspective quite different from that of the residents and interns at a university hospital, whose main concern, like that of their teachers, is with the functioning of the damaged heart, not with how its owner feels, or how he can learn to cope with his disability.

But the university hospital, with its platoons and companies of medical researchers, its elaborately equipped surgical suites, its crowded outpatient clinics, and its flying squads of interns, residents, and medical students, is also having more and more effect on the way medicine is practiced outside its immediate sphere of influence. For fifty years or more, most medical schools have had their own hospitals where students, under faculty supervision, first learn to question patients, and to listen to their hearts and feel their livers. But for much of this period a doctor's experience in a university hospital was ordinarily limited to his student days. After graduation, most young physicans spent a year or two as interns in a community hospital, and then went into private practice.

But after World War II the situation changed. More and more young doctors, as we have seen, chose to undergo two to five years of postgraduate training in surgery, or internal medicine, or some other specialty before going into practice. Many received this training at university hospitals, which, with the help of federal research funds, were able greatly to expand their teaching programs. Others were trained at municipal or community hospitals, where their services were eagerly sought after to take some of the work load off the shoulders of the regular attending staffs at a time when the treatment of hospital patients was becoming enormously more complicated and time-consuming. But there have never been nearly enough young doctors to fill all the internships and residencies that are offered, and hospitals have found that the best way to attract house officers is to offer them some of the advantages of a university hospital, such as regular contact with senior physicians engaged in interesting research. To this end, many hospitals without previous university connections have affiliated themselves with medical schools. Affiliation can bring about quite a change in the character of a hospital. In a community hospital, standards of medical care are left up to the attending staff—that is, to those physicians in private practice who have asked for and been granted the privilege of admitting their patients to the hospital. Under an affiliation agreement, however, a good deal of authority to set and enforce standards may be handed over to full-time, salaried chiefs of surgery, medicine, and pediatrics, who are appointed by, or with the approval of, the medical school with which the hospital has linked itself. In these circumstances, both the care that patients get, and the training of the hospital's interns and residents, come under the sway of academic views of medicine and medical practice.

As centers of biomedical research, American medical schools command worldwide respect. They are admired not only for their well-staffed and elaborately equipped laboratories, but for the free and nonauthoritarian style in which research is conducted. The authors of a 1964 survey of biomedical research in Western Europe noted that since World War II thousands of young Europeans had spent a year or two working in the laboratories of American medical schools, where they had been exposed to "what, for many, is a radically different and liberating atmosphere in medical research and education. . . ." In the opinion of the visitors, the authors went on to say, the most valuable elements of what they often referred to as the "American approach" included early independence for the young investigator, informal relations between students and professors, freedom to move from one institution to another, and "absence of academic hierarchism."

But distinction in research is no guarantee that a medical school and its affiliated hospitals will do a good job of preparing young people for medical practice. On the contrary, the transformation of medical schools into research institutes has widened the gap between academic medicine and what most people, most of the time, need from their doctors. Until quite recently, teaching at university hospitals was almost entirely by clinicians—that is, by physicians who were interested not only in studying disease, but in diagnosing and treating it in individual patients. Many professors of medicine and surgery were distinguished specialists with busy private practices, who spent part of their time making hospital rounds with students and house officers. But while there are still young faculty members who would like to combine teaching with practice, that is clearly no longer the way to get ahead in academic medicine. As time goes on, John Knowles has written, the clinician-teacher "enjoys less teaching responsibility, and his assignments are more in the outpatient department and less on the wards. He finds it progressively more difficult to understand 'grand rounds,' which used to be clinical exercises and are now an excuse for launching into the biochemical mechanisms of disease." Over the past fifteen years or so, practitioner-teachers have largely been replaced, as senior professors, by physicians who are happiest in their laboratories; who may be noticeably awkward and uncomfortable when dealing with sick people; and who, if one can believe a recent survey of medical-school faculties, may go days at a time without examining or treating a single patient.

This has disturbing implications for the education of the vast majority of young doctors who do not themselves end up as researchers. As Knowles points out, there is too much emphasis on the processes of disease, and on its diagnosis, and not enough on its management. Emily Mumford, in the course of her study of interns at "University Hospital," asked a number of the young doctors to explain what they meant by an interesting patient. "The really interesting case," one intern explained, "is the one who is a *challenge* to diagnose." Others "defined the interesting patient with attributes such as 'unusual disease,' 'unusual manifestations of a common disease,' 'a good diagnostic problem.'" Such patients are prized by young house officers, Dr. Mumford writes, because they may furnish material for a research paper, "or at the very least offer the intern or resident a chance to gain favorable attention on rounds."

In such an atmosphere, the young doctor being trained in internal medicine is not encouraged to spend his time learning how to deal with bronchial pneumonia, minor urinary infections, hay fever, chronic bursitis, rheumatoid arthritis, and other run-of-the-office ailments that he will mainly be called on to treat in private practice. The message he gets is that the treatment of such disorders is boring hackwork. Indeed, he may come to feel that practicing medicine in the world outside the university hospital is an occupation suitable only for physicians who are greedy for the money that can be made in private practice, or who lack the talent to make the grade in academic medicine—that is, to become medical-school professors themselves. Emily Mumford reports in this connection that former residents returning to University Hospital were often apologetic about their work, one of them remarking to a friend, "I'm just in practice." This is certainly not the attitude one looks for in one's family doctor. In any case, a student or young house officer is unlikely to learn very much about the art of caring for patients from teachers who don't know how themselves.

6

Some Notes on the Sociology of Healing

The character of medical care in any country is largely determined by the way its doctors are paid, and the way their work is organized and regulated. The most striking feature of medical practice in the United States is the rich rewards it confers on its practitioners. American doctors not only make a great deal of money and never have to worry about being unemployed, but they also enjoy an independence that is very hard to achieve in any other line of work. To a much greater degree than in most other countries, doctors in America have been free to practice medicine where and how they choose, without having to account for their actions to anybody but themselves.

Their independence is rooted in the entrepreneurial nature of American medical practice. It is true that more and more doctors in the United States are taking salaried jobs, as full-time emergency-room physicians, for example, or as employees of prepaid group practice plans. But more than three quarters of all American doctors, not counting those in training, still sell their services on the open market at so many dollars per consultation, injection, examination, or operation. From the doctor's standpoint this has great advantages. He does not have to work longer hours, or see more patients, than he wants to. If he does take on more patients, and therefore has to put in more time in his office, his income rises proportionately. In general he can charge what he likes and, unlike doctors in many European countries, who may have to take patients pretty much as they come, he can pick and choose his clientele. Unless he happens to be the only doctor in town he is at liberty to tell a whining, an ungrateful, or an overly demanding patient to take his ailments elsewhere. Furthermore, by virtue of the fact that his patients normally have to reach into their own pockets to pay his fees, the American doctor enjoys some protection against having to waste time on people who, in his opinion, don't really need a doctor. In England, by contrast, where anybody can see his general practitioner as often as he likes without paying a penny, GPs may feel put upon and complain, in the words of one English commentator, that they "are forced to spend most of their lives treating minor complaints, psychosomatic complaints they can't hope to cure, and long-term chronic illness they can do little to alleviate."

Family doctors in America have another edge over most of their European counterparts. In England, and in most European countries, there are two distinct classes of physicians. One consists of surgeons, cardiologists, internists, and other specialists who work almost exclusively in hospitals. The other consists of general practitioners, who treat patients in their offices, or in their patients' homes, but who are not permitted to have a hand in the more exciting (and more lucrative) medical work that goes on in surgical suites and in hospital wards. It is true that more and more American hospitals also are closing their doors to nonspecialists. But most family doctors in America, even if they have not been trained as specialists in pediatrics or internal medicine, still take care of their patients even when they have to be hospitalized. This not only makes the family doctor more important in his patients' eyes, and in his own, but it lets him escape for a few hours each day from colds and stomachaches and sprained ankles, and to confront illness in its more serious, unusual, and dramatic manifestations.

It is also relatively easy for an American doctor to specialize in any branch of medicine he likes. In most European countries a physician can practice as a surgeon, or a neurologist, or as any other kind of specialist only by undergoing years of formal postgraduate training, and then getting himself appointed to one of a limited number of hospital posts. In the United States, by contrast, there is no limit on the number of doctors who can set themselves up in specialty practice. Moreover, though few Americans may be aware of the fact, in the United States it is quite legal for a doctor to hang out his shingle as a specialist without having taken formal postgraduate training in his specialty, and without passing a special examination. All he has to do is to graduate from medical school, put in a year as an intern, and pass the same general examination that all would-be doctors must take to qualify for a medical license.

A doctor who has not been through a residency in which he has been specially trained in the diagnosis and treatment of eye disease is unlikely to hang out his shingle as an ophthalmologist. But many doctors who have not taken residencies in pediatrics or obstetrics nevertheless choose to specialize in the treatment of children or pregnant women, and a general practitioner is legally at liberty to do as much (and as complicated) surgery as he likes. And while some hospitals specify that certain operations may be done only by a doctor who has been through a four- or five-year surgical residency, and whose proficiency has been certified (after a special examination) by the American Board of Surgery, many hospitals are quite relaxed about who operates on their patients. A recent poll by the California Academy of General Practice indicated that nine out of ten of the Academy's members have access to a hospital where they can do any kind of operation they feel up to. In the United States as a whole perhaps one third of all operations are performed by doctors who have had little or no formal postgraduate training in surgery.

What is good for the American doctor is also, in many ways, good for his patients as well. Entrepreneurial, fee-for-service medicine may lead a doctor to do too much for his patients, but other systems of paying the doctor may tempt him to do too little. Many family doctors in America take and read x-rays and cardiograms, and some even consider it part of their job to counsel patients on emotional and family problems. Such services are seldom offered, however, by the British family doctor, who is paid a specified yearly sum for each patient who has signed up with him for regular care. Under this arrangement, the British doctor can gain more time for gardening or golf, without sacrificing any income, by referring patients to hospital specialists even when their ailments are simple ones that the doctor himself should be able to handle. Or, to look at his situation in a slightly different way, the English GP can make more money by taking on more patients, but not by doing more for those he already has. As a result, the average Englishman probably spends more time seeking out specialists than the average American—

the average American, that is, who is fortunate enough to have a family doctor.

There are distinct advantages, too, to a system that permits a family physician to treat his patients in as well as out of the hospital. A doctor who spends part of his time working in a hospital, where he observes (and is observed by) other doctors, is less likely to fall into sloppy habits, and more likely to keep up with changes in medical knowledge and techniques, than the doctor who, like the English GP, is limited pretty much to office practice. Moreover, assuming he is competent, and knows when to ask for expert advice, a doctor who already knows a patient well may be in a better position to deal intelligently with a severe illness than one who meets the patient for the first time in a hospital bed. Even when the family doctor must defer to the judgment of a surgeon or other specialist he can still act as the patient's adviser, interpreter, and friend at court. The frustration and despair that can overwhelm a patient who has no such guide has been described by Edward L. Brecher, a well-known medical writer, whose wife and collaborator, Ruth, entered a university hospital for diagnosis and treatment of a suspected cancer. The hospital was a hundred miles from the town where the Brechers lived (and where their family doctor had his office), and they knew no one on the staff. "Doctors came and went; no one of them was in command," Brecher wrote later. "One of them told Ruth one thing, the same doctor or someone else gave me an altogether different report, and there was no one to whom we could turn to tell us which version was true. Like many other patients we came to know during those stress-laden days and nights, we felt as if we were floundering in a quagmire of medical confusion. When things went wrong, as they not infrequently did, there was no one in authority to listen to me."

Being visited daily by one's own doctor may not do away entirely with such conflict and confusion. If they are to learn their trade properly, the interns and residents in training at a university hospital must be given responsibility for the care of patients, and this means that the physician in private practice who admits "his" patient to a university hospital finds his role restricted to looking over the shoulders of the house staff. But even so, he can interpret for his patient what the surgeon and the radiation therapist are saying (in Ruth Brecher's case, they said quite different things) and he can act as an advocate, or ombudsman, helping his patient cope with the often terrifying machinery of hospital medicine. Eventually Ruth Brecher found such an advocate, an internist on the staff of the hospital who became her personal physician. "When she asked a question, she now got a straight answer—and I got the same answer," Brecher wrote. "She knew that someone was thinking of her needs, planning in advance how to meet them, consulting her when important decisions were to be made. . . . Though her physical condition remained grave throughout the remaining year and a half of her illness (which was cancer), the real hazards and discomforts were no longer intensified by the struggle to extract good care from an impersonal medical-hospital system in which we felt friendless and powerless."

A further merit of private fee-for-service medicine, as it is practiced in the United States, is that people who can afford a doctor, and who live where they are in good supply, probably have a better chance than people in many other countries have of ending up with a doctor whom they like and trust. In England, for instance, while people are quite free to shop around for a general practitioner, the rules of the National Health Service do not ordinarily allow them to choose their own cardiologist or surgeon. In Russia and elsewhere in Eastern Europe, people are assigned to a physician, or, more commonly, a team of physicians, responsible for providing primary (that is, unspecialized) care to all persons living in a designated neighborhood or region. In seeking such care, which is free, one must ordinarily accept the doctor to whom one is assigned, and many people appear to find this a satisfactory arrangement. In Czechoslovakia, when people were asked what might be done to improve the quality of general practice in their country, fewer than 3 per cent suggested that patients be allowed to choose their own doctors. By contrast, 70 per cent said it would help if general practitioners' offices were better equipped. Yet in most of the socialist countries of Europe, including Russia, there are people who place so high a value on the privilege of choosing their own doctor that they go outside the official system for medical advice. Usually this means consulting—and paying—a doctor who conducts an after-hours practice in his apartment.

People who seek help on these terms are often moved to do

so not only by a desire to pick their own doctor, but also by a conviction that if they are paying a doctor directly he will try harder to find out why they are having severe headaches, or why they feel tired all the time. This points up what is perhaps the chief virtue of the American system of paying the doctor, namely that there is no doubt whom the doctor is working for. In countries where all doctors are salaried government workers, it is probably much less common than in the United States for people to have the kind of relationship with their doctors that Ruth Brecher had with "her" internist. "The [clinic] physician believes that he is professionally responsible to his head physician or director, not to his patients," two Czechoslovakian health-care experts, Emile Skrbkova and Milos Vacek, have written, adding that the result may be "a certain alienation in the physician-to-patient relationship," a tendency "to regard the patient as a subject of care, not as a live human being." This attitude, they note, may undermine the patient's confidence in the doctor and deprive the doctor of the patient's active cooperation, both of which "are indispensable for a successful therapy, or at least for relieving a patient's mental stress."

The same tendency has been observed in a prepaid group practice studied by Eliot Freidson of New York University, a specialist in the sociology of medical institutions. Some years ago, Freidson questioned members of the Health Insurance Plan of New York (HIP) who were getting all their out-of-hospital care, for a fixed monthly payment, from a panel of salaried doctors connected with Montefiore Hospital, a major teaching hospital in the Bronx. Most of the people covered by the survey believed that they had been getting better medical care since joining HIP. The Montefiore group, they pointed out, had excellent facilities, and specialists were readily available for consultations. But a fair number of people who made these points also said that the HIP doctors seemed less sympathetic, and less interested in their patients' problems, than the fee-for-service doctors to whom they had gone before signing up with HIP. Some complained that the HIP doctors took them too much for granted, or treated them like charity patients.

The difficulty is that doctors who are not directly dependent on patients' fees for their livelihood, and who regularly consult with one another and see each other's charts, may be less concerned with pleasing their patients than with demonstrating to their associates their diagnostic acumen and their mastery of new developments in medicine. This is particularly likely to be true of a group connected with a hospital like Montefiore, where there is a lot of emphasis on research and on the scientific aspects of medicine. Freidson notes that the people who had signed up with the Montefiore group were almost certainly right in their belief that they were getting care of a higher technical quality—with fewer diagnoses missed, fewer drugs inappropriately or unnecessarily prescribed—than ever before. But this advantage may have been at least partly offset by "a kind of uneasiness, an irritability, a sense of something lacking" that he detected in many patients. A patient in this frame of mind, Freidson goes on to say, may avoid going to the doctor when he should. When he does go, he may conceal things he should tell the doctor, and he may fail to carry out the doctor's recommendations. Repelled by the impersonality of group practice, he "will present the evasive, resentful but desperately demanding face to the medical world that all people present when confronted by forces they cannot control, which they know are sometimes indifferent to them, but which they cannot do without."

But while the traditional American style of medical practice has much to be said in its favor, the price we pay for its benefits is very high. Indeed, it is hard to see how medical care in the United States can be greatly improved, or its cost brought under control, without limiting the enormous freedom, both professional and economic, that has made the practice of medicine in America so gratifying to the practitioners. That freedom has meant, among other things, too much surgery, too many surgeons, too few family doctors, and wretched care for the poor. ("Why should I see poor patients?" a physician in Renton, Washington, asked the author of a recent article in *Medical Economics*. "My office is full of good, paying patients.") Moreover, because medicine in the United States is a business, it has attracted many people whose desire to comfort and heal is less than their desire to make a lot of money. Fifty years ago, in *Arrowsmith*, Sinclair Lewis described the ruling passion of Roscoe Geake, professor of otolaryngology at the University of Winnemac. "Roscoe Geake was a peddler," Lewis wrote. "He would have done well with oil stock. As an otolaryngologist he believed that tonsils had been placed in the human organism for the purpose of providing specialists with closed motors." Since *Arrowsmith* was written, American medicine has become not only more scientific, but probably more commercial as well. Outside the walls of medical schools and university hospitals, where salaries are excellent but where the entrepreneurial drive is muted, there is a preoccupation with making money that even some doctors regard as imprudent, if not improper. Not long ago, for example, a New Haven, Connecticut, physician named Charles Verstandig, in his farewell address as President of the New Haven County Medical Association, urged his fellow members "to quit strangling the goose that can lay these golden eggs." Without pausing to identify precisely what goose he had in mind, he noted that the "temptation to get rich while the getting's good is powerful," and went on to say, "A lot of our group have payments to make on their apartment house complexes, their shopping centers, their outside business interests. . . . You can't blame the average patient for thinking that we doctors are living much too high on the hog."

Quite apart from what all this can do to the doctor's image, it can also put a disagreeable chill on the doctor's relations with his own patients. Freidson reports that one HIP member, who had *not* liked his former doctor, complained that the doctor would "just sort of grunt when he examined you and then write out a prescription and not say anything. He really didn't treat you like a personality; he didn't seem interested. We felt we were just part of his business, like those ten garages he owned in the neighborhood which he was always renting to someone." Opinion polls have consistently indicated that Americans who feel this way about their doctors are in a fairly small minority. But if the characteristic sin of the clinic doctor in Czechoslovakia is bureaucratic indifference, the characteristic sin of the fee-for-service-doctor in America is a readiness to exploit his patients for financial gain.

Both individually and as a profession, American doctors have fiercely resisted any interference with their right to decide what is best for their patients. When the American College of Surgeons first proposed that every hospital should have a tissue committee, to check on whether tissue and organs removed in surgery had, in fact, been diseased, the suggestion was met, in the words of one historian, "with storms of disapproval, rejection, obstruction, and finally acceptance." More recently, many doctors have angrily denounced the leadership of the AMA for agreeing to cooperate with the government, albeit with extreme reluctance, in a scheme to have doctors themselves monitor the cost and the appropriateness of hospital care for the old and the poor for which the government is paying under Medicare and Medicaid. Their case has been succinctly stated by a Beverly Hills, California, doctor in a letter to Senator Wallace F. Bennett of Utah, who sponsored the monitoring law. "I oppose peer review," he wrote. "I have no peers."

Such attitudes reflect in part the fact that in an economy dominated by huge organizations that are run on bureaucratic lines, medicine as it is practiced in America appeals powerfully to people who are determined to be their own bosses. But the American doctor's insistence that he is the best judge of his own actions is also rooted, as Eliot Freidson points out in *Profession of Medicine*, in two notions that he has been taught to regard as fundamental to his calling. One is the notion of medical responsibility, which means that, once a patient has placed himself in his hands, the doctor is in sole command. The other notion is that nothing is quite so important to the doctor in exercising this responsibility as clinical experience. As medical students and young house officers are reminded again and again—and as they learn from experience—medicine is an art, and cures cannot be effected simply by looking up the right procedures in a textbook. Thus each doctor, Freidson writes, "builds up his own world of clinical experience and assumes personal, that is, virtually individual, responsibility for the ways he manages his cases in that world." In this way, the work of medicine "gives rise to a special frame of mind oriented toward action for its own sake. . . . Such action relies on firsthand experience and is supported by both a will to believe in the value of one's actions and a belief in the inadequacy of general knowledge for dealing with individual cases." The clinician, Freidson points out, "feels that his work is unique and concrete, not really assessable by some set of stable rules or by anyone who does not share with him the same firsthand experience. . . ."

This insistence that the work of a doctor, like that of a painter or sculptor, cannot properly be subjected to supervision or control has unfortunately allowed many doctors to practice medicine even though they are so incompetent as to endanger the health of their patients. Doctors have no quarrel, to be sure, with the existing licensing laws, which provide that before a doctor can practice medicine on his own he must graduate from an accredited medical school, put in at least a year as a hospital intern, and pass a series of long and stiff examinations. There is even a lot of support for a plan that would require young doctors to have a minimum of three years of postgraduate training before they could be fully licensed. But doctors generally have taken the position that once a doctor has undergone (and survived) the ordeal of being initiated into his profession he should never again, in the normal course of events, have to answer to any official body for his actions or competence. Thus even though many doctors fall into sloppy habits over the years, or fail to keep up with the new developments in medicine,* practicing physicians have strenuously objected to suggestions that their knowledge and competence should be subject from time to time to some kind of compulsory review.

As a result, while a few states now require doctors to be relicensed at regular intervals, about all that is asked of the applicant is evidence that he has spent, say, forty hours a year attending postgraduate lectures or seminars. In recent years several state medical societies and a few professional societies, notably the American Academy of Family Physicians, have also voted to make regular attendance at what are known as continuing education courses a requirement for membership.

Unfortunately, taking such courses may have little or no effect on how a doctor actually performs. Osler Peterson, in his investigation of general practice in North Carolina, found very little relation between the amount of continuing education a doctor had been exposed to and, say, the thoroughness with which he examined his patients. Similarly, the authors of a study of Kansas physicians could find no evidence at all that doctors who had taken postgraduate courses did any better by their patients than other doctors (including nearly half of the state's general practitioners) who hadn't been to a seminar or lecture for the past ten years or more.

* A sociologist who looked into the reading habits of midwestern physicians in the early 1950s reported that nearly half, by their own admission, did little more than leaf through the medical journals to which they subscribed, and 7 per cent said they rarely did even that.

The most plausible explanation for these discouraging findings is that continuing education consists mainly of listening to lectures, whereas everybody agrees that clinical medicine is best learned as it is learned by medical students and young house officers—that is, in the course of actually examining and treating patients. Too often, as Peterson noted in reporting on his North Carolina survey, "The extent or complexity of . . . lecture subjects [is] patently too great for many practitioners to absorb in a single session." The usefulness of lectures is further reduced when, as often happens, they are given by academic specialists more interested in talking about their own research, or in elucidating complex physiological processes, than in giving their listeners practical advice on how to deal with problems they face every day. "When I was a young faculty member at the University of Virginia," a professor at the Stanford School of Medicine recalled recently, "I used to go around the state lecturing to GPs about antibiotics. I cringe now when I think of the title of my talk. It was, 'Some Unusual Aspects of Antibiotic-Resistant Bacterial Endocarditis.' I got the message one night when an older doctor came up to me and said, 'It was sure nice of you to come all the way down from Charlottesville to talk to us. But what we really want to know is, is penicillin any good for the flu?'"

Failure to keep up with new developments is not the only reason why doctors bungle. Patients also suffer at the hands of doctors who, because of the generally permissive attitude of the medical profession, are legally free to undertake procedures they have not been trained to handle. Obviously five years of training as a resident in surgery, and a diploma from the American Board of Surgery, do not in themselves guarantee first-class surgical care. Conversely, there are general practitioners who do a good job as surgeons, limiting themselves to fairly simple operations, such as hernia repairs and Caesarean sections, and calling for expert help at the first sign of complications.

But it is significant that, if one may judge by a survey of members of the New Jersey Medical Association, when doctors need an operation they almost invariably choose to have it done by a fully-trained surgical specialist. Moreover, the temptation for a GP to overreach himself is strong. An hour or two in the operating room removing a patient's uterus, plus another hour or so spent with her before and after the operation, can earn a general practitioner a fee of four or five hundred dollars, a sum that it might take eight to ten hours to earn at regular office-visit rates. A general practitioner must also take into account the fact that many surgeons double as family physicians, and that if he refers one of his patients to a specialist for surgery he may lose the patient for good. For the same reason, GPs are often very slow to refer patients to a pediatrician or internist. No doctor, even one who has more patients than he can easily handle, likes to be abandoned for another doctor, and studies in both the United States and Canada have indicated that a GP, when confronted with a condition he is not really qualified to diagnose and treat, too often will try to muddle through instead of sending the patient to an appropriate specialist.

Obviously no one knows exactly how many incompetent doctors are practicing in America. By all indications the number is depressingly large. Malpractice claims against doctors are running at a rate of more than 18,000 a year, and a government commission that looked into the matter reported a couple of years ago that roughly half of all such claims are "legally meritorious." This greatly understates the real extent of malpractice, since many patients are understandably reluctant to sue their doctors even when they have reason to do so, and many others who might have a case are unaware that the injury they have suffered is a result of carelessness or incompetence rather than honest error. * Dr. Robert C. Derbyshire, a Santa Fe, New Mexico, surgeon who is a past president of the Federation of State Medical Boards, and who has made himself an authority on medical licensing and the disciplining of erring physicians, has estimated that at least 5 per cent, or more than 17,000, of the country's 350,000 doctors are unfit to practice medicine. In the course of a year, he noted recently, each of these doctors treats 7500 patients, and in their hands a license to practice medicine

---

* Occasionally the doctor himself will tip the patient off to what has happened. *Medical Times* recently carried the story of a gynecologist who performed a hysterectomy to remove a uterine tumor. The patient turned out not to have a tumor, but to be three-and-a-half months pregnant. The doctor was sued for malpractice after apologizing to the husband and confiding that he should have run more preoperative tests because the patient "did have signs of being pregnant." The lesson to be drawn from this sad tale, *Medical Times* said, was that a doctor should never allow "regret over mistaken judgment" to betray him into admitting he has goofed.

"becomes a license to kill." "I've seen lives lost because doctors haven't kept up with new techniques," he added.

Mechanisms of a sort do exist for calling to account a doctor who is dangerously incompetent, or who blatantly overtreats his patients. In principle, if his transgressions are sufficiently flagrant, his license can be taken away. But few state licensing boards have the staff they would need to carry out investigations on their own. They must therefore rely heavily on other physicians to build a case for suspending or revoking a doctor's license, and most doctors hate to point an accusing finger at another doctor, particularly in a public proceeding. (A few years ago, 214 doctors were asked, hypothetically, if they would be willing to testify against a surgeon who had set out to remove a diseased kidney and had taken out the wrong one. More than two thirds said they would *not* be willing.) In many states, too, the law provides that a doctor's license may be revoked only if he has been convicted of a felony, or has violated the narcotic laws, or if he has been guilty of certain other specific transgressions. "The appalling fact is that only fifteen licensure statutes enumerate professional incompetence as a cause for disciplinary action," Derbyshire pointed out not long ago.

All this can make it very hard to put a doctor out of business even when there is overwhelming evidence of his unfitness. Between 1954 and 1957, for example, the Michigan State Board of Registration in Medicine received twenty-five formal complaints about a physician, Dr. Ronald E. Clark, with a busy practice in the suburbs of Detroit. Clark was accused of, among other things, performing illegal abortions, molesting children, prescribing for nonexistent diseases, attacking patients sexually, and killing three persons by overdosing them with drugs. His license was repeatedly taken away, but each time he managed to persuade the board, or the courts, that it should be restored. It was not until 1968, when Clark was convicted of manslaughter (he was found to have caused the death of his own office assistant by giving her an overdose of sodium pentothal) that he was forced to give up the practice of medicine for good.

Not surprisingly, given the difficulties under which state licensing boards labor—and given, too, the fact that many of their members are themselves reluctant to blow the whistle on fellow doctors—the number of doctors who are actually disciplined is very small. Derbyshire has pointed out that in one recent ten-year period fewer than 2000 doctors had their licenses suspended or revoked, or were reprimanded by their state boards. Over a five-year period, from 1968 through 1972, seven states, with a total of more than 23,000 doctors, reported no disciplinary actions of any kind, not even reprimands. Moreover, even if a doctor's license has been revoked he does not necessarily have to give up the practice of medicine. If he already has a license in another state, as many doctors do, or if he can obtain such a license, which may not be too difficult, he can move there and start a new practice.

According to the AMA's code of ethics, "The medical profession should safeguard the public and itself against physicians deficient in moral character or professional competence." But beyond seeing to it that doctors get a solid education before they are licensed to practice, the AMA has done very little to make good on this pledge. "This is a preposterous situation," a member protested to the AMA's House of Delegates not long ago. "The AMA can assume unyielding positions before Congress. The AMA can commit the entire medical profession to wide-ranging courses of action. Yet the AMA can't proceed against some deadbeat in Podunk who's a disgrace to every doctor." The standard reply to such complaints is that it is not up to the AMA, but to its constituent state and county medical societies, to take action against erring members. While the local societies do occasionally suspend or expel a member, the occasions are very rare. "For several years the medical societies were asked to report their disciplinary actions to the AMA," Derbyshire told an international conference on medical ethics held in Washington in 1973, "but the project was abandoned as a waste of time. In 1968, the latest year for which figures are available, 33 state societies reported no actions taken whatsoever." The state societies have also been criticized sharply by Edwin J. Holman, a lawyer who is secretary of the AMA's Judicial Council on Medical Ethics. "Medical societies appear to have been reluctant to tackle tough problems relating to questionable actions by their members," Holman observed not long ago in an editorial in the *Journal of the American Medical Association*. "It is amazing how many excuses can be found for not conducting an investigation or for not taking action."

One way medical societies duck the disagreeable task of disciplining members is by keeping it pretty much of a secret that there is such a body as a grievance committee to which patients can bring complaints. Moreover, by undertaking to act only on patient complaints, which is how most of the societies operate, a society can avoid taking action against a doctor whose incompetence may be well known to other physicians (who are called on to repair the damage he has done) but which may not be so clearly recognized by his patients. Patients are in a poor position to judge their doctors' technical competence; in one of the investigations of the hospital care received by Teamsters' Union members and their families, three out of four patients whose treatment was rated as substandard by the reviewing specialists were convinced they had gotten the best possible care. Finally, medical societies seldom make their action public even when they do get around to expelling a member. His patients may therefore never learn that his ethics or competence have been judged and found wanting. To be sure, a doctor whose sins have been so egregious as to get him thrown out of his medical society may also lose the privilege of admitting his patients to the hospital where he regularly has been taking them. But, in such an event, he can usually find a less finicky hospital that will accept him on its staff, and where he will feel no real pressure to mend his ways.

This possibility exists, despite the activities of the Joint Commission on the Accreditation of Hospitals (JCAH), which spends a lot of time worrying about whether hospital patients are being cut open unnecessarily or otherwise exploited or mistreated by their doctors. The JCAH is a private body, most of whose members are appointed by the AMA and the American Hospital Association, and its stamp of approval is essential if a hospital wants to attract interns and residents, and to be eligible for Medicare payments. But many hospitals, including a good number of small hospitals that are run as profit-making ventures, are not interested in running training programs, and regard Medicare business as undesirable because it is relatively unprofitable. All together, the United States has nearly six thousand acute-care hospitals, not counting those operated by the Veterans' Administration or other federal agencies, or by state, city, or county governments. More than a quarter of these hospitals, containing about 9 per cent of the total number of beds, get along without accreditation.

Moreover, even though one is more likely to be operated on

unnecessarily, or to have one's case bungled, in an unaccredited hospital, the quality of medical care can be pretty bad even in institutions that have regularly passed muster with the JCAH. Some reasons for this were set forth in 1971 by a study group affiliated with Ralph Nader's Center for Study of Responsive Law. Reporting on an interview with the commission's assistant director, Joseph Stone, the group noted that "we learned that reinspections are now held every three years; that only one physician makes the inspection visit, either alone or occasionally accompanied by a nurse or administrator; that only part of one day is devoted to a review of the records of performance of the medical staff committees. . . ; that the turnover rate for surveyors is approximately 50 per cent every two years; that [the staff] must conduct around 2500 hospital inspections per year, i.e., about 11 per surveyor per month; that 'our basic approach to evaluation is not to look for mistakes, but for opportunities to be helpful'; . . . that 'we believe strict regulation stifles innovation.'"

To gain accreditation, a hospital must have formal procedures for reviewing the work of the doctors on its staff. But if a hospital has a tissue committee, and if the committee's minutes indicate that it meets regularly, the JCAH does not get too upset if they also indicate that a lot of normal appendixes are being taken out. A similarly relaxed standard has been used in passing on the work of other so-called internal-audit committees. Senator Kennedy has complained, for example, about the accreditation of a forty-bed proprietary (profit-making) hospital even though the commission's surveyor had reported that minutes of staff meetings "were stereotyped and do not give one the feeling that any serious work is actually going on," while hospital records "indicated that a high percentage of seriously ill elderly people had been subjected to elective operations without adequate clinical consultation." Giving a hospital and its doctors every benefit of the doubt has been justified by the Joint Commission's director, Dr. John Porterfield, on the ground that the only aim of accreditation is to foster "the optimum environment" for the practice of good medicine. "Dealing only with the environment has made some people mad at us," he added, "yet how can we approach medical care quality directly? We wouldn't be caught dead—or we'd be dead if caught—saying: 'You made the wrong decision, Doctor.'"

The requirements for accreditation have recently been made a little stiffer. Hospitals will now be surveyed every two years instead of every three, and many more surveys will be conducted by teams rather than individuals. But as two legal scholars who have made a careful study of hospital regulation have pointed out, the Joint Commission's view of its mission seems basically unchanged. Writing in the quarterly *Law and Contemporary Problems*, William Worthington and Laurens H. Silver observe, "So long as medical staff organization comports with the standards, surveyors are not to be concerned with the substantive findings of tissue review or necropsy committees, no matter how horrendous." Worthington and Silver also note that, in at least one respect, the JCAH has actually lowered its standards. In the past, a hospital desiring accreditation had to have a rule on its books requiring that a specialist be consulted in all complicated obstetrical cases, in all cases where surgery is proposed but the patient is a poor surgical risk, and in all cases where the attending physician has not been able to arrive at a clear-cut diagnosis. The new rules provide only that the use of consultants "should be reviewed as part of medical care evaluation." Furthermore, the commission's ability to put pressure on erring hospitals will continue to be weakened by its refusal to make public the reports of its surveyors. This is in keeping with the fact that the JCAH works for, and is paid by, the hospitals that seek its approval. When a consumer's group demanded to know why the reports were kept secret, Dr. Porterfield came back with a question of his own. "If we are a bought and paid for private consultant," he asked rhetorically, "can we go around talking about it?"

Some hospitals do a good job of protecting patients against medical bungling. University hospitals may have their shortcomings, but patients with acute organic disorders are relatively safe from mistaken diagnoses, unnecessary operations, or inappropriate treatment in a hospital where doctors—attending physicians and house officers alike—must routinely justify their decisions to their peers, and where status accrues to the doctor who impresses his colleagues as knowing exactly what he is doing. There are community hospitals, too, where a real effort is made to see to it that patients are treated in accordance with the best current standards. If some physicians on the staff turn out to be deviating from such standards, a special course may be arranged for them covering, say, the indications for a hysterectomy, or the proper use of antibiotics after an operation. If a doctor fails to mend his ways, the hospital's trustees and medical staff may take more drastic action. A general practitioner whose surgical reach exceeds his grasp, for example, may be restricted to a few simple procedures, and required to consult with a specialist before attempting even these. In extreme cases, a doctor may be told he can no longer treat his patients in the hospital at all.

The experience of the Chestnut Hill Hospital in Philadelphia, described in Chapter Three, shows how effectively such measures can work in cutting down on, for example, unnecessary appendectomies and excessive dosing with antibiotics. But there are many hospitals where doctors are free to do anything they like to, and for, their patients, and others where controls exist on paper only. Thus at one hospital being checked over by the Joint Commission on the Accreditation of Hospitals the surveyor sensed something odd about the minutes of the medical audit and tissue committees. When he questioned the secretary who had typed them, he found that she had made them up, and that the committees had not been bothering to meet.

Even when committees do meet they may be quite ineffective. Recently, for example, the magazine *Hospital Physician* carried an article titled "Is Peer Review a Force or a Farce in Your Hospital?" The author, who wrote under the pseudonym of Harry D. Crechner, and who was identified as the former chief of the medical staff of a 200-bed hospital in a southern state, reported that, despite the existence of a tissue committee, one of his colleagues at the hospital, to whom he gave the name of Riesford, had for years been cleaning up financially by performing unnecessary mastoidectomies. As an example of his colleague's chutzpah, Crechner recalled the case of a young boy with a minor ear infection on whom Riesford had performed a double mastoidectomy, earning $800 for his work. When the boy's symptoms persisted, Riesford repeated the operation, telling the parents that unfortunately it didn't always work the first time, and collected another $800. "The boy is still under treatment today," Crechner reported, "but his parents are out the $1600 they could ill afford. Had they taken their son to an otolaryngologist he would probably have put a polyethylene tube in his ear to drain it, and the bill wouldn't have been more than $80."

In a mastoidectomy a portion of the bone behind the ear is removed, and it is usually easy to tell by examining it later whether the operation was in fact necessary or not. Crechner reported that to avoid being second-guessed by the hospital's pathologist, or by the members of the tissue committee, to which the pathologist's reports were regularly sent, Riesford would simply fail to send the pathologist any bone or tissue, explaining that it had all been siphoned off accidentally in the suction bottle; when Crechner asked the pathologist why he put up with this, he was told, "I'm just a hired hand here, and I'm not going to stick my neck out." Crechner complained to the state medical society and to the JCAH, but apparently dropped his charges after Riesford, who had a flair for getting favorable publicity for the hospital, was elected to replace his accuser as its chief of staff.

One should, perhaps, hear Riesford's side of the story. But there is evidence that many hospitals have their Riesfords. A team of physicians who surveyed a suburban hospital in Southern California some years ago could find no justification for 98 per cent of the tonsillectomies performed by the doctors on its staff. Similarly, a study of appendectomies performed in nineteen hospitals in southwestern Michigan showed that the percentage of nondiseased appendixes removed ranged from 6.4 per cent at one hospital to 52.1 per cent at another. At one hospital three quarters of the appendixes removed by a particular doctor turned out, when looked at under the pathologist's microscope, to be quite normal.

The tolerance that hospital boards so often display toward doctors who make a botch of their work, or who consistently over-operate, reflects the fact that American hospitals, apart from those affiliated with universities or heavily involved in teaching, have been thought of simply as places where doctors could treat their patients when they were seriously ill. In proprietary hospitals, where it has been demonstrated repeatedly that patients are most likely to be incompetently treated or unnecessarily operated on, and in most nonprofit community hospitals as well, it is left up to the doctors who use the hospital to make and enforce such standards as they choose. Typically the chief of staff, and the chairmen of the departments of surgery, pediatrics, and the like, are elected by their fellows, serve without salary on a part-time basis, and have very little authority to make other physicians on the staff change their ways. The effectiveness of a hospital's arrangements for peer review is commonly undermined, moreover, by the fact that doctors practicing in the same community depend on one another for referrals—that is, for patients. A young surgeon serving on his hospital's tissue committee may therefore be most reluctant to criticize the work of a general practitioner from whom he is hoping to get patients requiring major surgery.

Hospital boards and administrators can press for effective quality controls, and some are doing so, partly as a result of a 1965 decision by the Supreme Court of Illinois. The case involved a malpractice claim by an eighteen-year-old college student who broke his leg playing football and had to have it amputated because the doctor who treated him put on too tight a cast, and gangrene set in. When the case was tried, the hospital defended itself on the traditional ground that it had done all that could be expected of it when it had verified that the doctor who had put on the cast was licensed to practice medicine in Illinois; whatever had gone wrong, the hospital argued, was his fault, not the hospital's. The jury, and eventually the state's highest court, were impressed, however, by the plaintiff's argument that the hospital *was* at fault in that, among other things, it had not seen to it that the doctor was qualified to treat serious fractures, it had not required him to take refresher courses, and it had not required him to call in an orthopedic consultant when complications developed. As a result, the hospital had to pay $150,000 in damages. And while the Illinois court's decision is not binding in other states, it is generally being followed, and hospital trustees are aware that they can no longer so easily disclaim all responsibility for the work of incompetent or careless doctors.

They are also aware, however, that they have to rely on the medical staff to keep the hospital's beds filled and its budget balanced, and their determination to enforce stricter quality standards may be vitiated by fear that a doctor who is told that he can no longer do hysterectomies without consulting a specialist may decide to take his patients elsewhere. Even when a hospital does conclude that a doctor's deficiencies are so great as to require dropping him from its staff, nothing is usually said to his patients. The blow is further softened, Robert Derbyshire has pointed out, by the custom of permitting "the errant staff member to resign voluntarily, placing nothing official in his record. If he moves to another locality, there is no way for officials there to learn of his past behavior beyond the 'grapevine.'" All this may explain in part how it could happen that a surgeon who was recently convicted of malpractice in Sacramento had found hospitals in which to practice his trade even though he admitted at his trial that he had performed at least thirty-seven unnecessary back operations—"with evil purpose . . . simply to line his pockets," as the trial judge put it—and that for a period of seven years he had been addicted to uppers and downers.

Just recently the way doctors treat their hospital patients—some of their patients, at any rate—has been made subject to formal outside scrutiny. In 1972, despite intensive lobbying by the AMA against what its spokesmen denounced as unwarranted bureaucratic interference, Congress voted to set up a network of so-called Professional Standards Review Organizations, or PSROs, to see to it that the huge sums the federal government now pays out for the care of the old and the poor when they are confined to nursing homes and hospitals is reasonably well spent. Each PSRO is made up of doctors practicing in a state, or a subdivision of a state, and is charged with seeing to it that Medicaid and Medicare patients confined to institutions in its area of jurisdiction are not subjected to unnecessary treatment, or to treatment that does not measure up to accepted professional standards. A doctor found to be billing the government for needless or inappropriate treatment can be required to return up to $5000 in fees, and can be declared ineligible for any future government payments. Under some national health insurance plans now before Congress, the PSROs would be responsible for monitoring all medical treatment, not only in hospitals but in doctors' offices as well. Their probable effectiveness (they have just begun to function) will be considered in Chapter Fourteen, along with other arrangements for improving the technical quality, and holding down the cost, of American medical care.

As things stand, a doctor who harms patients through ignorance, carelessness, or greed has really only one thing to worry about—that he will be sued for malpractice. Most doctors, of course, carry insurance against this contingency. But, even so, a malpractice suit can be a harrowing experience for the defendant. It is not just that legal conferences, the taking of pretrial depositions, and the trial itself can all consume enormous amounts of time. A doctor, having been taught to think of himself as accountable only to himself and, possibly, his medical peers, may find it excruciating to have to spend day after day in court confronting a lawyer bent on proving that he has, say, killed a patient by absent-mindedly giving her the wrong drug. The doctor's image of himself as a dedicated, benevolent, and even Godlike figure may be badly damaged even if, as happens in most malpractice suits that go to trial, the jury finds in his favor. If he loses—especially if the loss is not his first—the penalty is likely to be greater. His insurance premiums may be doubled or even tripled, thereby hurting him in his pocketbook as well as his psyche. Not long ago, for instance, an official of an insurance company told a Senate committee about a doctor whose record was so bad that the company's actuaries, calculating that there was a fifty-fifty chance that he would severely injure or kill at least one patient a year through negligence, fixed his annual insurance premium at $50,000. The doctor, who was reputed to have a very rich practice, said he would take his chances and insure himself. This is an extreme case, but in some states it is not unusual for a surgeon or obstetrician who has been successfully sued for malpractice to have to pay $15,000 to $20,000 a year for insurance.

Doctors have complained for years that the cards are stacked against them in the game of malpractice litigation. In 1975, in an effort to persuade politicians to straighten out the deck, specialists in some states, including New York and California, went on selective strikes, refusing to anesthetize or operate on patients except in serious emergencies. Their protests, which failed to bring about any major revision of the rules governing malpractice suits, but which did get them a better break on malpractice insurance, were touched off by staggering increases in the cost of such insurance. In New York, for example, standard rates went up by 93.5 per cent in July 1974. As a result, obstetricians, general surgeons, and anesthesiologists practicing in and around New York City were compelled to pay $9433 a year for a million-dollar policy. The rate for orthopedic surgeons and certain other specialists in high-risk categories rose to $14,324. Six months later the Argonaut Insurance Company, from which most doctors in the state were buying their coverage, asked permission to boost its rates by an additional 196.8 per cent. It later withdrew the request, announcing that it was no longer going to write malpractice insurance in New York. Although the state legislature took steps to make insurance available to doctors after Argonaut pulled out, it was clear that the price of insurance would quickly rise by at least 10 per cent, and perhaps by a lot more.

One reason why the price of malpractice insurance has been soaring—in Ohio, the principal insurer asked permission early in 1975 to raise its rates in certain categories by 747 per cent—is that juries have been getting increasingly generous in their awards to victims of malpractice. At the same time, more Americans have been accusing their doctors of malpractice, and more of them have been making the accusation stick. This does not necessarily mean that doctors are sloppier or less competent than they used to be. Rather, the volume of claims and the number of cash settlements and awards have risen because, among other things, the rules governing the trial of medical malpractice suits have been changing in ways that make it easier for a plaintiff to prove his case. The main difficulty that plaintiffs face in this connection is finding doctors willing to testify on their behalf. ("You wind up ostracized," a Los Angeles surgeon remarked recently. "We have referral practices; condemn a colleague and you lose his referrals. I personally testify, but I think I'm nuts: I have six kids.") This difficulty has now been eased by court rulings that permit a plaintiff to bring in experts from another state, or to use textbooks in place of live witnesses in order to show that the defendant deviated from standard medical practice.

Another reason for the rise in malpractice litigation has to do with the fact that as more and more care is given by specialists, doctors and patients are more and more likely to be strangers to one another. In such circumstances, patients seem less inclined to give the doctor the benefit of the doubt when something goes wrong. Also, the impulse to sue may be strengthened, or so many doctors believe, by an unwarranted faith in the efficacy of modern medical procedures, leading to a conviction that if a treatment miscarries, and the patient is hurt, somebody must be to blame. Finally, juries may be readier than in the past to award damages on humanitarian grounds to a patient who has, let us say, been horribly crippled by an operation on his spine, even when there is no evidence that the surgeon or anyone else was at fault. Lawyers who specialize in representing plaintiffs in malpractice suits have not been backward in exploiting this tendency.

The fear of being hit with a malpractice suit unquestionably has some salutary effects. One authority, Eli P. Bernzweig, who recently served as director of a special federal advisory group, the Commission on Medical Malpractice, has suggested that, at the present time, malpractice suits are "the most effective mechanism for coercing compliance with customary standards of care. . . ." Another authority, David Rubsamen, goes further. Rubsamen, who is both a doctor and a lawyer, and who edits a publication called *Professional Liability Newsletter*, has pointed out that in California, where patients are particularly quick to sue, the threat of lawsuits has brought striking improvements in certain aspects of medical care. "Anesthesia done by the general practitioner has not disappeared, but it is now a very small percentage of the total anesthesia in the state," he told a conference on malpractice in 1971. Because anesthesia exposes a patient to a lot more risk than, say, a course of penicillin shots, anesthesiologists have to pay a lot for malpractice insurance. "The general practitioner," Rubsamen added, "knows that his . . . insurance premium will be as high as that of the anesthesiologist if he performs any part of the practice of anesthesia. But, more important, hospitals are requiring that anesthesia be given by specialists. Hospitals have been nailed in the past when there have been anesthetic accidents." Rubsamen went on to speak of another way in which standards have been improved: "I also think that the malpractice threat has stimulated the willingness of physicians to obtain consultation, and that is good. Many physicians are growing more cautious; one gets the impression they feel they had better not try some of the big surgery. . . ."

Nevertheless, as a mechanism for upgrading the quality of medical practice the chief merit of malpractice litigation is that it is just about the only game in town. For one thing, it encourages what is known as defensive medicine. This consists of ordering tests, or carrying out procedures, whose only point is to protect the doctor in case he should be sued for malpractice. After examining a child who has fallen out of a tree, for example, a doctor may order a skull x-ray not because he suspects a fracture, and not because it would make any difference in the patient's treatment even if he did turn out to have a slight fracture, but because he doesn't want to be in a position of having to admit on the witness stand, in case something should go amiss, that he had failed to take all steps to establish an exact diagnosis.

Just how much of this goes on is impossible to tell. When the American College of Surgeons queried its members, more than half said they sometimes ordered x-rays and laboratory tests, or called in consultants, solely to protect themselves in the event of a malpractice claim. However, a study by investigators at the Duke University School of Law has produced persuasive evidence that doctors may be exaggerating the number of unnecessary x-rays and other procedures they call for in order to strengthen their case for outlawing or restricting malpractice suits. But defensive medicine does exist, and it can be dangerous as well as expensive. Prolonged exposure to x-rays may injure the germ plasm and the female gonads, causing congenital abnormalities to show up in a later generation. "By insisting on a lot of x-rays, often simply for the legal protection of the doctor, you can reap some short-term benefits," Mark Blumberg, an official of the Kaiser Foundation Health Plan, has observed. "But you are also causing unknown but almost certain adverse consequences to society. And how do you sue for that?"

Finally, a serious weakness of malpractice litigation is that it neither puts an erring doctor out of action nor compels him to improve his performance. There is no follow-up by state licensing boards, which ordinarily have no way of knowing that a surgeon has been hit, let us say, with three malpractice claims in the past year, and has been forced to settle them all out of court. Nor are a doctor's patients likely to find out, in the ordinary course of events, that he is being repeatedly (and successfully) sued for malpractice. As the case of the $50,000-a-year insurance premium suggests, a man can be proven again and again to be a horrible bungler and still enjoy a flourishing practice.

7

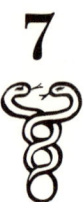

The Lingering Odor of Snake Oil

[The drug-company doctor] must learn the many ways to deceive the Food and Drug Administration and, failing in this, how to seduce, manipulate, or threaten the physician assigned to the New Drug Application into approving it even if it is incomplete. He must learn that anything that helps to sell a drug is valid even if it is supported by the crudest testimonial, while anything that decreases sales must be suppressed, distorted, and rejected because it is not absolutely conclusive proof. He must learn to word a warning statement so that it will appear to be an inducement to use the drug rather than a warning of the danger inherent in its use. . . . He will find himself squeezed between businessmen who will sell anything and justify it on the basis that doctors ask for it, and doctors who demand products they have been taught to want through the advertising and promotion schemes contrived by businessmen.
—*Dale Console, M.D., former Medical Director, E. R. Squibb & Sons*

There was a great deal of shocking testimony offered during these hearings. Four former industry detail men, working in four different parts of the country, and for four different companies, told essentially the same story: that they were under tremendous pressure to sell; . . . that they tended to minimize side effects and play up benefits; that they bribed their way into doctors' offices with gifts and gimmicks for doctors, nurses, receptionists, etc.; that they bribed pharmacists in similar ways in order to get their products stocked; . . . and that doctors often did what they, the detail men, wanted, and for admittedly unsound reasons.
—*Senator Edward M. Kennedy*

No aspect of medical care in America has been so painstakingly investigated, and none has so angered its investigators, as the making and marketing of prescription drugs. Over the past fifteen years, hundreds of witnesses have appeared before Congressional committees, notably those headed by the late Senator Estes Kefauver of Tennessee, by Senator Gaylord Nelson of Wisconsin, and by Senator Kennedy, to describe in rich detail the business strategies that have so handsomely rewarded the stockholders of the big drug companies. One reads the testimony of these witnesses, filling tens of thousands of printed pages, with the feeling that one has heard it all—or most of it—before, in another context. The sense of *déjà vu* arises from the striking similarities between the way these big companies do business and the methods used by old-time sellers of snake oil, potency restorers, and all-purpose nostrums. For it is clear that the miracle ingredient in the big drug companies' formula for sustained prosperity is not the prowess of its laboratory scientists. Rather, it is the techniques the companies have perfected for selling their goods at twenty, thirty, or forty times what it costs to manufacture them, even when other products that are just as good, or better—or, for that matter, identical—are available at one tenth or one twentieth the price. The feat is the more astonishing in that the makers of prescription drugs do not deal with a naive, uneducated yokelry. They must make their pitch to people—doctors—who are far better equipped, or so one might suppose, to evaluate the pitchmen's claims in a spirit of cool scientific skepticism.

The big drug companies obviously differ in one important way from the proprietors of medicine shows. They employ real scientists, who do real research in real laboratories, and whose work bears fruit from time to time in drugs that really ease pain, cure or prevent disease, and save lives. It is true that basic discoveries in pharmacology, such as Alexander Fleming's observation that penicillium mold inhibits the growth of staphylococcus germs, are more often made in academic than in commercial laboratories. But the work of transmuting such discoveries into safe, convenient, reliable, and effective products is ordinarily done by drug companies. Over a five-year period beginning in 1946, for example, Squibb scientists and technicians, following a lead provided by academic researchers, synthesized 5000 chemical compounds, and tested 1000 of these on tubercular mice, in a search for an antibiotic that would be specifically effective in treating tuberculosis. Another large firm, Hoffmann-La Roche, was working along similar lines, and in 1951 the two companies almost simultaneously discovered Isoniazid, a drug that has emptied tuberculosis hospitals and saved the lives of hundreds of thousands of people all over the world. Drug-company laboratories, using similar trial-and-error methods, also developed the broad-spectrum antibiotics, such as Aureomycin and Achromycin, that came into use after World War II. It was at Merck & Co. that researchers first identified and isolated Vitamin B_{12}, thereby providing doctors with a cheap, convenient, and highly effective means of controlling pernicious anemia.

But the discovery of a miracle drug like Isoniazid or Vitamin B_{12} is a rare event. A great many, perhaps most, of the thousands of new drugs marketed over the past thirty years belong in quite a different category. They are customarily the fruit of a tedious form of research called molecular roulette, in which the researcher plays with the chemical structure of an existing drug, typically, a patented product with which a competitor is cleaning up, in the hope of finding a variant with similar pharmacologic effects. Occasionally this process yields a new product that is significantly more potent, or has significantly fewer side effects, than the original. But more often the result is a so-called me-too drug whose only merit is that the company's marketing men believe they can profitably sell it in competition with its model. As Dale Console, whose reflections on the life of a drug-company doctor are quoted at the beginning of this chapter, once told a Senate committee, "with a little luck, proper timing, and a good promotion program, a bag of asafetida with a unique chemical side chain can be made to look like a wonder drug." On another occasion Console noted that in the 1950s, when he was Squibb's medical director, 75 to 80 per cent of the company's research money was spent on the development of me-too products or on other projects that promised no real benefits to the consumer.

Squibb and the other big drug companies have also flooded the market with a bewildering variety of pills and capsules in which two or more drugs are combined. Combinations are obviously convenient for the doctor, who has to write only one prescription instead of two or three, as well as for the patient, who has to take only one kind of pill. But their present widespread use is frowned on by most medical authorities, who point out that the fixed proportions in which a manufacturer elects to combine two drugs do not necessarily meet the needs of a particular patient at a particular time. Some combinations have also been criticized on the ground that one or more of the ingredients add nothing to the mixture except cost to the patient. In the past ten years, mainly because of changes in the federal drug laws, manufacturers have cut back on the introduction of new drug combinations. But more than a thousand combinations, many of them vigorously promoted by their manufacturers, are still on the market, and it has been estimated that at least 40 per cent of all prescriptions still call for drugs in combination form.

In an age when so much is made of medicine having at last been placed on a solid scientific footing, one might suppose that doctors, other than those conducting trials with new drugs, would be reluctant to dose patients with drugs whose makers cannot cite any hard—that is, scientific—evidence that they really work. But it has recently become clear that doctors do, in fact, prescribe vast quantities of such drugs. In 1962 the Pure Food and Drug Act was amended to require a manufacturer who wishes to market a new drug to show not only that it is safe, but also that it is effective. Four years later the Food and Drug Administration, which administers the law, decided to apply the effectiveness standard to old drugs as well as new, and as a preliminary to enforcing this provision of the new law the FDA asked for help from the National Academy of Sciences, an honorary body that is often called on by government agencies for scientific advice. At the FDA's request, the Academy assembled a group of two hundred pharmacologists and specialists in cancer, diabetes, and other diseases, and asked them to evaluate all claims made on behalf of all of the nearly three thousand drug products introduced in the United States between 1938 and 1962.

The Drug Efficacy Study Group, as it was called, worked at the task for more than two years, and then issued a report indicating that many of the claims that drug companies had been making for their products were based on evidence that differed very little from the testimonials traditionally featured in advertisements for bust-developers and hair-restorers. The study group said it had been unable to find any credible evidence at all to support some 2300 of the more than 16,000 separate claims it had examined. In the case of several hundred products, the manufacturers had been unable to come up with firm evidence that they were useful in treating anything. A much larger number of drugs were classified as "possibly effective" in treating one or more of the conditions for which their use was recommended—meaning that the study group had found hints in the material submitted by the manufacturers that further investigation might conceivably show these drugs to be of some value. Still other drugs were rated as "ineffective as a fixed combination." These included, for example, a pain killer called Zactirin, which got this rating because the study group could find no evidence that one of its two ingredients, ethoheptazine citrate, adds anything at all to the analgesic effect of its other ingredient, which is aspirin. (It does, however, add something to the price; Zactirin sells for about twenty times as much as the equivalent amount of plain aspirin.)

The study group made its final report in 1969, and since then most of the products that it classified as totally ineffective have been taken off the market. Eventually the manufacturers of drugs found to be only "possibly effective" will either have to prove that these drugs really do what they are said to do, or else stop making the disputed claims. A manufacturer who cannot produce evidence to support any of the claims he wishes to make for a product will have to stop selling it. But the FDA seems to be in no rush to crack down, and the pages of *Medical Economics*, for example, are filled with multi-page advertisements for drugs which, according to a small boxed notice that the FDA requires, have been found to be only possibly effective in treating bacterial rashes, or peptic ulcers, or mild depression, or low back pain, or whatever it is the writers of the ad are urging doctors to use the drug for.

The manufacturers of such products ordinarily do have some data purporting to show that the product really works. Usually this consists of reports from doctors who have been paid to try the drug on their patients. Such trials obviously can yield invaluable information about a new drug. But when a doctor reports that he has given Drug X to twenty-three patients, nineteen of whom seem to have been helped by it, it does not necessarily follow that Drug X is doing them any good at all. A patient may say he feels better—he may, in fact, feel better—simply because he wants to please the doctor, because he believes strongly in miracle drugs, or because he likes the idea of being part of a successful experiment. Also, when the doctor is being paid, and usually paid rather well, by the company whose product he is testing, his own objectivity is open to question. No matter how hard he tries to be impartial, he may unconsciously be influenced by the knowledge that if he is too hard on his sponsor's product he may not be given any more products to test.

The right way to find out if a drug is effective is to run what is known as a controlled double-blind test. In a test of this sort, one group of patients gets the real drug, while another, closely matched group is given a placebo (often a sugar pill) instead. As a further guard against bias on the part of the doctor, he is required to work "blind" from beginning to end, in the sense that he must have no way of knowing which of the patients are getting the real drug and which the placebo. The importance of such controls is shown by a recent analysis of 490 separate studies, most of them sponsored by drug manufacturers, of the effectiveness of certain antidepressants. With few exceptions, the weaker the controls, the better the drugs looked from the manufacturers' point of view.

Besides selling vast quantities of drugs that are probably ineffective, and certainly overpriced, the big drug companies have at times enthusiastically urged the use of their products in circumstances in which the risk of killing the patient, or at least of making him a lot sicker than he already is, far outweighs the potential benefits. This was true for years of Parke Davis's promotion of an antibiotic called Chloromycetin. Soon after its appearance on the market in 1949, evidence began to pile up that it could cause serious blood disorders, including aplastic anemia, a disease in which the body disintegrates and the victim eventually bleeds to death. Since the 1950s pharmacologists and specialists in infectious diseases have therefore issued repeated warnings that Chloromycetin should be used only to treat typhoid fever, Rocky Mountain spotted fever, and one or two other rare and dangerous infections that do not readily yield to other antibiotics.

Yet as late as 1967, when Senator Nelson's Subcommittee on Monopoly looked into the matter, Parke Davis salesmen were still reassuring doctors that it was quite all right to use Chloromycetin to treat a wide variety of minor ailments. Partly as a result, the committee was told, some three and a half million

Americans a year were being dosed with this highly toxic drug whereas there was no real need for doctors to expose more than ten to twenty thousand to its dangers. Over the years, witnesses testified, hundreds—perhaps thousands—of Americans had died of aplastic anemia after being dosed with Chloromycetin for such trivial disorders as colds, mosquito bites, styes, and infected hangnails. Relatives of the victims were understandably bitter. In a letter read to the committee, the father of a fifteen-year-old girl, who had died of aplastic anemia after her doctor had prescribed Chloromycetin for a sore throat, said he had a question he would like to put to the president of Parke Davis: "If he or his wife watched one of their children die a little bit each day for eleven weeks with a disease that struck our daughter like rat poison . . . could he take pride in his promotional prowess?" As a result of the hearings, sales of Chloromycetin, which is now sold by other companies besides Parke Davis under its generic, or official name of chloramphenicol, fell off by 75 per cent. But the Nelson committee's staff economist, Benjamin Gordon, estimated at the end of 1973 that for each case in which chloramphenicol was appropriately prescribed, seventy to eighty people were still taking it on their doctors' orders for conditions that could be treated just as effectively and far more safely with other antibiotics.

To win the hearts and minds of doctors, the indispensable middlemen of the prescription-drug business, the big drug makers entertain them lavishly at medical conventions, hire them as consultants, furnish them with research funds, pick up the tab for trips to company-sponsored symposia (often held in pleasant watering places in the United States and abroad), and shower them with free drug samples and other gifts. Certain gifts, like the black bags and stethoscopes that some companies give to medical students, are meant to create a general feeling of warmth toward a company and its products. (Older physicians, who already have stethoscopes, are likely to get such items as free golf balls stamped with the recipient's—and the company's—name.) Drug companies also cultivate the good will of physicians by inviting them to come and tour their plants. A Maryland physician told the Kennedy committee that he and his wife and another couple had twice accepted such invitations from a company that had the particular merit, in their eyes, of having located its laboratories and main plant just outside New

York City. "Twice we went to New York City, stayed at the Waldorf-Astoria, wined and dined at incredibly expensive restaurants, went to Broadway shows, and had a marvelous time, all at the expense of Lederle Laboratories," he testified. The witness added, seemingly as an afterthought, "Admittedly a tour of the drug company was pleasant and enlightening and of course we left with more gift boxes of samples."

Other gifts are made to promote specific drugs. Not long ago, for example, as a means of acquainting doctors with the virtues of a new tranquilizer called Sinequan, Pfizer Laboratories, at a cost of a quarter of a million dollars, gave each of ten thousand psychiatrists a set of ten classical records bearing the label "Sinequan Collector's Series." According to the Pfizer executive in charge of marketing Sinequan, this seemed an appropriate gift because "the psychiatrist thinks of himself as a Renaissance man. He's very much into art and music and appreciates these things." Other physicians, thought to be less into art and music, got a transparent plastic model of the human brain, filled with red and blue liquids that separated into layers like the ingredients of a pousse-café. The liquids, it was explained, represented anxiety and depression, which Sinequan was said to alleviate whether they occurred separately or in combination. Drug companies have on occasion offered colored television sets and similar big-ticket items to doctors who agree to stock up heavily on particular vaccines or other injectible drugs.

Drug-industry marketing men also see to it that doctors have plenty of informative reading material. A few years back a Tennessee physician who kept track of all drug-company mail that came to him in a single month reported that he had received, in addition to 44 drug samples, 125 direct mail advertisements, and 41 newspapers and magazines put out by drug companies—a total of 210 items that filled three shopping bags and weighed 35 pounds. Medical journals are filled with brightly colored and arresting ads that bear a strong family resemblance to television commercials for laxatives and headache pills. Recent advertisements have included paintings or photographs of a man walking a tightrope over a roaring stream ("NO TIME FOR ANTIHISTAMINE HAZE"); an appetizing young woman displaying a lot of thigh ("THE BARE FACTS . . . in many dermatoses the less they wear, the more they need . . ."); a sad-looking elderly man in slippers, carrying a portable radio and a newspaper, and trailing his suspenders ("THE IRREGULAR AMERICANS"); and the leaning tower of Pisa (in an ad for a drug said to be very good for treating impotence). Another ad, which took up four pages in a recent issue of *Medical Economics,* featured a photograph of a worried-looking woman, brows knit and hair awry, under a headline reading "LIFE BEGINS AT FORTY . . . but at 45, so do the early symptoms of estrogen deficiency." On turning the page, one finds another picture of the same woman, but now she is smiling, relaxed, and wearing a new hairdo, all of which are presumably results of having taken Premarin, an estrogen pill. "Tropical beaches, racing cars, and naked women," begins a disapproving editorial in *The New Physician,* the organ of the Student Medical Association. "All appeared last year in journal advertising for pharmaceuticals . . . titillating doctors with a sensory siege designed to tweak every neuron from crotch to frontal lobe."

This neuron-tweaking would be less disquieting if the information accompanying the naked women and tightrope walkers were accurate, complete, and presented in a balanced fashion. But even though the 1962 amendments to the Pure Food and Drug Act gave the FDA some control over drug advertising (a company can be made to modify or discontinue an ad that is found to be misleading), the agency's efforts to reform drug-company copywriters have been only partially successful.

Thus while the copywriters are now under increased pressure to give the bad news along with the good, the bad news is usually in small type, and often appears on a separate page from the selling copy. Recently, for instance, medical journals have been carrying a five-page advertisement for a drug, Atromid-S, that reduces the amount of cholesterol in the blood. The sequence begins with a painting of a group of slant-browed humanoids draped with the carcasses of dead animals. The headline reads: "One million years ago, a primitive ancestor of man assumed a meat-eating habit which he passed on to his descendants." On the facing page there appears a group of these descendants, in the guise of travelers at an airport, all of whom are noticeably overweight. It is only when one turns the page that one finds, wedged in among graphs and charts showing how effective Atromid-S can be in lowering cholesterol levels, a highly significant suggestion that this may not actually do the patient any good. "It has not been established," the reader is warned, "whether the drug-induced lowering of serum cholesterol or lipid level has a detrimental, beneficial, or no effect on the morbidity or mortality due to atherosclerosis or coronary heart disease. Several years will be required before current investigations will yield an answer to the question."

Another trick of drug-product copywriters, one that the FDA's reviewers can catch only by doing a lot of independent reading, is to quote selectively from the relevant medical literature. In the late 1960s, for example, Eli Lilly ran an advertisement for an oral contraceptive called C-Quens which stated that taking C-Quens required "no change in dress size." In fact, as the FDA pointed out, 15 per cent of the women taking C-Quens in a test program had gained an average of sixteen pounds in the first six months. Another firm, Wallace Laboratories, was required by the FDA to send out a "Dear Doctor" letter to all practicing physicians to correct what the FDA held to be misleading statements in an advertisement for a drug combination called Deprol. In the ad, Wallace had cited twenty-one clinical studies to support its claim that "three out of four nonpsychotic depressions respond to Deprol." It had failed to say, however, that the three-out-of-four claim was based on data from only ten of these studies, and that all but one of these were uncontrolled—that is, no placebos were used. Nothing was said, either, about the fact that most of the 323 patients covered by the ten studies had been getting psychotherapy as well as Deprol. The ad also neglected to mention that the authors of one of the studies it cited had later carried out another, better-controlled investigation, and that this one indicated that Deprol did nothing at all to relieve depression.

Many of the patients whom the average doctor sees each day have come to him because they are worried, or depressed, or sleepless, or are getting along poorly with their wives or bosses or children—in a word, because they are unhappy. Some doctors feel uncomfortable and put upon, and simply want to get them out of the office as fast as possible. Others recognize that what such patients probably need is counseling, but are reluctant to offer it because it takes up so much time—time for which, as a practical matter, the internist or general practitioner cannot charge at a psychiatrist's rate.

In either case, the drug industry's copywriters do everything they can to reassure doctors that the right thing to do in such situations is to give the patient a pill. Indeed, to a layman, and to many psychiatrists as well, they often seem to be urging tranquilizers and antidepressants not only for patients who are seriously disturbed, but also to help people cope with the pains and trials of everyday living. Richard Pillard, a psychiatrist on the faculty of the Boston University School of Medicine, furnished the Nelson committee with a number of advertisements that carried this message. One was for an antidepressant called Tofranil. It portrayed a woman in tears over her son's marriage, and the accompanying text read, in part, "Often in the mind of the lonely, widowed, depression-prone individual, she's not gaining a daughter, she's losing a son. The occasion may be marred by depression with such symptoms as feelings of sadness, incapacity, helplessness, and hopelessness. Tofranil often relieves symptoms of depression."

Pillard noted that the ad was open to criticism on the technical ground that a patient usually has to take an antidepressant regularly for two to four weeks before feeling any relief, and that over such a period of time the widow might well recover from her son's wedding without taking any pills. In a more serious vein, he went on to say, "Apart from the question of whether tranquilizers and antidepressants are effective in these 'situational' reactions—and there is not really much evidence that they are—there is a judgment to be made whether it is most healthy for people to be reacting to or chemically protected from these emotions which are an inevitable part of a full and normal life." Pillard added dryly, "I know of no studies on this issue."

A particularly brash specimen of the kind of drug-pushing to which Pillard objects showed up in medical journals in 1971. It was an ad for Serentil, a tranquilizer marketed by Sandoz Pharmaceuticals. The face of a woman, wearing the worried expression that so many women seem to have in drug-company advertisements, was shown as a piece of a jigsaw puzzle, under a headline reading: "FOR THE ANXIETY THAT COMES FROM NOT FITTING IN." The text went, in part, like this: "The newcomer in town who *can't* make friends. The organization man who *can't* adjust to altered status within the company. The woman who *can't* get along with her new daughter-in-law. The executive who *can't* accept retirement. . . ." This was too much for the FDA, and Sandoz was forced to run a retraction saying that the FDA considered the ad misleading because it suggested "unapproved use of Serentil for relatively minor everyday anxiety situations. . . ."

Possibly because of Sandoz's experience, manufacturers are generally careful these days to cover themselves by pointing out that tranquilizers and antidepressants should be used only when other methods fail. "If she calls you morning . . . noon . . . and night, day after day, to allay her chronic anxiety try her on Stelazine," a recent headline reads. The text goes on to say, "Excessive use of the telephone is often symptomatic of chronic neurotic anxiety. Because such patients are often immune to lasting reassurance, in addition to your counsel, supportive medication may be helpful." (Translation: if a patient bugs you, give her a fix.) A similar line is taken by an ad for Ritalin, a mood-elevating drug, which portrays a woman "who just doesn't respond to things"—in this case she looks bemused rather than worried—and suggests that if "counsel and reassurance" don't help, Ritalin may. Ritalin, the ad continues, "boosts spirits and brightens mood . . . helps the patient get moving again." The message is clear: Don't waste your valuable time on counseling—let Ritalin do the job for you.

Ritalin's ads themselves suggest some good reasons, however, for rejecting this advice. One reason is that Ritalin may get the patient moving in entirely the wrong direction. Drug manufacturers are required by the law to list possible side effects in their advertisements, and ads for Ritalin warn that it should be prescribed "cautiously" for patients who are emotionally unstable; the danger is that they may become addicted to the stuff—Ritalin acts rather like an amphetamine—and this in turn can lead to "varying degrees of abnormal behavior" and even to psychotic episodes. The ads note further that even when no dependence develops, Ritalin can cause nervousness, insomnia, skin rash, erythema (in which the skin turns red, as if sunburned), nausea, loss of appetite, dizziness, headaches, palpitations, abdominal and chest pain, irregular heartbeat, and weight loss. Such reactions are not terribly frequent, and might be worth chancing if Ritalin really did what it is supposed to do.

But even though it has been on the market for years, and has been prescribed for millions of people, it has been rated by the FDA as only "possibly effective" in treating mild depression.

The doctor's patronage is also solicited by the detail men who wait for him at his office. Spokesmen for the pharmaceutical industry often portray the detail man as a friendly tutor who offers the busy physician a balanced course in drug therapy. But recent testimony before the Kennedy committee paints a rather different picture. The language of the directives with which detail men are bombarded by their home offices suggests that they are expected to go about their work not like teachers but like door-to-door encyclopedia salesmen. Ortho-Pharmaceutical, for example, instructs detail men to remember the importance of "an emotional appeal, an appeal to the pride, ego, fear," while G. D. Searle tells them, "Sell the nurse; she is as important to moving your product as gas is to moving your car." Searle also urges its detail men to consider "each nonsold market a challenging 'must' project to be accomplished. The traffic sign 'Yield' does not mean 'Stop,' 'Turn Back,' or 'Give Up.'" (Kennedy asked Searle's president, James A. Buzard, if a detail man, in the face of such exhortations, might not forget that he was supposed to be an educator, and conclude that "the name of the game is sales." Buzard said this was unlikely, because the company was careful to send out its bulletins to detail men under a logo reading "RP/RP" "It means 'Right Pill, Right Patient,'" Buzard explained righteously. "That is the theme of our marketing program, Senator.") Again and again, Congressional investigations have shown that detail men have been instructed not to mention articles in medical journals that raise serious questions about the safety or effectiveness of the drugs they are selling. "Sure, maybe we will promote amphetamines as nothing more than 'diet pills,'" Ronald Serino, who spent three years detailing drugs for Lederle, told the Kennedy committee. "We really do not care how they are abused after they sell them. There is a good profit in speed. So we will promote the hell out of it until the FDA puts the brakes on, which they did."

It would be comforting to think that most doctors are too shrewd to be taken in by the detail men who call on them. But this is clearly not the case. Investigations have consistently shown that a great many doctors (in studies cited by witnesses before Senator Nelson's committee the proportion varied from 39 to 67 per cent) prescribe new drugs on the basis of what they are told by the manufacturer, either in print or via the detail man. "I have personally been very chagrined," a doctor who has done extensive research on drugs like Ritalin and Stelazine told the Nelson committee, "by the fact that even though I am known throughout the country and perhaps even over the world for my work with these drugs, I have really less influence in my own hospital on the prescribing habits of physicians than the next detail man who walks in the door."

One reason why detail men are listened to is that doctors are taught very little about drugs while they are in medical school, and much of what they learn is soon out of date. To be sure, a doctor who wants objective evaluations of drugs can get them by taking *The Medical Letter.* This authoritative guide to drugs and drug research was founded in 1958 by Arthur Kallet, who also founded *Consumers Union,* and it now goes out each fortnight to some 70,000 subscribers. But the editors labor under certain disadvantages. They are understandably hard pressed to keep up with all the new products that hit the market, and the detail man, arriving with his bag full of free samples, gets his licks in first. And while *The Medical Letter* is clearly and crisply written, reading it demands more intellectual effort than listening to the smooth and chatty presentation of the detail man. Detail men also lose few opportunities to remind the practicing physician that he (the physician) is the man on the firing line, and that no academic expert back at a rear base is in any position to tell him what drugs are best for his particular patients. This flatters the doctor's ego, soothes any anxiety he may feel when he contemplates the vast amount he doesn't know about drugs, and convinces him that the detail man, unlike the haughty and impractical purists who write for *The Medical Letter,* really understands his problems.

It is true, of course, that experience can provide a doctor with invaluable knowledge about differences among drugs, and about the best way to use particular drugs in treating particular conditions. But it cannot tell him anything very reliable about the relative effectiveness of Zactirin and plain aspirin, or about the odds against the possibility that Drug X will make his patients worse instead of better. Many a doctor prescribed Chloromycetin for hundreds of patients over the years without ever seeing a case of aplastic anemia develop. But neither his own clinical experience, nor the bland assurance of Parke Davis's detail men, really justified prescribing this dangerous drug for minor infections.

To make things easier for its copywriters and detail men, the drug companies have used economic and political pressure to keep doctors from having easy access to information that might conflict with what the industry wants them to hear. The Pharmaceutical Manufacturers' Association, or PMA, regularly lobbies against legislation opposed by the AMA, and the AMA returns the favor in kind. Thus even though a majority of doctors, according to a recent FDA poll, want reliable *comparative* information about drugs, the AMA has gone along with the PMA in opposing a plan to have such information published annually under government auspices. The industry would prefer to have doctors depend for guidance on the *Physician's Desk Reference*, an annual publication that is, in effect, paid for by the drug companies, and that is simply an uncritical compilation of their claims as to what their products can do.

The AMA's friendly feeling toward the drug companies may be fortified by the fact that more than a quarter of the AMA's income in 1973—$9 million out of $34 million—came from the drug industry, mainly in the form of payments for advertising in various AMA publications. (The AMA also owns some $28 million worth of drug-company stock.) Certainly the circumstances in which the AMA recently abolished its own Council on Drugs suggests an extraordinary sensitivity to the wishes of the drug companies. The council, a semiautonomous body whose members included a number of leading authorities on drugs, had from time to time taken it upon itself to challenge the industry's views on such matters as the safety and effectiveness of combination drugs. In 1971, having decided that something more was needed than sporadic bulletins and warnings, the council published the first edition of what was to be a yearly compilation of current information on drugs. It differed from the *Physician's Desk Reference* in that it compared similar drugs on the basis of how well they worked, and how risky it was to use them; in some instances drugs were ranked in order of their over-all effectiveness in treating certain conditions. This apparently struck the big drug manufacturers as an unpardonable display of lèse majesté, and they let the AMA's Board of Directors know how they felt. In 1972, while work was going forward on the second edition of the guide, and after the drug manufacturers had been shown a preliminary draft, the Board dissolved the council.

The official explanation was that the AMA could no longer afford to support the council's activities—especially, the Board said, now that many of its functions had been taken over by the FDA. But Dr. John Adriani, professor of surgery at Tulane University Medical School and a recent chairman of the council, had a different theory. "The fact that the council was dissolved as an 'economy measure' is laughable to one who knows the facts," he told Senator Nelson's Subcommittee on Monopoly. Adriani, whose testimony was supported by two other former officers of the Council on Drugs, went on to say, "The dilemma of the Board of Trustees is understandable. . . . They had no choice but to appease the pharmaceutical industry. There were only two solutions: (1) to either 'muzzle' the council to the point of abolishment if necessary, or (2) forgo income from advertising for its operating budget. As a result, the second edition of this well-received volume, which had reached the final stages of completion under the close surveillance of the Council on Drugs, will be completed by the staff of the [AMA's] Department of Drugs." The significance of this shift, Adriani said, was that the old Council on Drugs had been made up of "independent thinking scientists and practitioners" who were not paid by the AMA, whereas the Department of Drugs is staffed "by employees who are obligated to do the bidding of their superiors," and whose work was certain to be "emasculated and worthless." "Thus the AMA," he concluded, "has abrogated its responsibility of providing factual information on drugs to the physician in the public's behalf."

Drug manufacturers have accepted with poor grace the restrictions imposed on them by the 1962 amendments to the Pure Food and Drug Act. With support from a group of medical scientists and medical-school deans, they have complained that FDA bureaucrats have delayed the introduction of some useful new drugs, and have barred others permanently from the American market.

There is some foundation for such charges. A company wishing to market a drug in the United States has to put a lot more time and money into showing that it is safe and that it works than most other countries require. (The notable exceptions are Sweden and Canada, which screen new drugs in much the same way as the United States.) As a result, useful drugs developed by American manufacturers often go on sale in France or Germany or England months or years before they become available here. It is also true that the number of new drugs coming onto the American market has fallen from an average of several hundred a year before 1962 to eighty-three in 1971.

But all this is probably not very significant. A number of people who should be in a position to know have denied that Americans are being deprived of drugs they really need. They include James V. Warren, a past president of both the American Heart Association and the American Federation for Clinical Research, who said recently, "I do not know of a single new type of drug which represents a major breakthrough which is available in a foreign country and which is being withheld from the American people because of FDA policies." Even one of the FDA's chief critics, Dr. Robert D. Dripps, who is vice president for medical affairs at the University of Pennsylvania, has conceded that he cannot name a single significant new drug kept off the American market by the FDA. Furthermore, a falling off in the number of new drug products going on sale in the United States is not necessarily bad news. Much of the decline has been in the number of new me-too and combination products, while the number of new drugs classified by the FDA as "important therapeutic advances" has scarcely declined at all, falling from an average of seven a year to just under six in the years since 1962. (*The Medical Letter,* which uses a different and slightly tougher rating system, finds no decline at all in the number of new drugs it considers significant.) The FDA has been able, too, to cite evidence that its finickyness about new drugs has saved lives. A former director of the agency's Bureau of Drugs, Henry E. Simmons, recently noted with satisfaction that the FDA had refused to clear for sale in the United States an aerosol spray which English doctors were freely prescribing for patients with asthma, but whose use was later found to have brought about a sevenfold increase in deaths from asthma in England during the 1960s, resulting in the premature deaths of some 3500 persons, many of them children. Simmons also pointed out that drugs cleared for sale in certain other countries, but not in the United

States, included a tranquilizer "associated with suppression of blood formation, liver toxicity in dogs, increased mortality of the newborn in rats, cleft palate in rodents, and disturbance of liver function in 43 per cent of human patients."

This is not to say that the FDA is beyond criticism. The agency does take a needlessly long time to clear new drugs, and there have been plausible charges that some of the FDA's medical and scientific people turn down new drug applications because they are not really competent to evaluate the evidence submitted by the manufacturer, and are determined to keep their necks well pulled in. But what is called for is better regulation, not less. There is little in the history of the drug industry before 1962 to suggest that it can safely be left to regulate itself, and the way American drug companies do business in countries where the rules of the game are more relaxed than in the United States indicates that nothing much has changed since then. By and large, where drug companies are legally free to mislead, they mislead. To give just one example, *The Medical Letter* recently called attention to a two-page advertisement, in the Mexican edition of the magazine *Medico Moderna*, for a product called Winstrol Compound, which is marketed by one of the largest American drug firms, Winthrop Laboratories. The ad displayed a picture of a healthy-looking boy, about seven years old, and recommended dosing him with Winstrol "if he complains of poor appetite, fatigue, or weight loss." No adverse side effects were mentioned. *The Medical Letter* pointed out that the main ingredient of Winstrol Compound is a steroid, stanozolol, which is also sold in the United States, but with two important differences: the manufacturer is permitted to recommend its use only for treating aplastic anemia and certain serious bone and glandular disorders; and advertisements must include warnings about side effects. "Adverse reactions . . . include premature closing of epiphyses (which results in premature stunting of growth) and testicular atrophy," *The Medical Letter* noted. "In females this drug can produce hirsutism, male pattern baldness, deepening of the voice and clitoral enlargement that 'are usually irreversible even after prompt discontinuance. . . .'" These effects, *The Medical Letter* went on to say, "are not rare idiosyncratic reactions. . . . Every child who takes the drug in the recommended dosage for a long enough time will demonstrate these effects. The Mexican advertisement for

Winstrol Compound makes no recommendation for limiting the duration of treatment."

The high prices that Americans have to pay for so many drugs are a gauge of the shrewdness with which the big drug companies have taken advantage of this country's patent and trademark laws. In every other important drug-producing country except Belgium, any manufacturer can make and sell a patented drug simply by undertaking to pay the patentholder a reasonable royalty. In the United States, by contrast, there is no compulsory licensing. The holder of a drug patent enjoys an absolute monopoly. That monopoly runs out after seventeen years, to be sure, and at that point one might suppose that the manufacturer of a drug like Valium, for which druggists are now paying up to twenty-nine times what it costs to make the stuff, would be forced to cut the price drastically as competitors came into the market. But the big drug companies, as I have pointed out in Chapter Two, have been remarkably successful in getting doctors to prescribe a drug by its trade name even when it is available to druggists under its official, or generic, name at a very much lower cost.

One reason for their success is that they have made it easier for doctors to do so. Until recently, drug companies had a fairly free hand in choosing the generic names for new drugs they had developed, and they commonly picked names that were long and hard to pronounce. By contrast, trade names tend to be short, evocative, and easy to remember. A doctor is unlikely to write "chlordiazepoxide hydrochloride," the generic name of a best-selling tranquilizer, when he can write "Librium" instead. In this particular case, it would make no difference which name he used, since chlordiazepoxide hydrochloride is still under patent, and is sold by only one manufacturer, Hoffmann-La Roche. But it does make a difference to La Roche if the doctor gets so used to writing "Librium" that it will not occur to him to prescribe it under any other name. For trademarks do not run out with patents, and long after La Roche's patent on chlordiazepoxide has expired the company will still have the exclusive right to sell it under the name of Librium. And most states have laws, enacted at the urging of the big drug manufacturers, providing that if a doctor writes "Librium," the druggist cannot fill the prescription with the identical drug made by another manufacturer no matter how much money this might save the customer.

The big companies have used a number of other devices to keep doctors from switching to generic drugs. One obvious tactic is to avoid letting doctors know that the patent on a trademarked product has expired, and that the identical drug is now available at a lower price. (Detail men are instructed not to talk about prices at all if they can avoid the subject, and many doctors have little notion of what their patients pay for drugs.) News of this kind is unlikely, moreover, to reach doctors from the smaller firms that sell off-patent drugs under their generic names; such firms have to operate on margins that do not permit them to take out ads in *Medical Economics* or to send detail men around to doctors' offices. Companies like Hoffmann-La Roche, Squibb, and Winthrop also work hard to convince doctors that it would be short-sighted and boorish of them to throw their business to small firms that do no research and can't afford to hold symposia in Dubrovnik or Bermuda.

Finally, the big companies lose no chance to knock the safety and reliability of products that their detail men contemptuously dismiss as "junk drugs" or "schlock drugs." But although many doctors have been persuaded that trademarked drugs are superior to the same drugs sold under their generic names, as a general proposition this is simply not true. To begin with, one important group of drugs, the antibiotics, are tested by the government for purity and potency, batch by batch, before they are released for sale, and all manufacturers must meet the same standards. Other drugs are regularly spotchecked by the FDA, and it is not clear that most smaller firms are any more likely to turn out an unsafe product than the big ones. In one recent year, for instance, the FDA ordered the recall of nine batches of drugs found to be so contaminated, or of such substandard potency, as to endanger people's health. In every instance the manufacturer was one of the major companies.

The most telling argument against generic drugs, however, is not that they are unsafe, but that they may not produce the same results as the trademarked products on which they are modeled. Even though a generic drug may be chemically identical to its trademarked competitor—it has to be, or it cannot be put on the market—the inert substance with which the drug is compounded may be different, or the size of the particles may be finer or coarser, and it may therefore behave differently in the human body. To use the technical term, it may differ clinically from its model: it may, for instance, be much more slowly absorbed into the patient's bloodstream.

But major hospitals have been stocking their pharmacies with generic drugs for years, and the consensus of experts is that, with very few exceptions, they are in no way inferior to their trademarked competitors. This is the position taken, for example, by Massachusetts' new Drug Formulary Commission, which has compiled a list of drugs that doctors are urged to prescribe by their generic names. The commission is headed by Richard Burack, the author of *The New Handbook of Prescription Drugs,* who recently wrote that the members of the commission had "meticulously considered evidence (and lack thereof) for 'therapeutic nonequivalence,' and concluded without disagreement that it is a rare bird." The commission's view is shared by, among others, Alexander M. Schmidt, the present head of the FDA, and Edward G. Feldmann, who for ten years was director of *The National Formulary,* an authoritative volume, with quasi-legal standing, that lists a large number of drugs of proven efficacy, and sets forth the standards of strength, quality, and purity to which the manufacturers of these drugs must conform. Feldmann, who is also the editor of the *Journal of Pharmaceutical Sciences,* perhaps the world's leading publication in its field, has observed that the problem of nonequivalence "has been grossly overstated by those who would benefit by clouding this issue."

So long as differences exist, a physician may understandably hesitate at times to switch a patient from a trademarked product, on which he has been doing nicely, to a generic product that may conceivably not work as well. Such hesitation can and should be eliminated, however, by requiring all manufacturers to show that their products are clinically as well as chemically equivalent to the trademarked drugs on which they are modeled.

Although it is natural to be angry with the big drug companies, that anger is to a degree misplaced. For without the cooperation of the medical profession, it would not be so easy to sell sick people drugs they don't really need, at prices far higher than they should have to pay. Instead of acting as shrewd and skeptical purchasing agents for their patients, far too many doctors have let themselves be maneuvered into acting, consciously or unconsciously, as sales agents for the drug companies. It is hard to think of a more depressing indictment of American medicine.

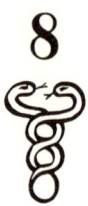

8

The Economics of Extravagance

The extravagance and inefficiency of American hospitals, and the fact that so many of their beds are occupied by people who don't need to be in a hospital at all, are defects that may prove hard to remedy, but that are easy enough to explain. They spring mainly from the peculiar way most hospitals in this country are organized, and from the peculiar workings of the market in which they sell their services. Elsewhere, even in such strongholds of private enterprise as the Netherlands and West Germany, most hospitals are built by the government and run by civil servants. In general, decisions as to how many hospitals a country needs, and where they are to be built, and how elaborately they are to be equipped, and how their doctors are to be paid—all these are political decisions, arrived at by the same pulling and hauling that determines how much money is to be spent on schools or highways or the military establishment.

The United States, too, has its public hospitals. They include military and Veterans' Administration hospitals and state-run hospitals for the mentally ill. They also include municipal and county hospitals that collect what they can from their patients—or, more commonly, from Medicare or Medicaid—but that are generally obligated to treat any patient who comes through their doors even though he may have to be treated cost-free. In addition, at the other end of the economic spectrum, the United States has more than a thousand proprietary hospitals—hospitals that are run as private business ventures like motels or Ford dealerships.*

* Some of these hospitals doubtless provide good care, but many are shameless in their exploitation of their patients, and their patients' insurance compa-

But municipal and county hospitals are patronized mainly by the poor, while proprietary hospitals are too few in number (and, on the average, too small in size) to accommodate more than perhaps 10 per cent of all middle-class and rich Americans requiring a hospital bed on any given day. The great majority of Americans, when they are seriously ill, are treated in voluntary hospitals, which are neither wholly public nor wholly private, but a mixture of the two. To the extent that they are owned by anyone, they are owned by their boards of trustees. Such boards are customarily self-perpetuating, and tend to be made up largely of bankers, lawyers, and businessmen. Responsibility for day-to-day operations is ordinarily delegated to an administrator appointed by the board. Together, trustees and administrator draw up budgets, borrow money for expansion, negotiate with unions, and hire and fire employees.

They also develop strategies for attracting customers—that is, patients—away from competitors. This may seem odd, inasmuch as the notion of competing for business is customarily associated with the notion of profit, and voluntary hospitals are, by definition, nonprofit undertakings, whose annual surpluses, if any, must be plowed back into the business. But this makes less difference than might be supposed. The trustees and the administrator of a voluntary hospital are often just as eager for new business as the directors and executives of IBM or the Hotel Corporation of America, even though they own no stock in the undertaking on which they can collect dividends or realize capital gains. They are motivated, rather, by the knowledge that the more money a hospital takes in, the better position it is in to buy new equipment, raise salaries, redecorate offices, build new wings, sponsor exciting research programs, hire new hands, and generally enjoy the fruits of institutional prosperity.

---

nies. "At a medical staff conference each patient's insurance coverage is studied," the administrator of a proprietary hospital in Southern California told the author of an article that appeared recently in *New Times*. "Then a 'treatment' program is mapped out to reap maximum available revenue. They get 'treated' for everything their insurance covers." The author, Roger Rapoport, added that at one Los Angeles hospital "specialists who just happen to be part-owners of the facility come in recommending expensive lab tests, x-rays and drugs. Next surgeons show up to suggest costly operations. . . ." To keep their beds filled, hospitals like this one may "buy" potentially profitable patients from their physicians. The standard fee, Rapoport reported, is $50 or $100 a head, or 10 per cent of the hospital bill, whichever is larger, for each suitable patient delivered into the hospital's hands.

But while running a voluntary hospital in some ways is like running a hotel, there are also big differences. The most important is that the trustees and their appointed administrator have only limited control over the character, quality, and cost of the main service the hospital is in business to provide—taking care of sick people. It is not they, but the doctors, who decide what patients are to be admitted, how they are to be treated, and when they are to be sent home. Doctors also influence, often decisively, the kind of equipment a hospital invests in, and the range of special services, such as open-heart surgery, it stands ready to provide.

Obviously doctors who work at public hospitals in England or Sweden or the Netherlands also have a lot to say about who is to be treated and how. But in these and most other industrially advanced countries the hospital specialist is a salaried employee who has to go along with policies laid down by his superiors if he wants to hold his job and get promoted. In the United States, by contrast, doctors who treat patients in voluntary hospitals are for the most part independent entrepreneurs who make use of operating rooms, nurses, x-ray equipment, orderlies, and laboratories that are placed at their disposal, free of charge, by the hospitals' trustees. Many American doctors have a choice of two or three hospitals in which they can treat their patients. If Hospital A fails to provide what its doctors want in the way of services and facilities, they may take their business across town to Hospital B, leaving Hospital A with empty beds and shrunken revenues.

Given this possibility, the medical staff of a voluntary hospital may understandably have a lot more to say about how it is run than the administrator who is nominally in charge, and who has often in the past been regarded by doctors and trustees alike as a sort of head clerk and housekeeper. It is true that hospital administration has become a recognized profession, whose practitioners are trained in special graduate schools. And it is true that, as the administrator's job has become more complicated and more important, his stock has risen on the status market. But even so, it may be dangerous for him to oppose plans for a new delivery room (even though fewer and fewer babies are being born in the hospital), or to push too hard for restrictions on incompetent or hyperactive surgeons. It is a near certainty that the doctors whose displeasure he incurs will take their case to the trustees, and it is not unlikely that they will win. The chief movers and shakers on the medical staff of the typical voluntary hospital not only make a lot more money than the administrator, but they usually outrank him socially as well. This puts the administrator at a serious disadvantage, since the trustees are likely to side with a prosperous surgeon who belongs to the right clubs—that is, the same clubs the trustees belong to—than with an administrator who is usually a servant of the local establishment rather than a member. "The establishment within the medical staff, and the establishment within the board of trustees, tend to be very closely associated," the administrator of a hospital in a rich New England town told me. "Decisions are often made on the cocktail party circuit, not in the board room. It's very hard for board members to resist the pressure they get from physicians—and from members of the local establishment who are influenced by physicians." In the circumstances, an administrator may conclude that the best way to get along is to avoid offending anyone. "Your typical administrator," another hospital director has observed, "is not organizationally in a position to do much of anything about anything really important. It is hardly surprising that we have bred a race of creampuffs and pantywaists. Such ineffectiveness is the price of survival."

Another distinguishing feature of the hospital business is that a hospital, unlike a hotel or a restaurant, can normally raise its prices without fear of losing customers. People who have to go into a hospital are rarely in a position to shop around for a good buy. They go where their doctor sends them, and the doctor's choice of hospitals, assuming he has a choice, is usually more influenced by where he thinks his patients will get the best care, and where he can treat them most conveniently, than by considerations of economy. In most instances this is perfectly all right with the patient. Three out of four Americans can now count on their hospital bills being paid, either in large part or in full, by Blue Cross, or by Medicare or Medicaid, and the size of the bill a patient runs up may serve mainly as a reminder of how lucky he is not to have to pay it himself. Most patients who cannot look to Blue Cross or the government for help are covered by commercial insurance policies. Their shock at being charged $170 a day for room and board, or 50 cents a pill for aspirin, is lessened by the comforting knowledge that even though they have to pay the bill, their insurance company will be reimbursing them for most of what they have laid out.

Blue Cross, Medicare, and other third-party payers, as they are known in the hospital business, obviously have a big stake in the cost of hospital care, for which they paid out around $39 billion in 1974. But it is the individual hospitals, not the third parties, who decide how much that cost shall be. The standard arrangement is roughly like this: Suppose that in the course of a year a hospital admits 5000 patients, who stay an average of six days each, thus requiring a total of 30,000 days of care. And suppose that in that year the hospital spends $3 million for food, laundry, nursing, bedpans, X-ray film, and other goods and services. This means that the hospital's per diem cost, which is the average cost of taking care of one patient for one day, will amount to $100. And after certain adjustments this is what the hospital collects from Blue Cross and most of the other third parties with which it deals.

The system described above is nicely adapted to the unnecessary expenditure of large sums of money. Some of this money, as we have seen, is spent on unnecessary surgery. In big teaching hospitals, especially those that are closely affiliated with medical schools, relatively little such surgery is performed. Cutting up patients for pecuniary reasons is frowned on in academic medicine, and university hospitals usually have full-time, salaried chiefs of surgery who share this point of view, and who have a great deal to say about the granting and withholding of operating-room privileges. But the trustees of the typical community hospital, however dim a view they take of needless surgery, and however keenly they may feel it is their duty to prevent it, are in a poor position to do much about it. Bankers and manufacturers are not qualified to interpret a pathologist's report, or to determine, by studying the medical records, whether a particular uterus, or a particular set of tonsils, should have been removed. And any move to hire a surgeon competent to make such judgments for them, and empowered to discipline offending surgeons, would be resisted to the point of rebellion by the medical staff. In the circumstances, the trustees have no choice but to leave disciplinary measures to the doctors who practice at the hospital (and who keep it supplied with patients); and most practicing physicians, as I have indicated, have very little stomach for cracking down on a colleague just because he is too quick with the knife.

Voluntary hospitals also have strong incentives to take in nonsurgical patients who don't really need to be hospitalized, and to keep patients in bed too long. To be sure, low occupancy rates are not as troublesome to hospital administrators as they are to the proprietors of hotels; as occupancy goes down, a hospital simply divides its fixed costs among fewer patients, and the per diem rate at which it collects from Blue Cross and Medicare and Medicaid rises more or less in proportion. But nobody connected with a hospital likes the layoffs and other disagreeable economies that may have to be made when too many beds regularly stand empty. "Like everybody else, we have our utilization review committee," I was told by the administrator of a small community hospital in Connecticut. "But until just recently it pretty much existed on paper. No one took it seriously except when there was a temporary shortage of beds. Then the committee would go on a housecleaning expedition and get rid of people who would be just as well or better off at home."

Overuse of hospitals is also encouraged by the fact that health insurance in America has mainly been hospital insurance. Half the population still have to pay out of their own pockets for x-rays, laboratory tests, or any other medical services they receive apart from those they get while confined to a hospital bed. As a result, doctors often put people into hospitals for diagnostic testing that the patient could just as well undergo at home or at work, but which he would then have to pay for. "Of course, Blue Cross won't knowingly pick up the tab for someone who's been put in the hospital purely for diagnosis," a New York internist told me. "So I fake the records to indicate that he was diagnosed before admission, and that he was admitted to the hospital for *treatment*. I perjure myself this way every week. Then, when the tests are done, I may keep him in the hospital a couple of days longer while I get him started on a restricted diet. That way the chart will indicate that therapy has been accomplished in the hospital." In a recent survey of doctors practicing in the Hartford, Connecticut, area, one out of three admitted that he sometimes admits a patient to a hospital solely because the patient would otherwise have to pay for diagnosis and treatment himself.

Doctors, too, may benefit financially by hospitalizing their patients. Blue Shield plans, which pay for surgery and certain other medical procedures, may allow a much bigger fee for a minor operation if it is performed in a hospital instead of in a doctor's office. In Southern California, for instance, Blue Shield's 1970 fee schedule allowed a physician to collect $75 for removing a simple fistula if his patient was hospitalized, and only $12.50 if he was not. The justification for this disparity is that the minor operation for which a patient needs to be hospitalized is likely to be more complicated than the operation that can be done in the office, and that the doctor is therefore entitled to a bigger fee. But the effect, obviously, is to reward the doctor who, when in doubt, puts his patient in the hospital.

Some hospitals have set up ambulatory surgical facilities, where minor operations like tonsillectomies, or dilations and curettages, or eye-muscle surgery can be done without hospitalizing the patient. This appears to have worked out well for both doctors and patients, but many hospitals are understandably less than enthusiastic about an arrangement which is likely to make it more difficult than ever to keep their beds filled. (The General Accounting Office has estimated that if doctors operated on their patients without putting them into a hospital whenever it was safe to do so the country would need twenty thousand fewer acute-care hospital beds, which is about as many beds as are to be found, all told, in a hundred medium-sized community hospitals.) The growth of ambulatory surgery may also have been held back by the fact that while Blue Cross and commercial insurers are quite ready to pick up the tab for a man who checks into a hospital for a cataract operation, they will not usually pay his hotel bill if he has the operation done on an ambulatory basis and then has to stay around for three or four days to be checked periodically by his surgeon.

The way American hospitals are run, and the way their services are paid for, also encourage inefficiency and the expenditure of huge sums of money on unnecessary services and facilities. One reason for this is that the trustees of a voluntary hospital do not ordinarily have to account to anyone but themselves for the way they spend the money the hospital takes in. Although most of that money comes from Washington, or from state and local agencies, or from Blue Cross plans which are themselves quasi-public institutions, trustees and administrators are permitted to run voluntary hospitals as strictly private organizations—which they once were—whose financial affairs are nobody's business but their own. Facts and figures of a kind that big corporations are required by law to make public as a matter of routine are sometimes kept secret even from members of a hospital's own board of trustees. The price that the community at large pays for this permissiveness has been pointed out by, among others, Gordon Chase, who served for several years as New York City's Administrator of Health Services. "Hospital professionals," Chase told a Senate committee, "sometimes use 'quality of care' . . . as a rallying cry that can obscure inefficiency, obsolescence, and traditional ways of operating which will not stand close scrutiny. Cost increases are simply passed on to the consumer and taxpayer through passive private and public insurance plans, which, by and large, reimburse hospitals for full costs."

To be sure, when a hospital informs Blue Cross that its costs per patient-day are $125, and that it expects to be paid at that rate for its services to subscribers, Blue Cross is entitled to ask how that figure was arrived at. But there is a good reason why this question has usually been asked in the mildest of tones. Most Blue Cross plans were founded, not by consumers, but by the hospitals themselves, who were struck with the notion, during the depression of the 1930s, that if they could arrange for people to set aside some money each month against the day when they would have to go into a hospital, they (the hospitals) would not be stuck with so many unpaid bills. Thus in 1936, when Illinois Blue Cross was incorporated, thirteen of the fourteen incorporators were affiliated with hospitals. And until quite recently, the governing boards of most Blue Cross plans have been dominated by hospital men. In the circumstances, Blue Cross auditors have generally gone about their work in a tolerant state of mind, accepting as fully reimbursable any costs that could be shown to have some relation to taking care of patients. As Sander Kelman, a medical economist, has sardonically observed, open-heart surgical units and the like do not come cheap, "and were it not for the ability of hospital officials to turn their uniforms inside out and—*Shazam!*—become Blue Cross officials, they might never be able to acquire them."

Voluntary hospitals, as I have said, are organized as not-for-profit undertakings. But because their finances are not subject to public scrutiny, and because they can charge pretty much what they please, hospital trustees and administrators are in a good position to line their own pockets at the expense of the hospital's customers. This seems to have been accepted practice, for example, at the Washington, D.C., Hospital Center, the largest voluntary hospital in the Washington area. In a series of well-documented articles, published in the fall of 1972, the *Washington Post* disclosed that for a long time the hospital had been giving away some $50,000 a year by keeping a million dollars or more on deposit in an interest-free bank account at the American Security and Trust Company, one of whose vice presidents also happened to be the treasurer of the Hospital Center. The newspaper also reported that a former controller of the hospital, while on the hospital payroll at $39,000 a year, had formed and assumed the management of a company called Space Age Computer Systems, whose business was providing hospitals with data-processing services. Space Age stockholders included the controller's boss at the hospital (who got his stock for nothing), and the company's first contract, under which it was paid $616,000 in 1971, was awarded to it without competitive bidding—Shazam!—by the Washington Hospital Center. Although the controller's job at the hospital was supposed to be full time, the *Post* quoted former employees of the controller as saying that he "spent the majority of his time on Space Age business, ignoring hospital problems for weeks or altogether because he was too busy flying around the country looking for new Space Age customers." The newspaper suggested this might explain why the Hospital Center was doing such a wretched job, in comparison with other large teaching hospitals, in collecting unpaid bills.

The *Post* further pointed out that in 1971 the Hospital Center provided $21,000 worth of free care to trustees of the hospital and to other "friends of the center." Many of these patients, the newspaper reported, had been accommodated in one of "a special suite of 12 rooms that other paying patients of the hospital subsidize by an additional $42,500, or $1.25 on the total average patient bill. The subsidy occurs because the rate of profit of the special suites is lower than that of other wards in the hospital." The *Post* noted that the VIP suites, as they were known, were built in 1967 for $500,000, the money coming from the hospital's operating fund, not from a special gift or bequest. "Each room," the newspaper continued, "is about twice the size of the average hospital accommodation and has fold-out sofa beds for overnight guests, wall-to-wall carpeting, balconies, floor-length picture windows and drapes, color television sets, kitchenettes, and Grecian baths. Food for VIP patients is prepared by a special gourmet chef in a separate kitchen. The menu features filet mignon and lobster tails, and patients can select from a wine list. Meals are served on chinaware with silverware and crystal glasses."

The hospital's administrator, Richard M. Loughery, told the *Post* that the suites had been built to attract wealthy patients who might otherwise go to Boston or New York for hospital care. After a stay in one of the VIP suites, he explained, such a patient might feel inclined to remember the Washington Hospital Center in his will. Loughery conceded, however, that in the five years since the suites had been built they had yielded only $50,000 in gifts to the hospital. The *Post* went on to say, "The free, luxury care contrasts sharply with the treatment given hundreds of poor patients who do not have Blue Cross or other means of paying for their hospital stay, and are turned away from the hospital center's emergency room for that reason."

There is, of course, no way of knowing how many trustees are doing themselves favors at the expense of the hospitals on whose boards they sit, or how many hospitals subsidize wealthy patients in the manner reported by the *Post*. The Washington Hospital Center is clearly not unique. Just recently *The Western Voice of Motorola*, a company newspaper, pointed out that in Phoenix, Arizona, where Motorola employs several thousand persons, one hospital was publicizing its $125-a-day, two-room deluxe suites, where patients were served cocktails, hors d'oeuvres, and breast of chicken Cordon Bleu at damask-covered tables set by former airline stewardesses in gold miniskirts, who also poured the wine and lit the candles. The paper reported that occupancy of these suites averaged less than 20 per cent, which meant that most of the cost of their upkeep was being borne by Motorola employees and other patients occupying ordinary semi-private rooms.

But even if one assumes that this sort of thing is fairly common, it cannot cost the public more than a fraction of the huge sums of money that are consumed by extravagance of a different variety—the building and staffing of new surgical units, new hospital wings, and even whole new hospitals for which there is no real need. Doctors understandably want the hospitals in which they work to be well staffed, and equipped with the latest and best instruments and facilities. And when a hospital's radiation therapist proposes the purchase of a $300,000 linear accelerator, which will enable the hospital to treat cancer patients with very high-energy radiation, it may do little good for the administrator or trustees to point out that a hospital across town already has such an accelerator that is in use only two or three hours a day. The doctor wants a machine for his own use, and he can argue that it won't really cost the hospital anything, since Blue Cross and other third parties will be footing the bill, along with those few patients who still pay for hospitalization out of their own pockets. Doctors can, and do, make the same kind of case for adding new wings, or against closing down old ones that have two or three times as many beds as patients.

As a rule, the doctors have had their way. "The hospital trustees are no match for the hungry demands of the doctors," Herbert S. Denenberg, a former Pennsylvania Commissioner of Insurance, said not long ago. Hospital boards, he added, "spend their time rubber-stamping the requests of doctors for an endless flow of new equipment, new services, and new buildings." Denenberg was recommended for his job by Ralph Nader. During the three years that he held it he was repeatedly accused by members of Pennsylvania's medical and hospital establishment of resorting to demagogic exaggeration. But in this instance (and, for that matter, in most of his criticism of doctors, hospitals, and health-insurance executives) he seems to have been on firm ground. In the late 1960s, for example, an economist, Edward Kaitz, took a close look at how six Massachusetts hospitals were spending their money. According to their own administrators, every one of these hospitals had developed facilities and services purely to satisfy the demands of physicians on its staff. One administrator told Kaitz that his hospital's charges were set at a level high enough to provide $350,000 a year for medical research; he explained that the physicians doing this research also provided the hospital with 90 per cent of its patients, and supporting their work was the price "that the hospital had to pay to maintain its near-capacity utilization." At another hospital visited by Kaitz, the trustees had voted to close down the pediatric and maternity units because three quarters of their beds were normally unoccupied, and plenty of pediatric and maternity beds were available at other hospitals nearby. But members of the medical staff objected violently, insisting that the units were essential to their practices, and the trustees gave in. More than that, they agreed to build a *new* maternity wing. At about this time a competing hospital, most of whose maternity beds also were normally unoccupied, made a similar concession to the gynecologists on its staff. "As a result of these two decisions," Kaitz writes, "sixty new maternity beds were constructed in an area where, based upon the calculations of the administrators, ten to fifteen beds would be sufficient."

In the last few years, growing irritation with the soaring cost of hospital care has brought changes, here and there, in the rules of the game by which hospitals play. More than fifteen states, including New York and California, now forbid the construction of new hospitals, or additions to old ones, unless the people who want to build them can prove they are really necessary. Also, some hospital trustees are developing a salutary resistance to unreasonable demands from doctors. "I've seen evidence of this on our own board," one administrator told me. "I can give you an example. We have three operating rooms, but we only staff two of them. Now our surgeons want the third room regularly staffed, so that all three can be used concurrently, and the surgeons can be sure of finishing up early in the morning. We did a survey, and we found that over a two-year period all surgery, on an average day, had been completed by 10:45 in the morning. Well, to staff a third room would cost at least $50,000 a year, and the operating room nurses, like the ones we have now, would really be working only part of a shift each day. I just don't think the expense would be justified. I'm aware that patients would just as soon get operated on first thing in the morning, but, basically, this would be for the convenience of the surgeons. Eight or nine years ago, the board would have said, 'Sure.' But this time I'm confident it's not going through."

This administrator observed that his board is finding it easier to reject such demands because of a new and tougher line being taken by the Blue Cross plan in his area. "For the first time, the hospitals and Blue Cross are butting heads," he said approvingly. Some Blue Cross plans have been putting more nonhospital people on their boards, insisting that hospitals justify the hospitalization of patients if they want to get paid, and generally behaving a little more like consumer organizations and less like collection agencies for hospitals.

One such plan is Blue Cross of Greater Philadelphia, whose new toughness can be credited mainly to the redoubtable Commissioner Denenberg. In 1971, Philadelphia Blue Cross asked the Pennsylvania Department of Insurance to approve a 50 per cent increase in its charges to the plan's 2,400,000 subscribers. Ordinarily when a Blue Cross plan asks for a rate increase the scenario is something like this: Blue Cross says that it is legally obligated to pay its subscribers' hospital bills, that these bills are going up, and that the plan will go broke unless it can raise its rates. Hospital spokesmen say they are doing everything humanly possible to control costs, and that their higher charges simply reflect better and more sophisticated medical care, and better pay for hospital workers. The Commissioner of Insurance, after due deliberation, issues a statement deploring the high cost of hospital care and simultaneously approves the increase.

Denenberg changed the story line, however. On the second day of a public hearing on Blue Cross's application, he announced there would be no rate increase unless and until Blue Cross cracked down on the hospitals. He thereupon ordered Blue Cross of Greater Philadelphia to negotiate a new contract with hospitals in its area. When a Blue Cross executive said, "You will confirm that direction in writing, I'm sure," Denenberg said, "Right. I'll give it to you right now. . . ." He reached for a pad, wrote "Blue Cross of Greater Philadelphia please move to negotiate in writing, H. S. Denenberg," tore off the top sheet, and had it handed to the official.

The new contract that went into effect a few months later included a number of changes for which Denenberg had been plumping. At the hearing, for example, he had pointed out that seventeen hospitals in the Philadelphia area had open-heart surgical units, although the amount of open-heart surgery actually being performed was sufficient to keep only four of these units even moderately busy. Under the new contract, hospitals are surveyed periodically by an independent Philadelphia planning agency, the Hospital Survey Committee, and Blue Cross will not have to chip in for the upkeep of services and facilities that the committee finds to be unnecessary. Philadelphia hospitals are also under much stronger pressure now to keep Blue Cross subscribers out of hospital beds unless they really need to be there. When a subscriber is admitted to a hospital, the physician who admits him must state how long he will probably have to stay. This forecast is then reviewed by the hospital's utilization committee, which can no longer be exclusively a doctor's show, but must include a nonphysician member of the hospital's board of trustees. If the patient stays longer than was predicted, an explanation must be provided before Blue Cross will pay the bill. The new contract further specifies that if Blue Cross concludes that a patient was improperly admitted to a hospital, or was kept there too long, the hospital itself will have to absorb the loss. In the past, when Blue Cross has balked at paying a bill, hospitals have been entitled to collect—or to try to collect—from the unfortunate patient.

The new contract, primarily because of its provisions for cutting down on unnecessary hospitalization, is already saving Philadelphia Blue Cross subscribers a lot of money. At a time when hospital administration rates in the United States were generally rising, the number of Blue Cross subscribers admitted to Philadelphia hospitals in 1972 was 9 per cent less than in 1970. In addition, subscribers who *were* admitted to hospitals spent 7 per cent less time there than they had two years earlier. As a result—or mainly as a result—the amount of money Blue Cross had to lay out on behalf of its Philadelphia subscribers, which had risen by a total of 67 per cent in 1969-71, rose by only 2.5 per cent in 1972. Denenberg, modestly describing what had happened as "the most successful hospital reform drive on record," calculated that the new hospital contracts, with a little help from the Economic Stabilization Program, had saved the plan's members $46 million in 1972.

Some hospital administrators have complained, justifiably, that in recent years they have been denied funds that they must have if they are to provide the services that the public rightly demands from them. The chief complainers are big-city teaching institutions, such as St. Luke's Hospital on Manhattan's west side, whose emergency rooms and outpatient clinics are jammed with patients who are too young for Medicare, too rich for Medicaid, and too poor to pay the full cost of the services they get. Such patients, the working poor, accounted for half of the nearly 300,000 visits to St. Luke's clinics and emergency room in 1972, and St. Luke's was able to collect from them only an average of $6 per visit for services that cost, by the hospital's reckoning, around $30 to provide. "We used to load this community service onto our inpatient costs when we worked out our reimbursable per diem with Blue Cross," I was told by St. Luke's vice president for finance, Edward A. Messier. "But under the new law that went into effect here in New York State in 1970, we can't do this any more." Mainly as a result of this change, he explained, St. Luke's quickly ran through a $6 million reserve fund, and, in 1973, anticipated a deficit of more than $3 million, most of it attributable to the emergency room and clinics. "We can't walk away from this situation," Messier said. "If we were to close down our clinics, or even materially shrink the services we are providing, I'm afraid the community would hit out at the handiest and most visible target, which is the hospital." He paused, and added, "Anyway, it's out of the question. If we cut down, where in hell would these people go? There's not a single municipal hospital on the west side of Manhattan."

But while cost-cutting has hurt some hospitals and some patients—mostly poor patients—the waste and extravagance that make Denenberg so angry are still largely unchecked. If Blue Cross refuses to help foot the bill for a third operating room, on the ground that it is not really needed, the trustees may go ahead with the project anyway, knowing that they can recover its cost by raising the hospital's charges to non-Blue Cross patients. Moreover, fewer than one third of the states have passed laws to keep hospital construction within reasonable bounds, and even where such laws have been passed they don't necessarily work. The bankers and businessmen who dominate the boards of most voluntary hospitals are often delighted with the notion of putting up huge, expensive new buildings, and their enthusiasm can be hard to curb. In California, planning agencies have repeatedly given in to pressure from hospital promoters. Overriding their own review committees, they have approved the putting up of new hospitals for which no real need has been shown. As a result, the *Los Angeles Times* reported in 1972, plans were under way to add 3831 more hospital beds in Los Angeles County by 1976, and 3143 more in neighboring

Orange County, even though more than 30 per cent of the existing beds in the two counties were normally unoccupied. "It seems clear to us," the *Times* commented, "that the Comprehensive Health Planning Agency system and the law as it now stands are not capable of coping with the problem."

The cost of maintaining empty hospital beds is very high. The *Washington Post*, in the same series of articles in which the Washington Hospital Center got its lumps, reported that average occupancy at Children's Hospital in Washington was only 62 per cent. The *Post* calculated that the hospital's per diem costs were 37 per cent higher than they would be if occupancy averaged 85 per cent. "This means," the newspaper said, "that each patient pays an average of about $45 extra for each day of hospitalization to cover the costs of the empty beds. During a year this extra payment comes to $2.3 million for all Children's Hospital patients." The *Post* added that even though the hospital's director, Dr. Robert H. Parrot, admitted there were already too many pediatric beds in the Washington area, Children's Hospital would soon be moving into a new $50-million building where it would have 15 per cent more beds than at its old location. In Philadelphia, the local Blue Cross plan has estimated that the area it serves could get along very well with 10 to 15 per cent fewer beds, and that their elimination would cut the community's hospital bill by thirty to forty million dollars a year.

A lot of money is still being wasted, too, on hospital services that could well be eliminated or combined with similar services at nearby hospitals. A particularly striking—and depressing—example of such duplication was reported not long ago by *Medical Economics*, in an article describing the pointless competition going on among three hospitals in Oakland, California. In this instance the villains were not doctors, but administrators and trustees. In 1972, the three hospitals, which are located within a block of one another in an area sometimes referred to as Pill Hill, were all operating so far below capacity that they could easily have accommodated one third again as many patients as they were actually caring for. In the circumstances, a group of doctors with staff privileges at one or more of the hospitals had urged that certain services should be consolidated. But this notion had been strenuously resisted by the hospital administrators, who continued to maintain "three laboratories, three x-ray departments, three nuclear medicine departments, two 24-hour emergency departments, two radiation therapy departments, and two OB [obstetrical] departments. And two similar and expensive laminar-flow operating rooms for hip surgery were recently installed." "The hospitals are pecking each other to death for the same patients," one doctor said bitterly.

Medical Economics reported that the Oakland physicians had been particularly galled by the recent establishment of the two emergency rooms. Doctors on the staffs of all three hospitals, convinced that there was a real need for a 24-hour emergency service on the Hill, had first suggested that it be provided by Samuel Merritt, the largest of the three hospitals. When Merritt rejected the idea, the doctors turned to Providence Hospital, which agreed to put it into effect. Possibly because of the patients attracted by its new service, Providence was soon reporting a slight rise in what is known in the hospital business as the daily bed census. Charles C. Jenkins, a trauma surgeon who had been a chief backer of the new emergency service, described what happened: "Merritt, watching this for a few months, couldn't stand it. It opened a competing emergency department right across the street even though a hundred of us physicians had voted that we didn't want competing emergency departments." Jenkins added, "So we end up with two second-class, competing, under-utilized facilities. We should have one that's top-notch."

The Business of Insurance

Leonard Woodcock, president of the United Auto Workers Union, recently complained that the American insurance industry "has failed to guide or improve the delivery of health care or to provide the financial protection that legitimately has been expected of it. There is nothing in its history or structure that suggests that private insurance can or will do appreciably better in the future. . . ." Not everyone agrees with Woodcock that what we need is a universal, compulsory health insurance system, run by the government, in which neither the insurance companies, nor Blue Cross and Blue Shield plans, would have any real part. The AMA sees things quite differently. Its view, and the view of the insurance industry itself, is that the system needs changing, but that there's nothing much wrong that can't be remedied by suitable injections of federal money. Specifically, the AMA would like the government to make it easy for people to get catastrophic insurance—insurance that would take care of all their medical bills above, say, fifteen hundred or two thousand dollars. It would also like the government to subsidize the purchase of private insurance by people too poor to pay for it themselves. But while such changes would be better than nothing, it seems clear that health insurance, as it has developed in the United States, suffers from congenital weaknesses so serious as to call for more heroic remedies.

Private health insurance in America dates back at least a century. In the years after the Civil War, mining, lumbering, and railroad-construction companies began hiring doctors to take care of their workers, and recouping the cost of the doctors' services by periodically deducting a small sum from each worker's pay envelope. But even though the flourishing Kaiser-Permanente Medical Plan evolved from arrangements of this kind, the sort of health insurance with which most Americans are familiar goes back only to 1929, when Baylor University Hospital in Dallas, Texas, undertook to furnish hospital care to a group of Dallas schoolteachers. For a yearly payment of $6 per teacher, the hospital agreed to provide up to three weeks in a semiprivate room, with no extra charge for laboratory tests, routine medication, or the use of an operating room. Soon afterward, as the country slid into the Great Depression, Baylor began signing up other groups on similar terms, hoping in this way to keep the hospital solvent at a time when many of its benefactors had lost their shirts in the market, and when few patients could pay their hospital bills.

As times got worse, forcing hundreds of hospitals all over the country to close their doors, many of the survivors followed Baylor's lead. Groups of hospitals formed nonprofit corporations that offered prepaid hospital care on a citywide basis, so that a subscriber could go to any hospital in town without having to worry about his bill. Enrollment in such plans, which chose the Blue Cross as their common symbol, grew rapidly after Pearl Harbor, when labor unions, prevented by wartime regulations from negotiating big wage increases, had to settle for fringe benefits instead. Chief among these benefits was health insurance, and by 1945 some nineteen million people had Blue Cross coverage. Ten million more were covered by life insurance companies like Metropolitan, Aetna, and Prudential which, having seen Blue Cross's success, had jumped enthusiastically into the hospital insurance business themselves. Unlike the Blue Cross plans, however, they did not undertake to pay hospitals directly, at cost, for such care as they might be called on to give a policyholder. Instead they contracted to pay the policyholder either a specified sum for each day in the hospital, or a specified percentage of whatever the hospital might charge him.

At first, Blue Cross and its commercial competitors stuck to paying hospital bills. This was largely to avoid stirring up the doctors, most of whom took the position that covering doctors' bills as well would destroy the close and—as the AMA has often reverently described it—sacred relationship between doctor and patient. In the view of the profession, a key element in that relationship was the doctor's freedom to charge his patients whatever he liked. And doctors were afraid, with reason, that once a third party began collecting money from patients, and paying it out to their doctors, that freedom would be undermined. Inevitably, the third party would try to put some limit on doctors' fees. From the doctors' point of view, this would be equally undesirable whether motivated by an ignoble desire to realize a middleman's profit, or by misguided zeal for protecting the patient's pocketbook.

But by the late 1930s there were ominous signs that, sacred relationship notwithstanding, Americans were bent on finding some way to avoid being stuck with doctors' bills they could not afford to pay. Many people were coming around to the idea that government insurance was the answer, and in 1938 California elected a new governor, Culbert L. Olson, who had promised to work for the enactment of a state-run health insurance plan. The California Medical Association thereupon changed its mind about medical-fee insurance, deciding that it might not be so bad after all, provided it was voluntary, and provided doctors ran the show. The result was the first of the Blue Shield plans. A nonprofit corporation was organized, with directors chosen by (and mainly from among) the California Medical Association's own leadership, and in 1939 it began enrolling subscribers to whom it undertook to provide, for a fixed monthly payment, a wide variety of doctors' services, both in and out of hospitals. The plan's directors soon discovered, however, that they had greatly underestimated the amount of out-of-hospital care that people would demand—and that doctors would order for them—if neither party to the transaction had to be concerned about the bill's being paid. They therefore decided to limit coverage to doctors' services for which the demand was somewhat less elastic—to surgery, and to nonsurgical care given by doctors to patients confined to a hospital. As other Blue Shield plans sprang up in the 1940s they generally followed California's lead.

Since World War II, health insurance has grown into a $20-billion-a-year industry. According to government estimates, 146 million Americans have health insurance of some kind, not counting those with Medicare coverage. About half this total are enrolled in Blue Cross or Blue Shield plans (or in both), and the other half have commercial policies. But, as pointed out, there may be as many as 41 million Americans under the age of 65 (and therefore too young for Medicare) who have no health insurance at all, and three or four times that number whose coverage would strike people living in most other rich industrial countries as a travesty of what health insurance should be.

One reason so many Americans are so inadequately protected against the costs of illness, or are not protected at all, is that those who have the least money to spend for health insurance ordinarily have to pay the most to get it. Most Americans are insured through their employers, who foot all or most of the bill. But a great many farmhands, casual laborers, domestics, and other low-paid workers can get insurance only by paying the full cost themselves. Moreover, it costs insurance companies a lot of money to sell and service a policy that covers only one person or one family. Ordinarily the buyer has to pay half again as much for a given package of benefits as they would cost an employer buying group insurance at what amounts to a wholesale rate. In the circumstances, individual coverage can be prohibitively expensive. Metropolitan Life, for example, sells an individual policy that offers fairly good protection, as such policies go. It does not cover ordinary visits to the doctor, but after certain deductibles, and up to a maximum of $25,000, it does pay $80 a day for hospital room and board, up to $1400 for surgical expenses, and 80 per cent of a variety of other in-hospital expenses. To buy this protection a husband and wife in their early forties, with two young children, would have to pay $838 a year. A family in which the husband earns $9000 a year would thus have to lay out roughly one ninth of his take-home pay of $146.32 a week for an insurance policy that would by no means cover all of the bills the family would run up in the event of a serious illness. Pondering these discouraging facts, a couple in this income bracket might well conclude that they couldn't possibly afford to take Metropolitan up on its offer.

The poor and the near-poor are at a further disadvantage because of the method now commonly used for calculating premium rates. For a long time Blue Cross used a method called community rating. That is, it charged everybody the same amount for the same coverage. This meant that the old and the poor, who tend to be in worse health than other people, were in effect being subsidized by younger and more prosperous subscribers.

But in the 1940s, when private, profit-making insurance companies began to compete aggressively with Blue Cross, they offered to calculate premiums by a different method, called experience rating. Premiums were to be based on the actual, or anticipated, use of hospitals by the members of the particular group of people to be insured. A company whose employees were young and well-paid was thus given a chance to buy insurance at a bargain rate. The managers of such companies were understandably delighted. And even though the national leaders of many unions complained that experience rating was unfair to the very people who needed health insurance most, local union negotiators, under pressure from their constituents to get the best possible deal on insurance, often went along with the employers when experience rating meant lower premiums. They did so even when the employer was committed to paying the entire bill, knowing that any money he might save on health insurance would be available, at least in theory, for other fringe benefits, or to be paid out in higher wages.

Blue Cross thus faced the disagreeable likelihood that its commercial rivals would sign up all the advertising agencies, airlines, and other employers of the young and healthy. And so, in the late 1950s, more and more Blue Cross plans began negotiating group contracts calling for monthly rates based on experience. One result has been to raise the cost of insurance to companies whose employees do work that is dangerous or unhealthy, or whose work force is elderly or consists mainly of poorly-paid service workers. This, in turn, has discouraged the owners of many small and insecure enterprises from offering health insurance to the people who work for them. Experience rating has also made many companies that do offer insurance reluctant to hire older people, or people who may be in less than perfect health. Such people, if hired, are likely to get sick, and thereby bring about a rise in the company's insurance premiums.

Many Americans who are not eligible for group insurance, and who can't afford the steep cost of a good individually-written policy, settle for cut-rate substitutes providing small cash payments—$20 to $30 a day is a common sum—for each day in the hospital. As I have said, this is, at best, a very expensive way to buy insurance. In recent years, advertising, sales commissions, the cost of handling claims, and profits have eaten up nearly 45 cents of every dollar paid in by the policyholders. Executives of companies that sell cut-rate hospital insurance, while admitting that the coverage they offer is scanty, argue that the people they sell to would otherwise have no coverage at all, and that they are therefore performing a worthy public service. Actually, people who buy such insurance often discover when sickness strikes that they would have been better off putting their money in a savings bank. National Liberty Corporation, which does a huge mail-order business in cut-rate policies, told a Senate committee in 1972 that in the previous two years it had felt obliged to turn down 30,000 of the 78,000 claims filed by owners of the company's most popular policy. Most were rejected on the ground that the policyholder's illness sprang from a "pre-existing condition" and was therefore not covered. Another leading mail-order house, Union Fidelity Life, has sold a policy that does not stop at ruling out pre-existing conditions; it specifies that, for the first six months the policy is in force, no payments will be made for tuberculosis, gall bladder disorders, diabetes, cancer, heart or circulatory diseases, hernia, sickness resulting in surgery, or diseases of the generative organs. About the only way a policyholder could collect would be to have an automobile accident bad enough to put him in the hospital, but not bad enough to require surgery.

The advertising that lures people to buy mail-order policies has often been deceptive. Copy may appear under a headline reading "$1000 A MONTH TAX-FREE CASH WHEN YOU GO TO THE HOSPITAL," but fail to state that the cash doesn't begin to flow until the policyholder has been in the hospital for five days. Union Fidelity Life advertisements have featured a claim that the company will pay "up to $50,000.00" in the event of a serious illness. While the claim is literally true, a Union Fidelity executive conceded at a hearing before Herbert Denenberg, when Denenberg was in charge of Pennsylvania's Department of Insurance, that the largest pay-out he knew of was $10,000. He also conceded that a patient would have to be in the hospital five years to collect the full $50,000. At another point in the same hearing Denenberg tongue-lashed Robert E. Slater, chairman of National Liberty, for making extensive use of an endorsement by Art Linkletter ("Dear friend, you know me. I wouldn't recommend anything I didn't honestly believe in. . . .") without disclosing that Linkletter, besides being a stockholder and director of the company, was being paid $50,000 to promote its products. "Maybe this Madison Avenue hogwash is acceptable in selling other products," Denenberg said angrily, "but we think insurance is too important a product for any sales techniques that don't meet the highest standards of honesty and fair disclosure." Denenberg did not point out, as he might have, that anyone who tried to sell stock by the methods routinely used in selling mail-order health insurance could end up behind bars.

Middle-class Americans, too, have in some respects been badly served by private health insurance. Even the best insurance schemes tend to have big gaps in their coverage. These gaps reflect the unwillingness of insurance men to underwrite risks that are not actuarially predictable. Thus on the theory that nobody can forecast how often a policyholder will go to the doctor if he knows that his insurance will pay the bill, the insurance industry—Blue Cross and Blue Shield as well as the commercial carriers—have been very reluctant to pay for routine out-of-hospital care. This can discourage people who are hard-pressed for money from seeking a doctor's advice as promptly as they should, and from taking their children to the pediatrician or eye doctor for routine checkups. Similarly, because no insurance executive in his right mind wants to assume unlimited liability for anything, insurers have put limits on the number of days of hospital care they will pay for, and on the number of dollars they will pay out on a policyholder's behalf. Admittedly, not many employers would be eager to take out a group policy that would pay all of a family's medical bills even if they ran up into the hundreds of thousands of dollars. Under the experience-rating system, an employer buying such a policy would be sharing with the insurance company unlimited liability for the medical expenses of his workers, and a run of bad luck could cost him millions. But this is simply another way of saying that under existing insurance schemes people cannot hope to get the protection against financially ruinous medical bills that most Americans now clearly want and are willing to pay for.

The insurance industry has also helped to drive up the cost of medical care in America. Partly because of Blue Cross's close ties to hospitals, and partly because of a conviction that there is no good way of determining whether the care received by a patient in the privacy of his doctor's office is necessary or not, health insurance has largely been hospital insurance. Two out of every three Americans have no coverage for any doctor's care they may require outside a hospital. Similarly, two out of three Americans have no coverage for care in a nursing home. As we have seen, this has encouraged unnecessary, and unnecessarily long, hospital stays. At the same time, the hospitals' natural propensity for extravagance has been fortified not only by the permissiveness of Blue Cross's auditors, but by the attitude of the private insurance companies, which have generally reacted to soaring hospital charges as though they were acts of God, to which the only appropriate response is another hike in premium rates.

Insurance plans have, in addition, encouraged doctors to boost their fees. A surgeon who is aware that the insurance company is prepared to pay $500 for a particular operation may elect to charge the patient $750, justifying his decision on the ground that, at an out-of-pocket cost of only $250, the patient is still getting a bargain. Many Blue Shield plans, to be sure, now undertake to protect their subscribers from this sort of economic thinking. These plans agree to pay a participating doctor whatever he chooses to charge, provided his fee is "usual, customary, and reasonable"; the doctor, in return, must agree not to charge subscribers anything over and above what Blue Shield will allow. But since Blue Shield plans commonly interpret "customary" to mean something like "not to exceed what the highest-priced doctors in the community charge," this arrangement tends inexorably to raise the general level of charges. A new doctor in town, even if he is fresh from his residency, has every reason, for example, to set his fees at a high level. Moreover, Blue Shield plans ordinarily permit a subscriber who goes to a non-Blue Shield surgeon for an operation to collect at least a large part of what the operation costs him. This means that a surgeon who feels the Blue Shield claims processors are leaning on him too hard in the matter of his fees can simply cut his ties with Blue Shield, and begin charging Blue Shield subscribers whatever he likes, without having to worry too much about losing Blue Shield business.

A few commercial insurance companies have also tried to enforce a usual-customary-and-reasonable rule, but with even less success than Blue Shield. In 1971 Aetna Life and Casualty, the leading commercial marketer of health insurance policies, decided to try taking a tougher line with doctors submitting exorbitant bills. Each policyholder receiving such a bill was informed that Aetna intended to pay only a reasonable portion of the total charge, and that if the doctor should sue the policyholder for the unpaid portion, Aetna would be happy to pay the legal costs of defending against such a suit. This sensible move outraged many doctors, however, and at the AMA's 1972 convention Aetna was angrily denounced for its effrontery and quickly backed down. The company agreed that if it got a bill that seemed on the high side it would first discuss the matter privately with the doctor. If the matter could not be settled in this way, Aetna further promised to eliminate all references to litigation from any correspondence it might have with the patient; and to leave it up to a local peer-review committee, made up exclusively of doctors, to decide if the disputed fee did or did not exceed the usual-customary-and-reasonable standard. Aetna also agreed that it would not step in to help a policyholder who had been stuck with an exorbitant bill if the patient had been told in advance what the doctor was planning to charge him. Final score: Doctors, 49; policyholders, 0.

Neither Blue Shield nor the commercial carriers have done much to discourage unnecessary surgery. "One thing we often feel uncomfortable about is, 'Was the surgery necessary at all?' " I was told by an executive of a leading insurance company. "But we are in no position to say, 'Doctor, you shouldn't have performed that hysterectomy." He sighed and added, "It's a very fuzzy and difficult area. We can act only when it is very, very clear-cut. I can look at a claim and be confident that the operation was unnecessary. But if we refuse to pay, we—or the patient—are going to be sued, and where are we going to find doctors to testify on our side?"

One of the most troublesome problems that Congress must solve before it can pass a national health insurance bill is what to do about the private health insurance industry. Most of the bills that Congress has been considering would either leave the industry pretty much intact (while fattening it with federal subsidies), or would have Blue Cross, Blue Shield, and the commercial carriers act, in effect, as fiscal and administrative agents of the government.

One way to get a line on how the industry might perform in this last role is to consider how well it has carried out the task, assigned to it by Congress in 1965, of processing claims from doctors and hospitals seeking payment under the Medicare and Medicaid programs. The record is not inspiring. On a number of occasions Blue Cross officials and their friends have been caught eating rather high on the hog at government expense. Government auditors found, for instance, that Virginia Blue Cross had billed Medicare for part of the cost of treating its clients (administrators of company-union welfare funds, for example) to "cocktails, beer, wine, alcoholic beverages, tickets for stage plays and football games, and golf fees." Part of the cost of a company picnic was also charged to Medicare, including the cost of 1050 buffet dinners, two bartenders, bingo prizes, and the rental of six ponies. The auditors took a particularly dim view of all the drinking for which the government had been billed, carefully explaining that "since alcoholic beverages are not considered stimulants of production and do not help to disseminate technical information, they cannot be allowable costs to the Medicare program." Virginia is not the only state where this sort of thing has occurred. One year, Louisiana Blue Cross billed Medicare for the cost of chartering a fishing boat for its board of directors, and Utah Blue Shield tried to collect from the government part of the $4000 its president had paid to join a country club.

There has also been a lot of bungling and inefficiency in the processing of Medicare and Medicaid claims. In 1970 the Senate Finance Committee dug into the records of the thirty-three Blue Shield plans, and the fifteen insurance companies, that were then in the business of handling payments to doctors under the Medicare program. Their performance, the committee staff reported, had "in the majority of instances been erratic, inefficient, costly, and inconsistent with Congressional intent." Again and again, both before and after the Finance Committee's study, government auditors have turned up evidence of doctors being paid twice for a single operation or office visit, or of being paid for services they may not have performed at all. Such revelations have not helped the industry's standing on Capitol Hill. Not long ago, for instance, a senior executive of Prudential Life, who had been giving the Senate Finance Committee the insurance industry's views on national health insurance, was roundly scolded by Senator Abraham Ribicoff of Connecticut. Referring to the industry's handling of Medicare claims, Ribicoff said angrily, "We thought we were going to get all the effectiveness and supervision of private industry, and it came as a shock to all of us when we found you were just as ineffective and inefficient and costly as any bureaucrat would probably be." He added, "We thought you would be looking out for Uncle Sam the way you were looking out for your own stockholders [but] in fact we found a general sense of indifference and very sloppy management."

The underlying weakness of health insurance in America is that it is better adapted to the needs of those who provide medical care than to the needs of those who receive it, and those who ultimately pay for it. Thus Herbert Denenberg, pointing out that eighteen of the twenty-seven seats on the board of directors of Blue Shield of Pennsylvania were occupied by doctors, recently asked, "How can Blue Shield protect the public from over-charging, fee-gouging, unnecessary surgery, and low-quality medical care when it is run by and for the doctors?" Insurance companies, of course, are not run by doctors, and one might expect to find them competing for the privilege of selling people what so many of them want—broad coverage at the lowest possible cost. But to do this, the companies would have to challenge the traditional assumption that what doctors do for their patients, and what they charge for doing it, is strictly their own business. And, as Aetna's rout by the AMA suggests, the insurance companies are of no mind to stand up to the doctors on this issue.

It is true that some companies have recently been helping to finance, plan, and sign up subscribers for prepaid group practices, which many doctors hate and fear. But this is mainly a hedge by executives who would much rather not get involved in the reorganization of arrangements for health care. They are more comfortable doing what they know how to do best, which is trying to get as much business as they can under the rules of the insurance game as it is now played. And as Walter J. Mc-

Nerney, President of the Blue Cross Association, observed some years ago, success in this game "too often depends on sharp underwriting and movement in and out of accounts or among individuals in quest of low loss ratios." He went on to say, "We need fewer carriers, better regulated and more actively participating in controls."

McNerney has an ax of his own to grind. It is fair to assume that he would like to see Blue Cross (perhaps in collaboration with Blue Shield) given exclusive responsibility for administering national health insurance. There is something to be said for this. The fact that some Blue Cross plans have used government (and their subscribers') money to rent ponies and buy country-club memberships is more significant as an indication of Blue Cross's freedom from accountability—until Medicare came along, Blue Cross plans, like voluntary hospitals, were under no compulsion to open their books to any regulatory body—than as an indication of widespread laxity and inefficiency. On the whole, Blue Cross has been efficiently run. Its administrative and marketing expenses, including the cost of servicing eight million subscribers who are not covered by group contracts, absorb only about 6 per cent of gross income, the other 94 per cent being paid out in benefits. This is somewhat better than the commercial insurers have done. "We were very critical of Blue Cross. . . ," Denenberg has said, "but we recognized that everything is relative and, as bad as they have been, compared with the commercial insurance companies they come on looking like angels." Certainly Blue Cross plans have shown more interest than their competitors in devising ways to lower the cost and raise the quality of medical care. And while they have taken their time about putting such methods into practice, the ties that have bound Blue Cross to the hospital industry are finally loosening. As McNerney is at pains to point out, consumer representatives, defined as people with no hospital connections, are now in a majority on the boards of most Blue Cross plans.

But except in a few places, such as Philadelphia, where seven members of the local Blue Cross board are now appointed by the governor of Pennsylvania or by other public officials, these consumer members do not truly represent anybody, being neither chosen by the public nor accountable to it. Only a minority of the country's Blue Cross plans have so far gone to the mat with the hospitals. As of 1973, only about one third of the plans required hospitals to have active utilization-review committees, and only one third required, as a condition for Blue Cross reimbursement, any proof of the need for new hospital services or facilities. Some Blue Cross executives still see their jobs mainly as running a collection agency for hospitals. Asked what he was doing to curb wasteful practices in hospitals, the president of one plan told a Senate committee in 1971, "I am not aware of our auditors ever uncovering wasteful charges, and I really wouldn't know what we would do if we ran into them."

Although such attitudes are no doubt less common now than they were in 1971, Blue Cross plainly is still a long way from being an effective purchasing agent for its subscribers. Where Blue Cross plans have stood up to hospitals, as in Philadelphia and New York, they have usually been under very strong pressure from state regulatory bodies. The lesson would seem to be that if we want to make use of Blue Cross's experience and technical expertise in the administration of a national health insurance system, we must see to it that Blue Cross plans are transformed into quasi-public organizations, accountable to the public in much the same way that the Social Security Administration, let us say, is accountable to Congress.

10

The Case for Health Maintenance Organizations

For the past twenty-five years or so a small but growing minority of Americans, now numbering some seven million in all, have been buying medical care outside the regular channels of trade. As subscribers to prepaid group practice plans they have, in effect, contracted with groups of doctors to furnish them with whatever medical care they need, both in and out of a hospital, for a fixed yearly payment. For their part, the doctors who provide this care do so on what amounts to a flat retainer. Instead of being paid like pieceworkers, they either work for a straight salary, or else divide among themselves, by a prearranged formula, the money the group is paid collectively for its services.

Arrangements of this kind have been made under a variety of auspices. Some plans are cooperative ventures, organized by groups of people who have chipped in to build a clinic and to hire doctors to staff it. Others have been organized by labor unions to care for their own members. The two largest plans—Kaiser-Permanente, with more than 2,700,000 members, and Health Insurance Plan of Greater New York (known as HIP), with 750,000—are both, like Blue Cross, run by not-for-profit corporations. These corporations act as middlemen, enrolling subscribers, collecting money from them and their employers, and contracting with groups of doctors to take care of the subscribers at a rate of so-and-so many dollars a head.

While a number of these plans have been in existence since the 1940s, and a few are even older, prepaid group practice has not, until quite recently, caught on very fast. The main exception is the Kaiser plan, whose membership has more than tripled since 1960. But as medical bills have soared, and as evidence has piled up that plans like Kaiser can provide good care for less money, group practice has looked better and better, not only to labor unions, but also to such spokesmen for big business as the Committee for Economic Development and *Fortune*. New plans have been started up by a number of medical schools, including Harvard, Yale, and Johns Hopkins. Insurance companies, uneasily aware that Kaiser has grown to its present size without their help, and eager to get a piece of the action if prepaid group practice should really take hold, have put up millions of dollars to get plans started in New York, Phoenix, the new town of Columbia, Maryland, and a number of other cities. Blue Cross has been busy too; by the end of 1974 it had helped to establish, and was recruiting subscribers for, fifty-four new prepaid plans, and was involved in the setting up of some seventy-five more.

The boom in prepaid practice has been fed by the prospect of generous federal subsidies. In 1970, the Nixon Administration, looking for a way to decelerate the rise in medical costs without getting the government too deeply into the medical-care business, discovered the virtues of plans like Kaiser, and invented a new name for them: Health Maintenance Organizations, or HMOs. (The term also applies to a somewhat different sort of plan, called a medical care foundation, that I shall come to presently.) For a time there was talk of the government's putting up enough money to help start 1700 new HMOs by 1976, enough to take care of forty million people. This scheme was energetically opposed by the AMA, whose leaders look on prepaid group practice as a heresy that may have to be tolerated, but that should certainly not be encouraged. As a result, the Administration's ardor soon cooled. Nevertheless, during the early 1970s Washington did make some money available, mainly in the form of planning grants, to groups intending to set up HMOs. And in late 1973 President Nixon signed a bill authorizing the government to make more such grants and, in addition, to make (or guarantee) loans to cover the losses that a new group practice plan ordinarily must sustain while it is getting under way and building up its membership. The bill further specified that if an employer had more than twenty-five employees, and if he offered them group health insurance, he must also offer them the option of membership in an HMO on the same terms, provided there is an HMO in their community that meets specified standards. This, of course, makes it much easier for sponsors of HMOs to sign up members.

The benefits of prepaid practice may be suggested by the experience of a hypothetical family I shall call the Thomases. George Thomas works as an assistant supervisor in the warehouse of a steel fabricating company in Seattle. Nine years ago he was given a choice of continuing his Blue Cross-Blue Shield coverage, or of enrolling in Group Health Cooperative of Puget Sound, which was highly recommended by his union. Mr. Thomas chose Group Health Cooperative. Group Health has two classes of enrollees, one of which is made up of people who pay their monthly dues out of their own pockets, and who are entitled to vote for the trustees who manage the plan. The other class, to which Mr. Thomas belongs, consists of employees of companies, or members of unions, that have contracted with Group Health for medical care. Mr. Thomas has a wife and three children, and Group Health collects $53.35 a month for their care. Of this sum, Mr. Thomas's employer pays $44 (an amount equal to the cost of conventional Blue Cross-Blue Shield coverage) and Mr. Thomas pays $9.35.

For this extra $9.35 the Thomases get, among other things, completely free medical care whenever they need it. When they want to see a doctor they go to the cooperative's Northgate medical center, about two miles from where they live. One of seven such centers, Northgate is a cheerful, modern building that contains x-ray facilities, a diagnostic laboratory, a pharmacy, and offices for eleven family doctors, five pediatricians, two optometrists, and a specialist in internal medicine. Group Health urges new enrollees to bring their children in for a checkup, and soon after the Thomases joined the plan Mrs. Thomas made an appointment with one of the Northgate pediatricians. As it turned out, she didn't particularly like him—he seemed too young to know what he was doing—and, after asking around, she switched to an older doctor, a woman, whom she liked very much. Since then the Thomas children have been seen regularly by this same pediatrician, or by the pediatric nurse who works with her, except on those occasions when one of the children had a bad earache or stomachache and the doctor was not at the center on the day Mrs. Thomas brought the child in.

At the time the Thomases joined Group Health they had only one child. When Mrs. Thomas became pregnant for a second time she arranged to be taken care of by the obstetrician who had delivered her first baby, even though this meant laying out nearly $800 for the obstetrician's fee and for a room in the hospital where he practiced. But over the next three years the Thomases both had occasion to visit one of the family doctors at Northgate, a general practitioner whom I shall call Dr. Moore. Like many of the family doctors who work for Group Health, he likes delivering babies. When Mrs. Thomas became pregnant again she decided to go to Dr. Moore instead of her former obstetrician, and the Thomases' third child was delivered by him in Group Health's 301-bed hospital in downtown Seattle.

Group Health requires its enrollees to put up part of the cost of maternity care, but the $250 the Thomases had to pay on this occasion is the only big out-of-pocket medical expense they have had since joining. Four years ago, Mrs. Thomas had a persistent back pain, and Dr. Moore, suspecting that it was of pelvic origin, sent her to one of Group Health's specialists in gynecology. Although she made several visits to the gynecologist's office at Group Health's downtown medical center, adjoining the plan's hospital, there was no charge either for his services or for the medication he prescribed. (The only prescription drugs that members have to pay for are tranquilizers.) The Thomases also have their eyes checked periodically at Northgate, and this, too, is free. Apart from psychiatric treatment, for which there is a charge of $5.75 a session after the first ten visits, there are no deductibles or co-payments. Not long ago the Thomases' oldest child, Cynthia, was badly burned when a small gasoline cooking stove exploded. She was in the hospital for five weeks, and had to go back twice for skin grafts. Between her stays in the hospital she was seen regularly at home by a visiting nurse. The total out-of-pocket cost to the Thomases was $77.50 for the rental of a television set.

People like the Thomases are clearly getting a bargain. In 1973, the cost of medical care provided by Group Health Cooperative of Puget Sound averaged out to $191 for each person enrolled. This was 38 per cent less than the $311 that was spent for a comparable package of medical services by, or on behalf of, the average American in that same year. Admittedly, the comparison is not altogether fair. It does not take into account the fact that people who belong to Group Health sometimes go to doctors who are not affiliated with the plan. And it does not take into account the fact that the plan's members, who include relatively few poor people, may be in slightly better-than-average health.

But even when allowance is made for such factors, it is clear that prepaid group practice lowers the cost of medical care. The most convincing evidence is contained in a study recently carried out under the direction of Dr. Milton Roemer, Professor of Public Health at the University of California at Los Angeles. Roemer and his associates took as their subjects some three thousand families living in Southern California, and looked closely into what these families (and their employers) were paying for medical care, and what they were getting for their money. One third of the families were covered by Blue Cross or Blue Shield, both of which, in Southern California, offer contracts covering both hospitalization and doctors' fees. Another third were covered by commercial group insurance. The remaining third were subscribers to prepaid group practice plans, either Kaiser-Permanente or another, unidentified plan that has a big enrollment in Los Angeles County.

The average cost of medical care for an average-sized family in each of these three categories, including all out-of-plan expenditures by group practice subscribers, was found to be as follows:

Type of Insurance	Average Premium Paid (by employer, employee, or both)	Out-of-Pocket Expenditures	Total Costs
Commercial Insurance	$208	$156	$364
Blue Cross/ Blue Shield	257	190	447
Group Practice	271	52	323

Thus, Southern Californians belonging to prepaid group practice plans appear to be paying 27 per cent less for medical care than those who are covered by Blue Cross or Blue Shield, and 11 per cent less than those with commercial insurance. It is very likely, too, that this comparison understates the savings realized by group-practice subscribers. As pointed out, insurance companies are happiest when they can avoid insuring sick people; and Roemer's study indicates that, at least in Southern California, they have reason to congratulate themselves on this score. Chronic illness—arthritis, hypertension, diabetes—was twice as prevalent among the group-practice subscribers as among the people with commercial policies. And it can therefore be assumed that the group-practice patients needed (and got) more medical attention. Blue Cross and Blue Shield subscribers fell between the two other groups on the healthiness scale.*

The savings achieved by plans like Kaiser and Group Health of Puget Sound are mainly a reflection of the plans' success in keeping people out of the hospital. Roemer and his associates found that families enrolled in prepaid group plans were spending only two thirds as much time in hospitals as families covered by commercial insurance, and less than half as much time as families covered by Blue Cross or Blue Shield. It is often supposed that the reason for such differences is that group-practice doctors can concentrate on keeping their patients from getting so sick that they have to be hospitalized. This, of course, is what the name Health Maintenance Organization suggests. And Roemer did report that members of prepaid plans in Southern California were getting a little extra, in comparison with people being cared for by fee-for-service doctors, in the way of complete physical examinations, immunizations, Pap tests, and other kinds of preventive care.

But preventive medicine has very little to do with the success of plans like Kaiser in cutting down on the use of hospitals. Obviously, group-practice doctors have a strong interest in seeing that children get their polio and measles shots. Most children, however, apart from the children of the poor, get their shots no matter what kind of insurance their parents have. And while

* Insurance companies themselves concede that prepaid group practice is a lot more economical than fee-for-service medicine. *Fortune* recently asked two large companies to figure what they would have to charge for a conventional group insurance policy providing the same complete coverage offered by plans like Kaiser. One company, Connecticut General, estimated the premium at 54 per cent more than the cost of membership in a prepaid group plan. The other company, Northwestern National, estimated the extra cost at 41 per cent. *Fortune* also reported insurance-company calculations indicating that families enrolled in a prepaid group plan in Columbia, Maryland, are paying about a third less for medical care than people in the same area who have conventional health insurance.

there are a few diseases that can be treated more effectively if they are detected before the victim is aware of anything wrong—hypertension and cancer of the uterus are examples—there is no vaccine or other medicine that a doctor can give his patients to *prevent* heart disease or cancer or arthritis or arteriosclerosis or most of the other diseases that are the principal causes of disability, suffering, and death. The most effective form of preventive medicine, as doctors like to point out, would be to convince people to eat less, drink less, exercise more, and stop smoking. There is no evidence that Kaiser doctors excel at this sort of persuasion.

The real reason why prepaid group practice plans use hospitals so little is that they reverse the motives that ordinarily work to put people in hospitals unnecessarily and to keep them there too long. There are no hospital administrators scheming to keep beds filled; and no patient stands to benefit financially by being hospitalized for diagnostic tests or for minor surgery that could just as well be done on an outpatient basis. When a patient does have to be hospitalized, the availability of home nursing care makes it easier to discharge him quickly. Finally, of course, surgeons in prepaid group practice, as I have already noted, have nothing to gain by the unnecessary removal of tonsils, uteruses, or vermiform appendixes.

There are several reasons why prepaid group practice, for all its advantages, has spread so slowly. For one thing, it takes time and effort and money to get a prepaid plan on its feet. For another, a great many Americans still have a family doctor whom they like and trust, and whom they are reluctant to give up even for the greater financial security and lower cost of prepaid group practice. This has become less of an obstacle as medical costs have risen and as family doctors have become harder and harder to find. But many Americans, even if they have no regular doctor at the moment, are nevertheless reluctant to give up the privilege of being treated by any doctor in town who will have them as a patient.

In disparaging prepaid group practice, spokesmen for the AMA and local medical societies have made much of the advantages that patients reap from the freedom to shop around for care. They have implied that many doctors who work for plans like Kaiser are unambitious hacks who could never make it in the bracing, competitive world of fee-for-service medicine, and who get by only because their patients are not free to take their business elsewhere. Yet Kaiser-Permanente has long required that members of groups with which it contracts must be offered a choice of insurance plans, and that those who choose Kaiser must be given a chance, at least once a year, to change their minds and sign up with, say, Blue Cross or Equitable Life. Most other prepaid plans have adopted the same policy, not only for reasons of equity, but also to keep from accumulating a lot of dissatisfied subscribers. In the circumstances, and considering that some prepaid plans make it quite easy to switch doctors, the freedom-of-choice argument seems a bit thin, and one suspects that many doctors who cite it are really worried that their own patients will abandon them if a prepaid plan comes to town.

This fear would account for the lengths to which doctors went to stamp out prepaid group practice when the first plans were set in motion in the late 1930s and 1940s. At the urging of state medical societies, many states passed laws prohibiting the furnishing of medical services by any organization not controlled by doctors. Under some of these so-called Blue Shield laws no prepaid group practice could be established without the specific approval of the state medical society. In states like New York and Washington, where the imprimatur of organized medicine was not a legal requirement, doctors joining prepaid group plans were expelled from their local medical societies, stripped of their hospital privileges, and generally ostracized.

In recent years the AMA's hard official line has softened. An AMA Commission on Medical Care Plans, headed by a Dr. Leonard Larson, a former president of the AMA, looked into the quality of care provided by doctors in prepaid group practice and concluded that it was just as good as—and sometimes better than—the care given by fee-for-service physicians. In accepting this report, the AMA's House of Delegates grudgingly amended its definition of freedom of choice to include the freedom to choose group practice. But state medical societies have lobbied hard, and in some instances successfully, to prevent the repeal or modification of Blue Shield laws. And while prepaid group practice has gained respectability in some areas where it has taken root (several doctors who work for Group Health Cooperative of Puget Sound, for instance, have served on committees of their local medical society) doctors in other parts of the country are still using some of the same old tactics to keep their communities safe for fee-for-service medicine. Recently, for instance, *Medical Economics* reported that doctors associated with a new prepaid plan in Nashua, New Hampshire, "had to fight for up to six months for hospital privileges—and they are still personally and professionally snubbed by many local men." The AMA itself has formally declared that prepaid group practice is "experimental and unproven," and that the government has no business putting a lot of money into HMOs, "prior to valid proof of [their] general effectiveness." Officers of the AMA have further warned Congress of the danger of "depersonalized, assembly line medicine," and hinted darkly that the real reason Kaiser subscribers spend so little time in the hospital is that they are not getting the medical care they need.

In putting down prepaid group practice as an untested experimental prototype, the AMA is clearly being disingenuous. For twenty years, researchers have been studying plans like Kaiser and Group Health of Puget Sound, and answers are available to most of the questions that skeptics keep raising.

The most serious question is whether prepaid group practice leads to undertreatment. The temptation obviously exists, particularly when doctors stand to get a year-end bonus if they succeed, as a group, in saving money for the plan by hospitalizing patients less frequently, and getting them out of bed faster, than the budget has allowed for. A group of doctors undertaking to furnish medical care at so much per head may also be tempted to boost its income by taking on more and more patients without hiring additional doctors to take care of them.

Some newly organized plans in California, mainly profit-making ventures established to furnish care to Medicaid recipients, have plainly been guilty of shortchanging their subscribers. People who have signed up with these plans, many of them at the urging of door-to-door solicitors wearing long white coats, have often been unable to get services that they had been promised, such as 24-hours-a-day emergency care, free transportation to and from the doctor's office, and pediatric care by certified pediatricians. Corner-cutting of this kind is not surprising in view of the no-nonsense spirit of commercial enterprise with which these plans have approached their task of caring for the poor—a spirit suggested by a recent advertisement in the *Los*

Angeles Times that read, in part, "Los Angeles-based HMO requires 30 physicians . . . profit sharing, stock options, malpractice, and other fringe benefits. Starting salaries $40,000 to $50,000."

But while this shows that doctors who are bent on exploiting their patients can do so under prepaid as well as conventional practice arrangements, it does not prove that prepaid plans achieve their economies solely by denying people care to which they are entitled. On the contrary, the overwhelming majority of plans, including the oldest and biggest, have strong built-in safeguards against undertreatment. To begin with, they are not operated for profit. No doubt the directors of the Kaiser Foundation Health Plan are delighted when they wind up the year with a surplus, which can be used to build new hospitals and clinics. But they are not under the same pressure to produce profits as, say, the directors of DuPont or General Motors; and they may be presumed to get their directorial kicks mainly from contemplating the size and importance of the organization over which they preside, and the respect that it commands. Obviously it is not in their interest to permit the plan's doctors to put patients on an overly lean diet of medical care. This would not only alienate subscribers—who are much more likely to detect or suspect undertreatment than overtreatment—but would bring down on them the wrath of medical reformers, mainly concentrated in schools of public health, who for thirty years have been defending plans like Kaiser against the AMA's attacks. As for the doctors themselves, they have been trained in a tradition that holds undertreatment to be a much worse sin than its opposite. A doctor who takes out tonsils or uteruses that could just as well stay in is held to be less of a menace than the doctor who neglects to order x-rays or an electrocardiogram when he should, or who fails to send a patient to a specialist when he gets out of his depth. Undertreating patients is also, of course, a good way to get sued for malpractice.

Another charge commonly brought against group practice is that it is hard to see a doctor, or even to talk to him on the phone, unless one is really sick. There is some truth to this. The Citizens Board of Inquiry Into Health Services for Americans, after looking into the Kaiser plan in Portland, Oregon, reported that people who were not acutely ill had to wait six to eight weeks to see a doctor, and that "the appointment system seems set up to deter all but those with the strongest resolve." Subscribers who don't want to wait six weeks can go to one of Kaiser's drop-in clinics or emergency rooms. But this can mean a two- or three-hour wait, at the end of which, a Kaiser subscriber recently complained, "you get one minute with a harried doctor who barely has the time to ask you what's wrong." Similar complaints have been made about other plans, including Group Health Cooperative of Puget Sound, which appears to try a good deal harder than Kaiser to make things pleasant and convenient for its members. At Group Health's offices in Seattle I looked through a batch of complaints, including a letter from a man who wrote that when he had called the appointment center he had had to let the phone ring twenty times before it was answered. When the phone was finally picked up, he added, he was not allowed to speak to the doctor; the nurse with whom he finally spoke took too much on herself; and the nurses and clerks seemed much too concerned with saving the doctor's time. "My time is valuable too," he concluded.

Long waits for a physical check-up, or to consult a doctor about insomnia or a tennis elbow, are probably inherent in prepaid group practices. (They are also common in fee-for-service practice.) "We can't be immediately accessible to everyone who would like to see a doctor without a big rise in our dues," Dr. Harold Newman, the director of Group Health Cooperative of Puget Sound, has pointed out. Most members of prepaid plans manage to crash the barriers and to see a doctor when they need to. Forty-three per cent of the people belonging to group-practice plans whom Roemer questioned said they saw a doctor *more* frequently because of their plan membership. Only 5 per cent said they saw a doctor less frequently. Roemer did find, however, that people working at unskilled jobs tended to see a doctor less often than other members. Noting that "it is common to hear in these plans that 'you get good care if you know how to work the system,' " he speculated that the least-educated and least-sophisticated members were also the least adept at getting around the appointment clerks.

But even though it is hard to imagine a group-practice plan that will not require its members to run a bureaucratic gantlet when they want to see a doctor, the ordeal need not be daunting. It seems to help if the members have a say in running the plan. They have no such role at Kaiser, where a dissatisfied subscriber's only recourse is to switch to another insurance plan. ("The Kaiser-Portland 'grievance procedure' is largely a sham," the Citizens Board of Inquiry reported. "We spoke to no consumer who was even aware of its existence. The woman in charge of the grievance office told us that 'We don't notify people about the grievance system because if we did, the office would be just a flood of complaints.'") At Group Health Cooperative of Puget Sound, however, complaints appear to be taken seriously by the elected board of directors. The author of the letter from which I have quoted will probably never be entirely satisfied with the way he is treated when he calls up the appointment center. But after receiving his letter, and a few others like it, the board did see to it that telephone-answering procedures were changed, and additional appointment clerks hired.

Although many doctors like to think that prepaid practice goes hand in hand with slipshod medicine, there is no ground for this belief. Most groups keep a new doctor on probation for a year or two before granting him what amounts to academic tenure, and there is an understandable reluctance to take on doctors whose competence is in doubt. Their mistakes will not only reflect on the other members of the group, but will also have to be rectified by them. Dr. Richard Handschin of the Puget Sound plan, whose job is to make a continuing study of the plan's own operations, concedes that not every physician who survives his probationary period, and is elected to the permanent staff, is an outstanding clinician. "But the system does make sure that we have fewer *lousy* physicians than you find on the outside," Handschin says modestly.

Moreover, as I have pointed out in connection with Eliot Freidson's study of a medical group at Montefiore Hospital in the Bronx, the conditions of group practice clearly foster technical proficiency. It is true that this particular advantage of group practice has sometimes been exaggerated. Dr. Richard Weinerman, a Yale professor who served at one time as Kaiser's medical director, noted sadly some years ago that "the self-sufficient work style of the solo practitioner" tends to persist in group practice. "Group conferences, medical audits, and informal office consultations," he added, "are, in my experience, common in the descriptive literature but infrequent in daily practice."

Still, doctors who have left individual for group practice are likely to argue persuasively that they can do a better job than when they were on their own. In Seattle, for example, I spoke with a doctor who, before joining Group Health Cooperative of Puget Sound, had practiced for ten years in a small town in Wisconsin where he was the only doctor. He had no wish, he said, to return to solo practice there or anywhere else. "In solo practice you're busy as hell," he explained. "You've got no time to read, no time to communicate with anyone. It's different here. I like the built-in quality controls. If some guy's ordering more blood sugar tests than all the rest of the staff put together, we ask him about it. Same thing if someone's over-dosing his patients with a particular drug. In Wisconsin it was ominous to work in a professional vacuum year in, year out."

In any case, such scant statistical evidence as exists tends to support the conclusion of the AMA's Larson Commission that members of prepaid group plans get medical care at least as good as other people in their communities. After going through the medical records of several hundred of the people covered by their Southern California survey, Roemer and his associates reported that subscribers to prepaid group plans not only were getting more preventive services, but were receiving care that was, on the whole, more "rational"—consultations, for example, were more likely to be obtained when needed—than people covered by conventional insurance. The ability of prepaid group plans to furnish superior care is more strongly suggested by a study, made in the 1950s, that focused on the perinatal mortality rate—that is, on the proportion of babies who were born dead, or who died before they were a week old—among babies whose mothers belonged to the Health Insurance Plan of Greater New York. The rate turned out to be significantly lower than for babies born to nonmembers. This was true even when the comparison was limited to mothers who, like those belonging to HIP, were delivered in private hospitals by their own physicians. The difference was particularly striking in the case of nonwhites, the perinatal mortality rate for babies born to nonwhite mothers in the HIP sample being 23 per cent less than for babies born to other nonwhite mothers in New York City.

As Freidson's investigations have indicated, the warm, personal relationship that most people would like to have with their doctors—and that some people still enjoy—is less likely to flourish in the setting of a group-practice clinic than in the office of the traditional fee-for-service doctor. When members of HIP were surveyed some years ago, a fair number had the same complaints that are commonly voiced by people who get their medical care in hospital clinics and emergency rooms. One out of six members agreed that HIP doctors "don't give you a chance to explain exactly what your trouble is." One out of four agreed that the doctors "don't take enough personal interest in you."

But HIP is something of a special case. Doctors who work for Kaiser and the other big prepaid plans, apart from a few specialists, give all their time to group practice. By contrast, at the time the HIP survey was made, a great many HIP doctors were spending only part of each day seeing HIP patients. The rest of the time they were in their own offices seeing private patients on a fee-for-service basis. In this situation, the way for a doctor to maximize his income is to spend as much time as possible with those patients who pay him by the visit, and as little as possible with his HIP patients. Over the years, indeed, many doctors have considered their work in a HIP clinic as a temporary arrangement, to be discontinued as soon as they have built up a sufficiently large practice of their own. Those who have gone on working for HIP have sometimes come to look on their HIP patients with the same mixture of condescension and impatience often displayed by doctors working in the outpatient clinics of large city hospitals.

Most soundings have indicated that people who belong to prepaid plans are generally very happy to be members. For example, the Southern Californians who received questionnaires from Roemer and his associates were asked how they felt about the financial protection their insurance gave them. Ninety-one per cent of the people belonging to prepaid plans, as compared with 75 per cent of those with commercial coverage, and only 65 per cent of those covered by Blue Cross and Blue Shield, said they were "satisfied" or "very satisfied" on this score. More significantly, when people were asked to say how they felt about the medical care they were getting, 92 per cent of the group-plan members, as against 82 per cent of the people with other kinds of insurance, described themselves as satisfied or very satisfied.

Roemer points out that the high degree of satisfaction with the prepaid group plans may be due, in part, to the fact that unhappy members can always switch to another form of coverage, whereas most people with conventional insurance are locked into whatever plan their employer happens to offer them. But however one chooses to interpret Roemer's findings, they offer no comfort to those defenders of fee-for-service medicine who tell themselves that Americans will never accept prepaid group practice unless it is forced down their throats by the federal government.

Doctors who hate the idea of prepaid group practice have lately turned to a new technique for preventing its spread. Fighting fire with fire, local medical societies have been organizing medical-care programs of their own that are a cross between traditional fee-for-service medicine and the prepaid group variety. These hybrid programs are called medical care foundation plans, and they work like this: A county medical society, working through a nonprofit affiliate (the foundation), arranges with one or more insurance companies to market a policy, carrying the imprimatur of the foundation, that provides a specified set of benefits. Typically these benefits include coverage for routine out-of-hospital expenses, such as taking a child to a pediatrician for periodic checkups, that can ordinarily be obtained only by joining a plan like Kaiser. But whereas the Kaiser subscriber has to go to a Kaiser clinic, the holder of a foundation policy can go to any doctor in the county who has signed up with the foundation. The doctor, for his part, sees the patient in his own office, and bills the foundation for his services. In a few instances, foundations have bypassed insurance companies and, like Kaiser and other prepaid group plans, have entered into direct contracts with employers or unions. Thus the San Joaquin (California) Foundation for Medical Care, an early prototype of the foundations now springing up around the country, has been under contract for more than twenty years to provide medical services, for a flat yearly sum, to members of the International Longshoremen's and Warehousemen's Union. This same foundation has recently made a similar arrangement covering federal workers in San Joaquin and three neighboring counties.

Foundations undertake to save money for their subscribers by persuading doctors to accept, from their own peers, stricter controls over how they treat their patients, and what they charge for treating them, than doctors are willing to put up with under conventional insurance schemes. A doctor who signs up with a foundation must not only agree to charge his foundation patients no more than is reasonable and customary in his community. He must also consent to having his bill reviewed by a rotating panel of doctors who can withhold full payment if they find he has been overcharging. The San Joaquin Foundation is using the same review system to discourage sloppy or inappropriate treatment. For each of a large number of illnesses, general guidelines for treatment have been laid down, and the foundation's computer is programmed to winnow out claims for payment containing indications that these guidelines have been violated—that the doctor submitting the claim gave the wrong drug for the condition under treatment, for example. Such claims are then gone over by the panel, which may decide, after questioning the doctor, not to pay his bill, or to pay only a portion of it.

Foundations have also devised machinery for keeping hospital costs down. Under one scheme, called CHAP (Certified Hospital Admissions Program), registered nurses are employed to monitor hospital care. If a monitor suspects that a patient for whom a bed has been reserved doesn't really need to be hospitalized, she notifies a doctor whose job is to look into the matter at once. After he has gone over the patient's medical chart, and discussed the case with the attending physician, he may refuse to certify the admission as necessary. This means that if the patient is admitted anyway the foundation will not pay the bill. (However, a physician who feels strongly that his patient is getting a bad deal can appeal to a kind of medical court that will hand down an immediate decision.) Similarly, a doctor who wants to keep a patient in the hospital for a longer time than is customary for patients of the same age, who are suffering from the same condition, may be required to justify his decision to the foundation before further payment will be authorized.

Foundations have a number of attractions. There are no bureaucratic straits for the patient to navigate. He simply goes to his own doctor, ordinarily the same doctor he went to before joining the plan. Moreover, there is evidence that foundations can, in fact, cut hospital costs. In Phoenix, Arizona, Motorola employees were recently reported to be spending 17 per cent less time in hospitals since Motorola signed up with the Maricopa County Medical Care Foundation. There is also persuasive testimony that foundations are having some success in curbing greedy doctors and in straightening out careless and incompetent ones. Foundation plans have the further advantage that they can be set in motion much more quickly, and at less cost, than a prepaid group practice, since the doctors simply keep on doing business at the same old stand.

But foundations have not shown that they can reduce the use of hospitals, or reduce the over-all cost of medical care, as effectively as plans like Kaiser have. One reason is that a doctor who joins a foundation is still open to the temptations of pecuniary surgery, and if he is discreet about his transgressions there is not much the foundation can do to keep him honest. Furthermore, unlike a group plan which owns its own hospital or hospitals, and limits the number of beds to the actual needs of the plan's membership, a foundation has no good way to keep the hospitals with which it deals from putting up new buildings, or buying expensive new machines, that they don't really need. Another weakness of foundations is that the kibitzing that goes on in group practice is more likely to keep a doctor from falling into sloppy habits than a system that allows him to go on working in isolation, subject only to such controls as can be applied by scrutinizing his bills.

While many doctors, particularly those who dominate county medical societies, are still passionately committed to what a Texas medical foundation has referred to as the "dear principle" of fee-for-service medicine, attitudes in the profession are changing. The growth of prepaid group practice is unlikely to be hindered, as it has been in the past, by the difficulty of attracting good doctors. It is true that while group practice pays quite well—a young family doctor or pediatrician may start at $30,000, plus fringe benefits, while a specialist in his forties or fifties may make twice as much—the money is not as good as it is in private practice. "Probably doctors here make on the order of 25 per cent less than they would net on the outside," I was told by Dr. Richard Nesson, who is the medical director of the Harvard Community Health Plan in Boston. "But there are offsetting advantages in more regular hours, educational opportunities, and life style. Of course you can't earn anything like $100,000 a year, even though we do pay bonuses for people in certain specialties. Specialists is where we can run into difficulty, but money is no problem in recruiting people to deliver primary care."

Nesson went on to say that even though more and more prepaid group plans will be competing for doctors, he has no fear that the demand will outstrip the supply. "My impression is that in the next decade we're going to get a bonus from the decade of the late sixties and early seventies," he said. "We're going to see people coming out of medical school and finishing up their residencies who want to deliver their services in the best way possible, who want to have reasonably stable hours and a reasonably stable income, and who want to work with bright colleagues. Of course, anyone who comes into a group like this has to be willing to be exposed. Not everyone is going to want to work in this kind of fishbowl, but the percentage will be a lot higher than in the past." (Nesson's optimism would appear to be borne out by the results of a 1970 poll of medical students at Chicago, Duke, and the University of Florida. More than half said they would like prepaid group practice.)

Nesson also argues that a plan like Harvard's has advantages for a young doctor who wants to take care of poor people. "For years I watched young people going out to do their thing in neighborhood health centers," he said. "They worked very hard for two or three years, but they would get very depressed and leave. It's bound to be depressing when almost everybody you see has terrible psychosocial problems that you can't do much about." Pointing out that the Harvard plan takes care of both rich and poor people—the poor have their dues paid wholly or in part by the government—Nesson said, "Here, it's different. You're going to see lots of poor people, but you're going to see lots of others, too, and the variety of problems is greater."

Given the demonstrable advantages of prepaid group practice, its rapid growth seems assured, no matter what Congress does about national health insurance. At the same time, as more and more fee-for-service doctors join together in groups of their own, and as more and more such groups elect to march under the banner of a medical care foundation, fee-for-service medicine will take on, for better or for worse, some of the characteristics of prepaid group practice. Doctors will inevitably become brisker and less personal in their dealings with patients. And this development will come about not because of the scheming of power-hungry health planners in Washington, as some doctors will doubtless charge, but because of the changing technology of medicine itself.

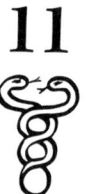

11

The Trouble with Medicare and Medicaid

In the late 1940s and early 1950s, the American Medical Association, confronted with President Harry Truman's determination to pass a national health insurance bill, spent tens of millions of dollars to arouse Americans to the deadly peril of what it labeled, incorrectly, as socialized medicine. The AMA's main argument was that if politicians and bureaucrats were ever to get into a position to regulate the terms on which medical care was provided—and the AMA was quite right in its conviction that some regulation would be inevitable once the government began underwriting people's medical expenses—the quality of American medicine would go into a disastrous decline. The AMA's leaders claimed to be concerned only about preserving the patient's freedom to choose his doctor, and the doctor's freedom to use his best medical judgment. Neither of these was, in fact, threatened by the bill for which Truman was pushing. But it can be assumed that the AMA was at least as deeply concerned about preserving the doctor's freedom to charge what he liked for his services, a freedom which might indeed be harder to maintain if the bill were passed. In any case, organized medicine carried the day. By 1951 national health insurance had been shelved, and for nearly fifteen years Washington's involvement in medical care consisted mainly of putting up money for new hospitals and for medical research, expenditures that were acceptable to the AMA because they did not cramp the entrepreneurial style of the practicing physician.

But in the 1960s the AMA faced another major battle, and this time it was beaten. President Kennedy had proposed broadening Social Security benefits to include health care for the elderly. Congress failed to take him up on this suggestion, but, in 1964, the voters who gave Lyndon Johnson his huge margin over Barry Goldwater also sent to Washington a larger group of liberal senators and congressmen than had been seen there since the early years of the New Deal. One of the first items on Johnson's agenda for realizing the Great Society was a limited form of national health insurance, covering people sixty-five and over. And within a few months of his inauguration, Congress, brushing aside the AMA's contention that old people were making out fine just as things were, enacted the program that came to be known as Medicare. At the same time, it enacted Medicaid, and during the remaining years of Johnson's administration dozens of other bills dealing with medical care were passed and became law.

Many of these bills differed from Medicare and Medicaid in that they were not simply financing arrangements, intended to help people obtain from doctors and hospitals in their communities medical care they needed but couldn't otherwise afford to pay for. Federal agencies in these years also got into the business of actually delivering medical care, especially to the poor. By the early 1970s, several million Americans were being cared for, mostly free of charge, at a wide variety of federally-supported medical facilities, including neighborhood health centers that undertook to help poor people cope not only with disease but with such nonmedical problems as contaminated water supplies, flaking lead paint, and the indifference of welfare departments. Between 1965 and 1974, federal spending for health programs rose from $2.6 billion to $22.8 billion a year, not counting the additional billions of dollars that were spent on the huge, self-contained medical-care systems maintained by the Veterans' Administration and the armed services. When these expenditures are included in the reckoning, the share of the nation's medical bill that is footed by the federal government now stands at 27 per cent.

There are many doctors who argue that Americans, by and large, get all the medical care they have coming to them, and that everybody would be better off if politicians would refrain from further tampering with the market in which doctors' services are bought and sold. "Some people think that people are entitled to health care as a matter of right, whether they work or not," Edward R. Annis, a former president of the AMA, remarked not long ago. "This is just as absurd as saying that food, clothing, and shelter are a matter of right—one step further than that is a revolutionary system bordering on Communism. . . ."

But doctors like Annis, although they may win a battle here and a skirmish there, are fighting a rearguard action. The central issue in the politics of medical care is not whether there should be national health insurance, whose inevitability is conceded even by its most intransigent opponents. The issue is, rather, what the government can and should do to make reasonably good care available to all who need it, at an acceptable cost to them and to society at large. Reforming the country's huge and complicated medical-care system is, of course, a formidable job, and as we go about it there is much to be learned from the programs that were launched in the 1960s with the flag of the Great Society flying bravely at their mastheads—programs that have changed the terms on which tens of millions of Americans get medical care, even though the changes have not always been precisely those intended by the programs' architects.

In 1961, with Medicare looming on the political horizon, the AMA furnished its members with a poster intended for display on the walls of their waiting rooms. It was headed "Socialized Medicine and *You*," and read, in part, "Freedom is what we all stand to lose. Your freedom to choose the doctor *you believe is best for you*. And your doctor's freedom—his freedom to treat you in an individual way, adapting his knowledge and skills to your particular problems. These freedoms are bound to be lost when the Federal Government enters the privacy of the examination room—controlling both the standards of practice and the choice of practitioner."

Since the advocates of Medicare were asking only that social security benefits be broadened to include the payment of a portion of the medical bills run up by old people, this was all nonsense. As it has turned out, Medicare has given old people *more* freedom to choose among doctors, not less. It is easier now for those who are living on small incomes, and who might otherwise have to look around for a doctor willing to take them on as charity patients, to buy the medical care they need at the going rate. Medicare has also left the doctors' professional freedom quite intact. It is true that in the last two or three years the government has been increasingly reluctant to pay for the hospitalization of elderly patients who might just as well be cared for at home. And some of its decisions—or some made on its behalf by Blue Cross administrators and other middlemen—have rightly struck doctors as arbitrary and unfair. But most doctors would probably concede that the trouble is not so much with the government's intentions as with its ineptitude in carrying them out. The privacy of the examination room has, in any case, remained inviolate.

The AMA poster did not mention, as a freedom worth defending, the doctor's right to set his own price on his services. But this freedom, too, has survived under Medicare. It has, in fact, flourished. Although Medicare applies the usual-customary-and-reasonable test to medical fees, there is nothing to stop a doctor from charging more than the formula permits and collecting the difference from the patient. Given these ground rules, and given the stepped-up purchasing power of millions of people who had previously felt they could not afford to go to a doctor except in a case of dire necessity, or who had been charity patients, getting treatment free or at a reduced rate, doctors could hardly fail to prosper under the new law.

Prosper they did. By 1970 Medicare was costing the taxpayers $7 billion a year, twice as much as the government's planners had predicted, and one reason the planners had been so far off was that they had failed to anticipate what a good thing doctors would make of Medicare. In 1968, according to a tabulation by the Senate Finance Committee, eighteen doctors each collected $150,000 or more from Medicare, and more than four thousand collected $25,000 or more. There was clear evidence that some of these doctors were fattening their earnings by billing the government for unnecessary injections, blood tests, and x-rays. Some doctors also fell into the lucrative habit of making what the committee called "gang visits" to nursing homes, seeing forty or fifty patients in a single sweep, and billing Medicare for their services at five to ten dollars a head. Most doctors, of course, did not cheat the government. But most did take advantage of the new money coming into the market, and of the gratifying flexibility of Medicare's payment formula. In the four years after Medicare was enacted, a period when the general price level rose only moderately, the average family doctor raised his fees by nearly one third.

Hospitals also found a rich lode in Medicare. Some had been

treating some old people free, passing on all or part of the cost to their paying patients; now, every hospital could collect from Medicare the full cost of caring for the elderly, including depreciation charges, plus a 1.5 per cent bonus to help pay for new facilities and equipment. In the circumstances, many hospitals went on a buying spree. "Medicare is the computer manufacturer's friend," the trade journal *Electronic News* observed in 1968, a year when companies making electronic blood-cell counters, X-ray equipment, and hospital computer systems were reporting record earnings. All this worked to push up the cost of hospital care, which rose by an average of 12 per cent a year during the late 1960s, as compared with an average rise of 7.5 per cent a year between 1950 and 1960. Medicare also eased the problems of hospital administrators who had been having trouble keeping their beds occupied by paying patients. Hospitals getting Medicare money were required to have utilization review committees, charged with preventing unnecessary use of hospital beds at government expense. In 1970, however, a report by the staff of the Senate Finance Committee concluded that the work of these bodies was, by and large, "of a token nature" and "more form than substance."

In 1972 Congress tightened the government's control over Medicare expenditures. A hospital that installs a new surgical unit that has not been approved by the local hospital planning council may now be denied the right to include any part of the unit's cost in the bills it submits to Medicare. Since almost a third of the money that hospitals collect for inpatient services comes from Medicare, this may put a damper on some of the extravagances described in Chapter Eight. Moreover, the cost, quality, and appropriateness of hospital care paid for by Medicare and Medicaid are now being monitored, as I have pointed out, by Professional Standards Review Organizations, or PSROs. But the PSROs are just getting down to their work, and it is too early to tell whether the government has hit on a formula for holding down the cost of Medicare without further chipping away at the protection it offers its beneficiaries.

Indeed, the worst fault of Medicare is not that it has been too generous with doctors and hospitals, but that it has been too stingy with their patients. To limit the cost to the taxpayers, and to appease those doctors who complained that unless old people were required to pay at least a part of their medical bills they would demand too much of their doctors' time and attention, Congress, in 1965, surrounded Medicare's benefits with a hedge of exclusions, deductibles, and co-payments. As a result, Medicare actually pays only 43 per cent of the total cost of medical care received by people who are sixty-five or over, and an elderly patient who has a serious illness can easily run up a bill of a thousand dollars or more.

Consider, for example, the out-of-pocket costs incurred by a man who is operated on for the removal of his prostate gland; who suffers from complications that require his remaining in the hospital for two weeks; and who is then transferred to a nursing home, where he spends an additional thirty days before going home. He must contribute $84 toward the cost of his stay in the hospital. He must also pay part of the cost of the operation, his share being $60 plus 20 per cent of all charges in excess of $60; if we assume that the surgeon's and anesthesiologist's bills add up to $1100, the patient's share comes to $268. Finally, the patient has to pay $9 a day for the last ten days of his stay in the nursing home, only the first twenty days being paid for in full by Medicare. Total cost to patient: $442.

In arriving at this figure I have assumed that the surgeon's and anesthesiologist's fees were judged by Medicare to be usual, customary, and reasonable. But the National Council of Senior Citizens has complained that only two out of five doctors consistently stay under the Medicare ceiling when billing old people, and in New York City doctors' bills for treating the elderly in 1973 exceeded the Medicare level by an average of 21 per cent. In the hypothetical case I have just given, if the bill for surgery and anesthesia had come to, say, $1250, and Medicare had found this to be 21 per cent more than the maximum it was prepared to underwrite, the patient's out-of-pocket expenses would have totaled not $442, but $694.

There are other gaps in Medicare's coverage that expose its beneficiaries to heavy expenses. Medicare pays for nursing-home care only if skilled medical attention is in order—if the patient is just learning to walk after a stroke or an amputation, for example, or has complicated dressings that must be changed at frequent intervals. But a bedridden patient recovering from a major operation who needs mainly to be fed, bathed, watched, and medicated must pay for such care himself. Furthermore, Medicare pays for only such medication as a patient gets while in a hospital or a skilled nursing home. An elderly person who has emphysema and heart disease (a not uncommon combination), or who suffers from inflammatory bowel disease, may have to spend $40 or $50 a month of his own money for drugs.

Many people simply do not have the means to meet the expenses that they are left to pay by Medicare. In New York City, for example, nearly one third of all households headed by persons sixty-five years old or older (most of these were one-person households) had incomes of $2000 or less in 1973, and old people living on such slender incomes cannot pay even a very modest medical bill without starving themselves. All told, perhaps five or six million old people, some of whom are on welfare but most of whom are getting by on small pensions and social security, are in this situation. In most states, an old person who cannot pay his medical bills can sign up for Medicaid. But Medicaid medicine is welfare medicine, and, quite apart from its other shortcomings, getting on Medicaid—and staying on it—can be a hard and degrading ordeal.

Just how degrading it can be was made clear in a talk I had not long ago with a New York community worker named Elma Harris. Mrs. Harris, a black woman in her late thirties, works for the East Harlem Committee on Aging. The committee is housed in an old school building, part of which now serves as a social center for old people. In the empty classroom where we talked we could hear music of the 1930s and 1940s, played by a three-piece band in a room near the main entrance where, as I came in, some twenty old couples had been dipping and jitterbugging. Mrs. Harris said that sooner or later most old people in East Harlem have to go on Medicaid if their health is poor. This means, to begin with, filling out a ten-page form, and she said she and her associates spend a lot of time helping people with this task. "If we didn't, they would all end up like they were doing at the beginning," she said. "They would be going down to the Medicaid Center on 34th Street three or four times a week, trying to get in that office so someone could fill out that damned form for them. And then they would wait three or four months before they knew whether they were eligible or not."

She went on to speak of the way old people are sometimes humiliated at the 34th Street center. "They've had old people in a line, and when they've gotten to the door, they've closed the door in their faces. The people that are hired for those jobs have no consideration for anybody. They're just *there*. Sometimes they will fill the form out wrong, and then you have to go back. They are God, and if the clerk decides, well, you've got nineteen cents over the income limit, you can't get Medicaid. When you do get your card, it is usually good for a few months, and, with senior citizens, they usually send a recertification letter. But often the senior citizen doesn't understand it, so his Medicaid card runs out, and he has the whole hassle all over again."

Many old people in East Harlem, Mrs. Harris continued, would rather not go to the doctor than to go through all this. "Last year we had a health fair here, and we must have had four hundred seniors," she said. "We got people who hadn't seen a doctor in twenty years. The minority races, and the poor, and this means all races, have been promised so many things that once they get to be sixty-five they don't trust anybody. They are ashamed to go on welfare. They think Medicaid is welfare. Most of them can't afford to go to a doctor under Medicare, so they stay home and they suffer." She paused, and added in a harsh, angry voice, "Another thing: Medicaid and Medicare, neither one does a thing for the homebound senior, if there's no family to take him out—and remember that you've got, say, 50 per cent of the seniors that are living alone. I don't see Medicare or Medicaid get any health counselors, any doctors, any nurses, or anybody else to go into these families, into these homes, to see that these old people really get the treatment that they should. If it wasn't for the visiting nurse service, and other voluntary agencies, then you would have them dying by the hundreds alone in these apartments."

When Medicaid was enacted in 1965 there were optimists among its backers who predicted that, in time, it would do away with the catch-as-catch-can medical care for which so many Americans, living on welfare or small pensions, or working at marginal jobs, had previously had to settle. The essence of the new law was a commitment by the federal government to reimburse individual states for up to 83 per cent of whatever they might spend on medical care for people too poor to pay for it themselves. The law specified that Medicaid's benefits need not be confined to people on welfare, some of whose medical expenses were already being defrayed by Washington, but could be extended to the medically needy. While this term was not precisely defined, Congress clearly had in mind the working poor: people making enough money to feed and clothe and house themselves and their families, but not making enough to pay doctors' or hospital bills. These were the people who, in larger and larger numbers, were showing up in the emergency rooms and clinics of municipal and county hospitals, where free care was available if one waited long enough; or who were presenting themselves to university hospitals as teaching patients, obtaining free or low-priced care in return for their willingness to be practiced on by medical students and interns. Under Medicaid, it was commonly said, these people would now be launched into the mainstream of medical care. Armed with a Medicaid card, they would be able to command the services of doctors and hospitals on the same terms as middle-class Americans.

But such hopes were quickly dashed. Underwriting decent (i.e., middle-class) care for the poor turned out to cost a lot more than had been anticipated—and a lot more than politicians had reason to think their constituents would stand for. The first alarms were sounded when New York enacted a Medicaid law hailed by its governor, Nelson Rockefeller, as "the most significant social legislation in three decades." The most striking feature of the New York law was the number of people it covered. Congress had left it to the states to decide who should be eligible for Medicaid, and most of them took a rather narrow view of what constituted medical neediness. Illinois, for example, set $3600 a year as the maximum income a family of four could earn and still qualify for Medicaid. In New York, however, the ceiling for a couple with two children was set at $6000; a family of six, in which the mother and father both worked, could earn as much as $8550 a year and still get Medicaid.

This meant that some eight million people, nearly half of the state's population, would be eligible to get their medical care at public expense. When the implications of this sank in, there were loud protests not only from taxpayer groups but from a number of county medical societies. The latter had no objection to doctors getting paid for taking care of people who were really destitute. But there was strong opposition to a scheme that would put half the average doctor's patients on Medicaid, forcing him to treat them—if he wished to go on treating them at all—for fees that would be set by the Medicaid authorities, and that, unlike Medicare fees, he would be forbidden to supplement by extra charges. Such an arrangement, the Suffolk County Medical Society protested angrily, would "deprive physicians of their constitutional rights to practice medicine in a free society."

In Washington, too, there were second thoughts about Medicaid. Congress had been told that Washington's share of its cost would come to $950 million a year, or only about $350 million more than the federal government was already spending in 1965 for various medical assistance programs that Medicaid would supplant. But less than a year after the new law was enacted the Social Security Administration's chief actuary, Robert Myers, warned Congress that Medicaid would soon be costing the federal government at least $3 billion a year, more than three times as much as he himself had forecast. Soon afterward Congress took steps to limit Washington's liability by writing into the law a complicated formula that would deny federal Medicaid funds to any family whose income exceeded by more than a thousand dollars the level at which that family would be eligible for welfare. In New York the eligibility ceiling for a family of four was lowered from $6000 to $5000. Most other states, as I have said, were soon restricting Medicaid to people on, or eligible for, welfare.

The removal of millions of the working poor from the Medicaid rolls met with little opposition. The euphoric mood in which Lyndon Johnson and the Congress had declared war on poverty had been soured by the war in Vietnam. Moreover, support for Medicaid had quickly been undermined by revelations that, in far too many instances, the program's chief beneficiaries had been doctors, dentists, podiatrists, and nursing-home proprietors. Within two years of the new law's enactment doctors all over the country were collecting huge sums from Medicaid by whisking the poor through their offices at a rate of one every two or three minutes. While some people were getting hasty and superficial care, others were getting care that they didn't need. Since 1965, thousands of group practices, of a kind known as Medicaid clinics, have been established in low-income city neighborhoods, and at some of these clinics it is standard procedure for a doctor to pass each new patient on to his associates for additional examination and treatment. This is called ping-ponging. "There was a group like that on 119th Street and First Avenue," Elma Harris, the East Harlem community worker, told me. "If you walked in that office, and you said you had a stomachache, that meant you were going to see an M.D. After you saw the M.D., they sent you to the dentist. After you saw the dentist, then you had to see the podiatrist." Mrs. Harris conceded that this might have made good sense for some people, but that the podiatrist in the group seemed to find a remarkably large number of foot defects. "There were never so many shoes prescribed for children that were not needed," she said. "Because you know that *every* child that is born of a poor family does not have something wrong with his feet. But every child that went in that office got a prescription for shoes. My husband and I were paying fourteen dollars and seventy-five cents for Dr. Posners, and my little daughter refused to wear them. She said, 'Those are welfare shoes.' Because everybody was getting Dr. Posner shoes from the Medicaid."

People who make a business of catering to Medicaid enrollees have found other ingenious and shoddy ways of exploiting them. Doctors have accepted kickbacks from laboratories to which they regularly refer patients for tests that they may or may not need. (In New York City, the Health Department has reported several instances in which tests for sickle cell anemia had been ordered for white persons, and one instance in which a man was sent to a laboratory for a pregnancy test.) Pharmacists have kited Medicaid prescriptions by raising the number of pills called for on a prescription blank from, say, 100 to 200, and billing Medicaid for the larger amount. Dentists falsely claiming to have done work on one patient have supported their claim with x-rays of work done on another. Medicaid patients, as everyone knows, have also been shamelessly mistreated by greedy nursing-home proprietors. To give just one example, Senator Frank Moss of Utah called the Senate's attention in 1971 to the owner of a nursing home in Illinois who was feeding his patients on 54 cents a day each while realizing a pre-tax profit of $185,000 on the $400,000-a-year business he was doing with Medicaid. Moss went on to hint at exploitation of an even more shocking variety. In Illinois, he pointed out, the amount of money a nursing home could collect from Medicaid was determined by a point system based on the physical condition of the patients. "To my great dismay," he said, "I learned that large bedsores once developed by the patient are worth eight points, and at $6 a point the reimbursement to the nursing home increases $48 a month." Moss said he had been told that nursing-home operators in Illinois commonly referred to bedsores as "being worth $48 a month."

Doctors who callously milk their patients are, of course, in a small minority. Dr. Lowell Bellin, New York City's Health Commissioner, recently estimated that no more than 5 to 10 per cent of the city's doctors who have big Medicaid practices are, as he put it, "scoundrels." Some poor people have unquestionably gotten more and better care because of Medicaid. One indication is the sharp rise in the number of pregnant women in poor families who consult a doctor during the first three months of pregnancy. Poor people are seeing doctors more often than they used to, and they are likely to have a greater choice of doctors to go to, partly because Medicaid has brought doctors into poor neighborhoods who would not otherwise have set up practice there.

But in many parts of the country the poor are not much better off than they were before 1965. Five years after Medicaid's enactment, Pierre de Vise, assistant director of the Hospital Planning Council of Metropolitan Chicago, complained that Medicaid had had "no perceptible effect on encouraging more hospitals and physicians to serve Chicago's poor." De Vise went on to say, "The main result is that the same few welfare physicians and hospitals are now making much more money." In 1968, he pointed out, "73 physicians (out of 6000) dished out cafeteria-style medicine to 170,000 Medicaid recipients, at a cost to the taxpayer of $50,000 per physician. And one hospital, out of 80, serves half the city's black inpatients, two thirds of its black outpatients, and three fourths of its black emergency patients." Even in cities like New York and Boston, where the poor make out much better than in Chicago, Medicaid has conspicuously failed to rescue them from the depressing backwaters of American medicine.

To be sure, there are doctors in poor neighborhoods who take time and pains with their patients, and who practice good medicine. Not long ago I talked with one, a young man who had just enrolled in a family-practice residency after working for two years in a Medicaid clinic in East Harlem. During those two years he saw an average of fewer than twenty-five patients a day—about the same number, he said, as he would have seen if he had been conducting a busy practice in the suburbs. He conscientiously attended postgraduate seminars and lectures for practicing physicians, and even took Spanish lessons so that he could communicate better with his patients, most of whom were Puerto Rican. The other doctors in the clinic, he told me, had impressed him as being highly competent, except for two who were quickly replaced. "There was absolutely no ping-ponging," he said.

Most Medicaid doctors, however, feel that seeing only twenty-five patients a day is a luxury they cannot afford. If Medicare has been too generous in the matter of doctors' fees, Medicaid has been too stingy. In New York City, for example, Medicaid allows only $6 for a visit to a general practitioner and $7.50 to $20 for a visit to a certified internist; in both instances, this is less than half the going rate. As a result, a doctor whose patients are almost all on Medicaid, and who sees no more than twenty-five of them a day, has to settle for half the money he could make if he were seeing an equal number of middle-class patients paying him out of their own pockets. In the circumstances, and given a heavy demand for doctors' services from people who are not in a position to be choosy, doctors who specialize in treating Medicaid patients tend to get them in and out of their offices rather fast.

Admittedly there are valuable services a doctor can render even when he is seeing sixty or seventy patients a day. With routine screening tests he can spot diabetics and people with high blood pressure. He can prescribe Butazolidin for a sore shoulder, Gantrisin for a urinary infection, or bismuth and paragoric for diarrhea. He can reassure a mother that there's nothing wrong with her four-year-old that time and aspirin won't repair. But there is no time to tackle complicated problems of medical management, such as helping a patient whose diabetes he has diagnosed to live with his disease. There is no time to do anything about emotional distress and its consequences other than to write a prescription for Miltown or Librium. And as Dr. Mildred Morehead, an expert on the evaluation of medical care, has pointed out, there is likely to be no time for careful record-keeping. After visiting the offices of twenty doctors with large Medicaid practices, all of them in rural areas, Dr. Morehead wrote, "Are the deplorable record-keeping practices observed in these few offices typical of the average practitioner? How many physicians keep their records solely for billing purposes, where entries consist only of charges and drugs distributed?"

The quality of care available to the poor also suffers from the fact that doctors who treat large numbers of Medicaid patients often have no hospital connections. Many voluntary hospitals don't want to be overrun by poor people, even if the government is ready to pay all or most of the cost of their care, and may be reluctant, as I have said, to give staff privileges to doctors practicing in poor neighborhoods. The big medical centers do need poor patients as teaching material, but they are not at all eager to share them with local practitioners. "The snobbery of the hospital establishment and the medical-school establishment is incredible," a New York City public health officer remarked not long ago. "As far as they're concerned, the local doctor doesn't know zilch—he's just out there ripping off the community. They don't want him. He's not part of the team."

This attitude not only tends to cut the Medicaid doctor off from what is going on in medicine, and to allow him to slide more easily into sloppy work habits. It also deprives his patients of the kind of advice that most Americans count on from their family doctor when they are seriously ill. A Medicaid patient who may require surgery is likely to be told by his doctor to go to the emergency room of the nearest municipal or university hospital. If the admitting physician decides the patient should be hospitalized, he will be taken care of by interns and residents. When the time comes for his discharge, no one will bother to tell his doctor what the hospital learned about his condition, or what was done about it. Nor can his doctor ordinarily arrange to see the patient's hospital chart except at the cost of a lot of time and trouble. The patient thus has a choice of returning periodically to the hospital for follow-up care, or of returning to a doctor who may not know enough about his condition to treat it intelligently.

When Medicaid was enacted there were hopes that it would enable hospitals to do more for the poor and the near-poor who would continue to use emergency rooms and outpatient clinics as their family doctors. Here and there hospitals are trying to offer such patients the kind of prompt, compassionate, and technically competent care that is available to middle-class Americans who belong to a good prepaid health plan. When I visited the new Martin Luther King Hospital in the Watts district of Los Angeles, shortly before it was opened, I was told that the phones in its acute-care pediatric clinic would be manned twenty-four hours a day by nurse specialists whom parents could consult about their children; that the clinic itself would be open sixteen hours a day, seven days a week; that minibuses would be sent to pick up children and parents needing transportation to the hospital; and that every pediatrician on the hospital staff, including the chief of pediatrics, would take his turn at night duty in the clinic.

But providing this kind of service requires, among other things, money. A great many people who look to hospitals for all their medical care are ineligible for Medicaid, and yet are living on so little money that it is unreasonable to expect them to pay the full cost of the treatment they get. Many hospitals charge such patients less than the standard clinic fee, or waive the fee altogether. At one time it was possible for hospitals to make up for losses incurred in this fashion by tacking an extra two or three dollars onto the daily rate for bed patients. Medicare and Medicaid—and, in many areas, Blue Cross as well—have put a stop to this, however, and the outpatient departments of hospitals that make a regular business of caring for the poor are generally far more strapped for money today than they were before Medicaid.

In the circumstances, few such hospitals have shown much enthusiasm for schemes to make things pleasanter and more convenient for the people who use their emergency rooms and clinics. The clinic visitor must still, as a rule, put up with long waits, inefficiency (nothing can be settled by phone), and the kind of stop-and-go processing to which a recruit is subjected on his first day in the army. Moreover, Medicaid has done nothing to change the widely held notion that seeing poor people in a hospital clinic is a boring and intellectually unprofitable way for a doctor to spend his time.

This point was stressed by a doctor with whom I talked not long ago in a tiny office on the ground floor of a famous New York teaching hospital, where she is director of ambulatory services. She said that her position, a relatively new one, had been created with the aim of improving conditions in the hospital's fifty-four clinics and in its emergency department, which are visited by as many as two thousand patients on a busy day. "It's a slow, tough job," she said. "Some doctors here couldn't care less. They take the position, 'The community be hanged.'" She explained that it is the chiefs of medicine and surgery and pediatrics and obstetrics—rarely seen in the hospital's outpatient clinics—who decide which doctors shall work in the clinics, and when. "I have no control over anyone here except the clerical staff," she said. "All the people around town in my position are in the same boat. If we're going to improve things, we must have authority to plan and organize. We must have control of physician attendance." She added, smiling, "At least the chiefs of service have begun to invite me to their monthly dinners, and I suppose that's progress. But it's clear I'm not their equal in the hierarchy."

12

Killing Rats in Mound Bayou: New Styles in Missionary Medicine

To some of the strategists of the War on Poverty that Lyndon Johnson declared in the mid-1960s it seemed obvious that providing decent medical care for the poor involved more than just paying the bills. Accurately foreseeing the shortcomings of Medicaid, they proposed setting up health centers that would offer millions of low-income city dwellers, as well as people living in rural slums like those of Appalachia and the Mississippi Delta, a kind of medical care that would be quite new in their experience. For one thing, there was to be no probing into the financial status of patients; the centers' services were to be free to everyone in the neighborhood who cared to make use of them. For another, while Washington was to foot the bill, collecting what it could from Medicaid to defray operating costs, control was to be exercised to a large degree by the centers' patients. Local boards or councils would settle such questions as what services a center should offer (eye examinations? birth control advice?), and who should have first claim on dental services (children? old people?). Most important, the boards would have the final word on the hiring and firing of personnel, including doctors. Neighborhood residents were to be involved in the work of the centers in another way as well. They were to be hired and trained as appointment clerks, medical assistants, and family health workers, whose jobs would combine elements of nursing, social service, and something new called patient advocacy. Another distinctive feature of the new centers was that responsibility for the care of patients would be vested not in doctors alone, but in teams whose voting members might include two or three doctors, an equal number of public health nurses, and half-a-dozen family health workers.

The first of the new centers was opened in Boston in 1965. Founded by members of the faculty of the Tufts University School of Medicine, it was established to serve people living in Columbia Point, a large public housing project built on an isolated peninsula that had once been a city dump. Public transportation between Columbia Point and the rest of Boston was so poor that a resident might have to waste half a day on a routine visit to a doctor. "Prenatal care meant being at the Boston City Hospital at eight o'clock," Conrad Herr, one of the doctors who founded the center, has recalled. "By nine you had to be sitting there with your urine specimen and your panties in your purse, waiting for the OB man. Then at eleven or twelve, perhaps, a forty-five-minute trip back home."

The residents of Columbia Point found the new center much to their liking. According to a door-to-door survey made in 1967, they liked it not only for its convenience, but also because it offered care that seemed more personal than they were likely to get at hospital clinics or even in the offices of doctors in private practice. The survey also turned up the fact that people using the center were spending much less time in hospitals than they had before the center opened. In the case of the project's poorest families, the decline in hospital use was an almost incredible 80 per cent.

The same Tufts physicians also founded another center, in Bolivar County, Mississippi, a cotton-growing area where the average family income in 1966 was only about $900. Doctors were scarce, and the health of the population appalling. "We found everything one would expect and more," the center's first director, Dr. H. Jack Geiger, has said. "Infections, malignancies, an especially high rate of hypertension in adults and infectious diarrhea in children." But it was apparent to Geiger, and to the doctors and nurses who went to Mississippi with him to staff the new center (and it was even more apparent to the center's local advisory council) that medicine and medical care were not what was most urgently needed. Geiger has described the plight of people living in and around Mound Bayou, the small, all-black community where the center's staff had set up shop in a church parsonage. Most of them, he has written, "lived in an unceasing, and often losing, struggle against disaster. They were hungry; there was no food. They were unemployed; their skills had been made obsolete by the mechanical cotton picker. . . . They lived in crumbling patchwork shacks with leaking roofs, rotting floors, buckling walls, gaping windows, newspapers for insulation, and crude stoves for heating and cooking—when there was firewood. Many drank contaminated water from drainage ditches and used dilapidated surface privies for personal sanitation. Infants under such circumstances often ingested their own excrement. . . ."

To help meet the need for food, the center borrowed and leased 120 acres of land, and worked with 800 of the poorest families in the area to form a farm cooperative that harvested, in its first year, more than a million pounds of collard greens, okra, onions, lima beans, and sweet potatoes. Crews were organized to build privies, repair and fumigate houses, dig wells, kill rats, and, in general, bring sanitary conditions at least up to the level of a big-city slum. At the same time the center was giving medical care to some 12,000 persons. Judging by the commonly used standard of infant mortality, all this had a strikingly beneficial effect on the health of the community. In the mid-1960s, infant mortality in northern Bolivar County was running at around seventy per thousand births, or more than three times the national average. Two years after the Mound Bayou center opened the rate had fallen to thirty per thousand.

Few if any of the more than one hundred other health centers that have been established since 1965 have had so dramatic an impact as these two. That is not surprising, since few if any of the communities where other centers have been opened were so peculiarly isolated as Columbia Point, or so desperately poor as Mound Bayou. But there is persuasive evidence in the form of surveys and medical audits that the doctors who staff these centers have been skillful and conscientious, offering patients a brand of care that is, by and large, a little better from a technical standpoint, and a good deal more personal and sympathetic, than they would be likely to get in the outpatient clinic of a university hospital.

More important, the family health workers employed at the centers have given poor people kinds of help that are rarely to be had from hospitals, and never from doctors in private practice. There are ways, to be sure, in which the health worker's job resembles that of the familiar visiting nurse. In the course of her daily rounds she may check the blood pressure and pulse of a patient being treated for hypertension; show the daughter of a bedbound woman how to bathe her mother; make sure that a recently diagnosed diabetic knows how to test his urine; and show a new mother how to deal with diaper rash. But the health worker does other things as well. Drawing on what she has come to know about a family whom she visits regularly, she may work out, with other members of her health-care team, a plan for helping the family to cope with a retarded child, a senile grandmother, or an alcoholic father. She—or he, for some family health workers are men—may also spend a lot of time helping patients to set in motion the bureaucratic machinery that exists, in principle, to serve the poor. "A family of eleven lived in a dilapidated apartment with only six beds," the director of a health center has written. "The three-year-old had been eating large quantities of broken plaster. The family health worker persuaded the fearful mother to have the child hospitalized for examination and explained the dangers of lead poisoning. She also helped her to get a special grant for new beds from the welfare department, showed her how to shop economically, and helped her to contact a local group which would arrange to have repairs made in her apartment."

Family health workers are usually ready, too, to lend an ear to patients who are anxious or depressed. "A lot of people just need someone to talk to," one worker told me. "About half of what I do is sitting and listening." I was told much the same thing by another worker, a square-built, soft-voiced man in his late thirties who had worked as a cook and as a film technician before going to work at a health center. I had been with him to visit one of his patients, a towering middle-aged immigrant from Yugoslavia who was suffering from multiple sclerosis, and who occupied a relatively bright and pleasant room in an otherwise dark and malodorous building on the upper West Side of Manhattan. Much of the visit had been taken up by an account of our host's recurring impotence. The health worker had listened closely, and finally had suggested in a tentative way that the impotence might be connected with the patient's readiness to settle for paid sexual partners whom he really despised. "I get a person's life history, I let him unwind," he said later. "It's a little like a psychiatrist: I reflect problems back to people."

The family health workers I have just quoted were both employed at the Neighborhood Health Services Program, a health center on West 100th Street in Manhattan. I spent some time there in 1971, sitting in on staff meetings and talking with doctors, nurses, health workers, and patients. About twelve thousand people are enrolled as patients at this center. Most are black or Puerto Rican, although the center also serves a good number of elderly white people, some of whom live in what are known as SROs—dark, warren-like apartment buildings that have been converted to single-room occupancy, and that cater mainly to welfare clients, many of whom are alcoholics. The center occupies quarters on the second floor of a modern city-owned building, quarters that are much too cramped to accommodate properly the hundreds of patients who visit the center every day. The tiny waiting room is usually packed with patients ranged on rows of folding wooden chairs, and there are a pervading clutter and confusion not unlike that of an overtaxed emergency room or the general medical clinic of a municipal hospital.

It seemed to me, however, that the people working at the center, most of whom, with the exception of the doctors, were black or Puerto Rican, were warmer and less condescending in dealing with patients than their counterparts in many hospitals. Dr. Harold Wise, the former director of the Dr. Martin Luther King, Jr., Health Center in the Bronx, has warned against the sentimental fallacy of assuming that poor people installed in positions of authority will continue to empathize with other poor people. "The 'half-life' of the subprofessional, during which he still identifies with the consumer, may last less than 24 hours," Wise has written. "Unless carefully supervised, he may begin to talk about 'my clients' and 'these people,' and to act in the same way as he had been acted 'upon' when he was on the other side of the establishment's desk." But although many of the people at the center seemed to be highly charged with energy and confidence, they did not seem to have forgotten what it is like to be poor. "When I'm in doubt about how to handle myself," a family health worker told me, "I ask myself what my caseworker would have done when I was on welfare. Then I do the opposite." And in going about the neighborhood with this woman and some of her associates I saw for myself that many poor people were getting sympathetic and practical help that was greatly needed and appreciated.

But it also became obvious that, in other ways, things were not working out at this particular center in quite the way the planners had hoped. I learned, for one thing, that the center's local advisory body, the Mid-Westside Neighborhood Health Council, had very little to say about how the center was run. This was not only because of the members' lack of experience in coping with complicated administrative and budgetary problems, although that plainly was part of the trouble. More importantly, the Council's impotence reflected the fact that important decisions were all made in Washington by the Office of Economic Opportunity, whose officials determined how much money the center was to get each year, and how that money was to be used. The only real power the Council had was over hiring and firing. Although this power was sometimes used to good purpose—for example, to screen out doctors who seemed likely to prove insensitive and condescending in their dealings with patients—much of the Council's energy went into acrimonious wrangling with the center's director over the qualifications and work habits of employees whom the director wanted to fire, but who happened to be protégés of Council members.

There was also trouble about the doctors. Although the pediatricians were by all accounts dedicated and conscientious, people at the center were not so happy with the internists who made up the balance of the full-time medical staff. At meeting after meeting I heard doctors criticized for their inability or unwillingness to accept the family health workers as collaborators, and accused of being lazy and perfunctory in their work. "The problem is how to get the doctors as enthusiastic about the program as most of the rest of the staff," the center's director remarked after one meeting. "I'm talking about the kind of commitment that we expect of our family health workers." At another meeting there was a long argument about a doctor who had been scheduled to see a patient, an elderly woman, at three-thirty in the afternoon. When she failed to show up until four (through no fault of hers, but because the miniambulance sent to pick her up had been delayed) the doctor kept her waiting for an hour while he took a nap on his examining table. A colleague argued that the doctor had not taken any time off for lunch that day, and that if he wanted to use his lunch hour for a nap instead of to eat that was his privilege. This defense failed to mollify the angry nurses and health workers, and it was obvious that a long procession of such incidents had made easy forgiveness out of the question.

Another source of frustration for the staff was its inability to give most of the center's patients the continuous care, in and out of the hospital, that the new centers were intended to provide. The difficulty lay in the center's relations with St. Luke's Hospital Center, fourteen blocks to the north, with which the center is formally affiliated, and through which it gets its money from Washington. Ideally, a health center patient should remain under the care of his team doctor even when he has to go into a hospital. If the hospital is a major teaching hospital, like St. Luke's, this may not be feasible. But even in a teaching hospital the team doctor could be encouraged to consult with the house staff on the care of his patients, just as he would if he were an attending physician who had hospitalized one of his private patients. This was, in fact, the arrangement for the hospital care of children enrolled at the center. But I was told that St. Luke's chief of medicine had refused to give the center's internists any special status at the hospital—or to pay any attention to their recommendations—and that, as a consequence, an adult patient requiring hospital care was likely to be treated pretty much like someone walking in off the street and presenting himself in the emergency room. "I had a patient with an acute gall bladder incident," one doctor at the center told me. "We sent her up to St. Luke's, with her history and records, and even so she was made to wait three hours so that she could be examined by an intern and a resident before they decided to admit her."

Not long ago, after an absence of two-and-a-half years, I went back to West 100th Street. The director's office was now occupied by a young black woman, Janice Robinson, who had been supervisor of public health nursing, and of the family workers, when I had visited the center in 1971. She seemed depressed, and when I asked her why, she said the problem was money. The center had been transferred from the Office of Economic Opportunity to the Department of Health, Education and Welfare, which was insisting that it become self-supporting. Miss Robinson explained that this would mean requiring at least half the center's enrollees—those not qualifying for Medicaid—to pay for care they had been getting free. Moreover, she said, since Medicaid would not reimburse the center for the salaries of its family health workers, some of them would have to be let go, and this, she added, was what was really depressing her.

I asked her how good a job she thought the center was doing. "Fairly decent," she said. "We've at least provided a place where the patient knows his doctor by name, a place where people come in and feel comfortable." She added that she had been reassured of this by a preliminary report from a Columbia University graduate student who had been interviewing patients at the center. "The big thing people zero in on is a feeling of comfort," Miss Robinson said. "They know the people on the staff, and the staff speaks their language." I asked if the center was still having trouble getting good doctors, and she said it was. "We began to attract younger doctors who went in for militant rhetoric about community control," she said bitterly. "We had two of them, and both left after a while for traditional jobs where they could concentrate on a specialty and do research. Still, some of the doctors here have changed. I've seen them ask family health workers not just for information, but for *conclusions*."

After leaving the director's office I stopped in to see the center's child psychiatrist, Eli Messinger. A friendly man with a bushy beard, Messinger is a former chairman of the Medical Committee for Human Rights, an organization dedicated to bringing about radical changes in American medical care. I asked him how things were going. "Every institution becomes self-perpetuating, self-protective, rigid to a degree," he said. "This one is no exception. It's getting more like a typical civil-service office: people shooting the breeze, drinking coffee. The community has been ineffective in flexing its muscle and giving direction to the program. The Council's presence should be felt here, but it isn't." He paused, and continued. "Still, it's a good place. Most patients get pretty good care. The difference from two years ago is that I don't expect it to change much for the better. I don't see any real push for improvement and change. It's just another project. We won't be wiped off the face of the earth, but we'll become more and more like everybody else offering medical care—more forms for people to fill out, more fees to be paid, more waiting."

The history of most other centers is not unlike that of the Neighborhood Health Services Program. Some centers have been able to get money to build or buy adequate facilities, but many have not. And all the centers are reluctantly having to give up their aim of giving free medical care to everyone living in their neighborhoods. Many centers, too, have been treated with indifference and condescension by the medical staffs of their affiliated hospitals. Most of these hospitals are teaching institutions, run by academic physicians who have little interest in patients with routine disorders and little interest in doctors who spend their time caring for such patients. What this can mean for the doctors at a health center, and for their patients, has been described by Dr. Samuel Standard, professor of clinical surgery at the New York University College of Medicine, an academic physician who does not share the prevailing attitude of his colleagues. Writing in the magazine *Medical Care*, Dr. Standard noted that he had had occasion to look into the arrangements for hospitalizing patients of a health center affiliated with Beth Israel Hospital, on New York's Lower East Side. On certain days, he had found, the chief surgical resident at Beth Israel went to the center to review cases requiring hospitalization, and to pick those that would be admitted by Beth Israel. "The rest must fend for themselves," Standard reported. "I have had long experience with Chief Residents and I can envisage this scene as a kind of slave market at which he can pick and choose the delectable surgical procedures that interest him and leave the others." Standard added, "The Center personnel must feel like mendicants standing hat in hand, head bowed, knees bent, waiting for a hand-out of a surgical bed from the mother hospital . . . the rat race the patients are subjected to in the effort to place them in a hospital is a disgrace."

It has been hard, too, for most centers to find and keep the kind of doctors they want. Many doctors cannot put up with having their judgments and actions challenged by nurses and community workers. A further difficulty is that doctors are taught to expect gratitude from their patients, and they do not always get it at a health center. The doctor working in a ghetto clinic, one observer has written, is "irritated, and his pride wounded, when patients to whom he has given much thought and attention break scheduled appointments and then come in unscheduled and demand to see him." Much the same point has been made by Dr. H. Jack Geiger. The professional, he has written, finds it "painful and stressful . . . to be involved and challenged; to have his half-conscious needs for gratitude and subservience go unmet." Not surprisingly, many young doctors who have gone to work in neighborhood health centers have quit after a year or so and fled to the suburbs; there is plenty of work for them there, and the patients know their place and are properly appreciative. Some doctors have left health centers for another reason. They have felt emotionally overwhelmed by the terrible afflictions of the poor—afflictions which medicine alone is, of course, often powerless to cure.

Many people connected with health centers share Eli Messinger's regret that they have failed to demonstrate the feasibility of a new relationship between poor people and the institutions that are meant to serve them. Transactions between the professionals manning the health centers and the local residents on the centers' community boards have been marked by paternalism and benevolent arrogance on one side, and by bitterness and apathy on the other. Board members have angrily complained, sometimes with reason, that the new missionaries descending on their neighborhoods really wanted their gratitude, not their collaboration. Doctors and other professionals, for their part, have been impatient with people who are not used to thinking very far ahead (long-range planning is a luxury beyond the means of the very poor) and who seem to approach problems with their emotions rather than their intellects. Collaboration has been made harder by the difficulty many doctors and nurses have in accepting black mothers on welfare, or Puerto Rican busboys, in decision-making roles. One physician who helped to found a health center, Dr. Eva J. Salber, has written that doctors see such people only "as patients, or as people whose children may be emotionally disturbed, or delinquent, or school phobics, or bedwetters, or neglected." Members of health-center boards have also been resentfully aware that even if the money for their center were to come directly to the board, instead of being funneled through a sponsoring hospital, the important decisions—for example, decisions as to whom the center should serve, and on what terms—would still be made in Washington.

This is not the place to analyze and pass judgment on the notion, written into law by the planners of the War on Poverty, that there should be "maximum feasible participation" by the poor in everything done on their behalf. But it can be said with certainty that the neighborhood health centers, with some exceptions such as the center at Mound Bayou, have not had the galvanizing effect on their communities that their founders, perhaps naively, had expected. Disappointment on this score has been expressed by, among others, Dr. William Lloyd, director of the Martin Luther King, Jr., Health Center in the Bronx. Martin Luther King is at once one of the most innovative and one of the best-managed of the health centers, and Lloyd, who gave up a career as an academic specialist in kidney diseases to become its first medical director in 1966, is highly enthusiastic about team medicine as it is practiced there. "Working with a team is a fantastic experience," he told me. "I think the care we've developed here has gone light years beyond what has been done before." But he went on to speak with irony and regret of some of the hopes with which he had begun his work at the center. "We have been unable to have any real impact on social conditions," he said. "We're a very small institution shaped by enormous outside forces. Like Don Quixote, we thought we were going to change the way the Welfare Department treats our patients. Hah!" Lloyd continued, "I also had a feeling that, at the personal level, the combination of personalized services, community organization, and community control would reinvigorate our clients, change the welfare dependency syndrome, remedy the lack of black pride. But I don't think we've affected all this very much. I don't think we're breaking the welfare-poverty cycle. If anything is going to change this around here it will be things like the black-is-beautiful movement, not what we do."

Some of the lessons to be drawn from Medicare and Medicaid, and from the history of the neighborhood health centers, are obvious enough. Medicare has shown the folly of injecting billions of dollars of new purchasing power into the medical-care market without adequate cost controls. Medicare's history would also seem to argue against any plan for national health insurance that requires people to pay a large part of their medical bills out of their own pockets, and that forces them to undergo the humiliating ordeal of a means test when their pockets are empty. The way to save money on medical care is to devise more economical ways of delivering it, not to put the squeeze on sick people.

Finally, Medicaid and the neighborhood health centers have both shown clearly that devising special programs for the poor is not the best way of seeing to it that they get better medical care. Medicaid has failed so dismally mainly because it is a welfare program, a form of compulsory charity that furnishes handouts to the poor and (presumably) shiftless at the expense of the hard-working taxpayer. People on Medicaid are given cut-rate services on the theory that they don't deserve anything better, and they are made to pay for these services in the same coin—humiliation—that doctors and hospitals so often in the past have exacted from the poor. The health centers have been unable to realize their potential effectiveness because they, too, offer handouts to the poor, handouts that the government can reduce or do away with any time it wants. All this strongly supports the arguments, which I shall be making in the next chapter, for the passage of a national health insurance scheme that is not only unencumbered by deductibles and co-payments, but that also gives the poor and the near-poor, as a matter of right, exactly the same claim on doctors and other providers of medical care as everybody else.

National Health Insurance: The Need for Heroic Therapy

In 1969 the AMA, whose official spokesman had once described national health insurance as "perhaps the most virulent scheme ever to be conjured out of the mind of man," unveiled a national health insurance plan of its own. Calling its scheme Medicredit, the AMA proposed that the federal government, through tax credits and cash subsidies, should make it possible for every American to buy comprehensive health insurance at a price he could afford. Coverage would be provided by insurance companies, or by Blue Cross or Blue Shield, and critics were quick to point out that the AMA seemed bent on rewarding the health insurance industry for its shortcomings by handing it a blank check on the federal treasury. But the defects of the AMA's plan were less significant than the fact that the association had offered a plan at all. Twenty years earlier, the AMA and other opponents of President Truman's health insurance plan had been able to contend, with some show of plausibility, that the insurance industry was well on its way to furnishing Americans with all the protection they needed. In the unlikely event that it should fail to reach this goal, they argued, it would be time enough for the government to step in. By the late 1960s, that time was clearly at hand. By then, anyone who thought about the matter, including the leaders of the AMA, could see that there was an irreducible gap between the coverage that private insurers could provide and the coverage that most Americans felt they ought to have.

The rising sentiment for national health insurance was fortified by the results of what had already been done to patch up the worst holes in the existing system for financing medical care. Medicare, for all its faults, had been a popular program. It had meant more and better care for older people, and it had made it easier for them (and for their children) to pay their medical bills. Inevitably it struck many people that what was good for the old might be good for the young as well. The failures of Medicaid, like the successes of Medicare, also converted many politicians to the cause of national health insurance. Some saw it as the only way to provide something better for the poor than the dreary poorhouse medicine that Medicaid usually offered. Others had more direct and pressing reasons. "City and state governments are terrified by the pressure put on their already strained budgets by the galloping inflation of medical costs," Dr. George A. Silver of the Yale School of Medicine, who was then serving as an officer of the National Urban Coalition, pointed out in 1970 in the *American Journal of Public Health*. As a consequence, he wrote, local and state officials "were terribly anxious for the government to take over the health insurance business." Other people, too, were angered and dismayed by the way medical bills soared after the passage of Medicare. "Just as fast as we could negotiate money to provide more and better health services for our members," George Meany of the AFL-CIO observed bitterly, "the doctors raised their fees and the hospitals boosted their charges." In the circumstances, more and more people grew skeptical of the notion that things would work out for the best if only doctors, hospitals, and insurance companies were left to themselves.

The AMA, of course, has not been alone in putting forward a detailed plan for national health insurance. In 1974 and 1975 Congress had before it bills reflecting the views of, among others, the health insurance industry, the American Hospital Association, the United States Chamber of Commerce, the AFL-CIO, and the Nixon and Ford Administrations. Some of these bills differed greatly from one another in the extent to which they would modify existing arrangements for medical care. At one extreme was the AMA's bill, a modification of its original Medicredit plan, which would leave doctors free to charge pretty much whatever they liked; would forbid the federal government "to exercise any control over the practice of medicine or the manner in which medical services are provided"; and would, in general, limit the government's role to pumping billions of dollars a year into the buyers' side of the medical market. At the other extreme was the so-called Health Security bill, enthusiastically backed by organized labor and, for many years, by Senator Kennedy. If enacted, a bill written along its lines would enormously stimulate the growth of prepaid group practice, and would put doctors remaining in fee-for-service practice under heavy pressure to accept government-imposed ceilings on their fees. It would also give the federal government a considerable say in deciding what kinds of operations a doctor may perform, what kinds of postgraduate courses he takes, and even what brands of drugs he prescribes. In 1974 Kennedy tried to find some common ground among all these proposals on which Congress and the Administration might both be willing to take a stand. Breaking with his labor supporters, he joined with Representative Wilbur Mills of Arkansas (who was then still chairman of the House Ways and Means Committee, and whose support was thought to be indispensable if any health insurance bill was to pass) in backing a new bill of their own. This attempt at compromise bogged down rather quickly in Mills's own committee, however, indicating that disagreement over the form that national health insurance should take runs so deep that it may be years before any bill is enacted into law.

Although drawing up a detailed plan for national health insurance is a complicated business—the Kennedy-Mills bill ran to 254 pages—it is not hard to list the ingredients such a plan should contain. To start with, everybody should automatically be covered. One of the chief defects of most of the bills before Congress in 1974 was that coverage would be optional. Thus under the plan backed by the Nixon and Ford administrations (which I shall refer to for brevity's sake as the Nixon bill) insurance would be compulsory only to the extent that employers would have to offer all full-time, regular employees a specified package of benefits. The package would include catastrophic coverage, limiting a family's liability for hospital and doctors' bills to a maximum of $1500 a year. Seventy-five per cent of the cost—more, if he agreed—would be borne by the employer, and the rest by the employee. But no employee would be forced to accept coverage. Similarly, while the government would pay all or part of the cost of individual policies taken out by self-employed or part-time workers with incomes of less than $7500 a year, no one would be forced to buy such a policy.

An arrangement of this kind appeals to most people on the sellers' side of the market. They tend to see compulsory insurance as a threat to their independence, fearing that if the government forces its citizens to buy health insurance it will inevitably insist on having a lot to say about what they are getting for their money.

But apart from the fact that cost and quality controls should be written into any health insurance scheme, voluntary or compulsory, there are sound reasons why coverage should be compulsory—or, to put it another way, universal and automatic. So long as coverage is optional, some people will choose to buy cut-rate, inadequate policies, and others will choose not to buy any insurance at all. Under a plan such as Nixon proposed, the number of such people would have run into the millions. Small employers would have had strong incentives to farm out as much work as possible to part-time or temporary employees, for whom they would not have been required to lay out any money for health insurance. (An employer could also save money by making prospective employees promise that they would turn down the insurance coverage that he would be legally required to offer them.) Moreover, under the scheme put forward by Nixon—and most other voluntary plans are quite similar in this respect—people who are self-employed, or who are working only part-time, could get standard coverage for themselves and their families only by buying individual policies, for which families earning more than $7500 a year would have to pay the full cost. That cost would come to at least $75 a month for a family of four, and a man averaging, say, $800 a month as an odd-job man or seasonal laborer might well decide this was too stiff a price, and settle for a cheaper policy that would leave him with huge bills in the event of a serious illness.

Opponents of compulsory coverage argue that this is fair enough, that it is a man's own risk if he passes up a chance to provide for his own and his family's care. But of course it is not entirely his own responsibility. No one any longer contends that a person who has been run over by a car, or has suffered a heart attack, or is about to have a baby, should be denied a hospital bed or a doctor's care even if he (or she) lacks means to pay for them. Under any of the voluntary plans that Congress has been considering, doctors and hospitals would still be expected to take care of seriously ill people who had exercised their option not to buy insurance. Each year, hundreds of thousands of people would be the beneficiaries of a grudging institutional charity—charity that could be largely done away with, at very little extra expense to society, by putting everybody under the umbrella of national health insurance.

National health insurance should not only be compulsory, but it should be paid for by taxes. A major objection to the Nixon bill, and to several other bills before Congress in 1974, was that while insurance for people in low income brackets would be heavily subsidized by tax money, other people would have to pay the full, actuarially-determined cost of coverage. It is true that most people would be insured by their employers, who would pay most or all of the necessary premiums. But the money would really come out of the employees' pockets. A company that employs ten thousand people, and that spends $7 million a year for health insurance, is, in effect, deducting $700 a year from the pay of each employee. And unless an employee is permitted to take the $700 in cash if he prefers, an alternative that none of the plans now being considered would offer him, he is actually being subjected to a regressive tax, one which takes a much bigger bite, proportionally, out of the paycheck of a file clerk than it takes out of the president's salary. Under the Kennedy-Mills compromise plan, by contrast, benefits would have been paid for by a new 4 per cent payroll tax: 3 per cent to be paid by employers, and 1 per cent by employees. This would have made a big difference to people with low-to-middle incomes. Assuming that the entire cost is really borne by the employee, an $11,000-a-year bookkeeper with a wife and two children would have paid $440 for his health insurance under the Mills-Kennedy plan (4 per cent of $11,000), as against $600 to $700 under the Nixon Administration proposal.

People who take the Nixon and Ford Administrations' approach to national health insurance, as well as those who support the AMA and insurance-industry bills, see nothing wrong with requiring most Americans to pay the actual cost of their insurance. Their attitude is reasonable enough if one considers medical care to be in the same category as groceries or shoes or housing. But if it is to be considered as a public or community service, which should be available without stint to everyone who needs it, then it seems fairer to ask everyone to contribute to the cost of medical care—his and other people's—in proportion to his ability to pay, and make that contribution obligatory.

With the important exception of the plan backed by labor, which would dispense entirely with deductibles and co-payments, all the health insurance plans that have been urged on Congress in recent years would require people to pay some part of their medical and hospital bills with their own money. Under the 1974 Mills-Kennedy proposal, for example, a typical family would be liable for the first $300 of medical expenses in any year, and would have to pay 25 per cent of bills in excess of that amount. There would be a limit of $1000, however, on the total sum that a family would have to lay out, after which all further expenses would be paid by the government.

The trouble with cost-sharing, as it is called in the insurance business (the term is thought to fall less harshly on the ear than "deductibles" and "co-payment"), is that it may discourage people, especially those with little money to spare, from seeing a doctor when they should. Deductibles and co-payments can, of course, be scaled to income. Under the Mills-Kennedy bill, families earning less than $4800 a year would pay nothing at all for most kinds of medical care, while the out-of-pocket expenses of a family earning $7000 would be limited to $550. Kennedy and Mills further proposed that certain kinds of preventive care—well-baby checkups and prenatal examinations, for example—should be covered in full whether the patient was rich or poor. Provisions such as these would obviously mitigate the harmful effects of cost-sharing. But by the same token they would tend to defeat its main purpose, which is to make people think twice before going to a doctor. If medical care were entirely free, it is often argued, American doctors, who are already overworked, would be overwhelmed, not just by people with legitimate medical problems, but by chronic worriers with trivial complaints that do not really require medical attention.

It is possible to get a pretty good fix on the validity of this argument by considering the present state of medical practice in Montreal. Montrealers, like most Canadians, have for some years had their hospital bills paid by the government. But until more recently, unless they were getting public assistance, they paid their own doctors' bills (in some cases with the help of private insurance). Then, in November, 1970, all residents of

Montreal, and of the entire province of Quebec, became eligible for free doctor's care at government expense. There had been dire predictions about what the new system would do to the quality of medical care in Quebec, and well before it was to go into operation a group of researchers at McGill University in Montreal, and at the University of Pittsburgh, had made plans to measure some of its immediate effects. In 1969 and 1970 they interviewed some 11,000 residents of Montreal and its suburbs. Later, after the new law—known in Canada as Medicare—had been in effect for a year or so, they interviewed many of the same people again, along with some 5000 persons who had not been seen the first time around. The researchers also had before-and-after interviews with several hundred Montreal doctors.

They found, among other things, that in late 1971 and 1972 it took almost twice as long to get an appointment with a doctor—an average of eleven days instead of six—as it had taken two or three years before. They also found that poor people were going to doctors much more frequently, and rich people somewhat less frequently, than before Medicare. Unskilled laborers, for example, had increased the frequency of their visits to a doctor by 68 per cent, while executives, owners of large businesses, and "major professionals" had cut the number of their visits by 25 per cent.

As had been predicted, some of the new patients who were crowding the waiting rooms of Montreal's doctors probably didn't need to be there. Doctors reported that the proportion of their patients who had "sought medical advice without reasonable cause" had risen slightly since Medicare—from 1.1 per cent to 1.9 per cent. The researchers had also made plans to get a line on how Medicare would affect people really needing medical advice. In both rounds of interviews, each interviewee was presented with a list of common symptoms generally considered serious enough to call for a doctor's attention. The list included, for example, chest pains coupled with shortness of breath; an unexplained loss of weight; and a cough lasting more than two weeks. Before Medicare, 38 per cent of the people interviewed who reported having had one or more of the symptoms during the previous twelve months said they had not consulted a doctor about them. After Medicare the proportion dropped to 27 per cent.

The greatest change was reported by people with annual incomes of less than $3000. But at every income level except the highest, people suffering from one of the designated symptoms were more likely to see a doctor than they had been before the government had undertaken to pay the bill. For people with annual incomes of $15,000 and over, who had generally been quick to consult their doctors even before the new law went into effect, Medicare made no difference. Putting all the evidence together, the picture looked like this: Since Medicare, people with low and moderate incomes had been taking up so much of the time of Montreal's doctors—mainly for quite legitimate reasons—that the city's more prosperous residents, forced to wait ten days to two weeks for an appointment, were letting minor complaints run their course instead of seeing a doctor about them. This, of course, is what the poor had always done.

Both patients and doctors were asked by the McGill and University of Pittsburgh researchers what effect they thought the new law had had on the quality of medical care. One out of four patients, including one out of four of those with the lowest incomes, said they thought the treatment people were getting from their doctors was "worse than it used to be." Only one in eight said they thought treatment had improved. But there were indications that some people were basing their negative opinions on irritation over long waits for appointments, and on hearsay, rather than on their own encounters with doctors. When people who had seen a doctor during the preceding year were asked whether they had received "the best possible care," 91.4 per cent said they had. This hardly differed from the 92.8 per cent who had answered "Yes" to the same question in the pre-Medicare round of interviews. As for doctors, only 18 per cent said they thought the new law had lowered the quality of medical care. An almost equal number—17 per cent—were of the opinion that patients, by and large, were getting better care than before Medicare. Fifty-nine per cent said the law had made no difference.

The implications for Americans are quite clear. Making medical care free would be most unlikely to damage its quality. On the contrary, care would greatly improve in the sense that many more people than now—not all of them poor—would go to a doctor as promptly as doctors would like them to. (A few more people than now would also seek medical attention that they don't really need, but Montreal's experience does not suggest that doctors' offices would be overrun by an army of hypochondriacs.) There would be a price to be paid for the benefits of free care: the demand for doctors' services would increase and, given the present supply and distribution of physicians, many middle-class and upper-middle-class people who can still get in to see their doctors on fairly short notice would find it much harder to get an appointment unless their symptoms were serious. Over a period of years this situation could be eased by training more doctors, and by inducing them to go into useful specialties—family practice, for example—and to settle in communities where they are most needed. But in the short run, there is no getting around the fact that while free medical care would be good for the poor and the near-poor, it would be bad—anyway, annoying and inconvenient—for the rich and the near-rich. The only way to avoid the annoyance and inconvenience is to burden national health insurance with deductibles and co-payments high enough to keep many people away from doctors' offices except in case of dire necessity.

The AMA has taken the remarkable (though not surprising) position that even under national health insurance a doctor should be quite free to decide for himself what he is to be paid for his work. Given the surge in the demand for doctors' services that would follow the enactment of a health insurance bill—even one requiring a lot of cost-sharing—doctors' fees, if uncontrolled, would be likely to shoot up even faster than in the early Medicare years. The drafters of plans other than the AMA's have therefore generally proposed some limits at least on some fees. The Nixon bill, for example, would have permitted doctors, when treating most patients (those covered by employer plans), to charge whatever they liked. As under Medicare, if a doctor had chosen to charge more than the patient's insurance company considered reasonable, the patient would then have been expected to make up the difference out of his own pocket. But in the case of patients who were old or poor, a doctor would have had to accept, as full payment for his services, specified fees established by negotiation between his local medical society and a designated state agency. This would have been a little less inflationary than the AMA's scheme, but inflationary nonetheless. Moreover, applying a double standard to doctors' fees is not a good idea. Under a plan like the Nixon Administration's, treating the old and the poor would have tended to be less profitable, on a dollars-per-minute basis, than treating the young and prosperous. As a result, many doctors would have avoided taking as patients people who were old or poor, or else would have treated them, as many doctors now treat people on Medicaid, as semicharity cases, deserving neither the time nor the consideration due to higher-paying patients.

In their 1974 bill, Kennedy and Mills set forth a somewhat better scheme for regulating fees. In each city or county, the local medical society would have drawn up a fee schedule, and any doctor signing up with the national health insurance plan would have been bound to follow it whether his patient was on welfare or making $100,000 a year. This did not mean, however, that doctors could collectively set their own price. A medical society would have had to set fees at such a level that total payments to doctors in its area would not exceed, over the coming year, a specified total. That total would have been equal to the sum of all fees collected by doctors in that area in the year 1973, adjusted to take into account such factors as population growth and changes in the general price level. If a proposed fee schedule appeared to violate these guidelines, the government could turn it down and, if necessary, impose a schedule of its own.

But even under the proposed Mills-Kennedy plan a doctor could elect to stay outside the health insurance system, and to charge whatever he liked. If he did so, he would not have the privilege, available to participating doctors, of sending the government a consolidated weekly bill for his services. Instead, he would have to go to the trouble and expense of billing patients individually, and of helping them to fill out the claims they would have to file in order to get back some of the money they had paid him. Nevertheless, and despite the cost to patients in time and money, even if the Mills-Kennedy proposal were put into effect it is likely that many doctors would choose to take their chances outside the system unless the standard fees were boosted every year or so. This obviously would raise the average cost of doctors' services and, at the same time, tend to perpetuate the present arrangement whereby one kind of doctor treats the poor, and another kind treats everybody else.

Perhaps the best way to avoid such difficulties would be to

follow the line taken by organized labor. The Health Security bill, which labor is backing, provides that the government will pay no portion of a doctor's bill unless he has agreed never to charge more for his services, no matter how grateful and well-heeled a patient might be, than is specified by an official fee schedule. A doctor could refuse to sign such an agreement, and undertake to earn his living by treating only those patients able and willing to pay him with their own money. But the total number of such patients—and the total number of doctors catering to them—would obviously not be large. The great majority of people, under this system, would be treated by doctors whose fees would be regulated, and who would earn exactly the same amount of money for treating a migrant farmworker as they would for treating his employer.

National health insurance should, finally, be designed so as to reward efficiency and penalize extravagance and profiteering (just how this might be done will be considered presently) and the necessary controls should be in the hands of the federal government. By contrast, most of the insurance schemes recently urged on Congress call for state regulation.

Under the Nixon Administration's plan, for example, it would have been up to each state to pass on the reasonableness of hospital charges and insurance premiums. The authors of the plan were vague as to just how a state would carry out this mandate, or what would happen if it should fall down on the job. The bill that the insurance industry has been pushing is more specific. Each hospital and nursing home would have to draw up a schedule of charges and submit it for approval to a special state commission. This body, which would function something like a public utility commission, would also be empowered to pass on the insurance plans that each state would establish to cover the poor and the near-poor; each such plan would be administered by an insurance carrier, or by a group of carriers, on a cost-plus basis, with the size of the "plus" to be determined by the state. The Department of Health, Education and Welfare would be charged with regulating the regulators. Insurance coverage for people with low incomes would be heavily subsidized by Washington under the insurance industry's proposal, and, if HEW concluded that a state commission was too soft on the insurance companies or hospitals under its jurisdiction, it could withhold federal funds until the commission mended its ways.

The trouble with such schemes is that many states would not be up to the job of coping with the formidable economic and political power of the health-care industry. There would, of course, be exceptions: New York, for example, is already quite successfully curbing the exuberance of hospital promoters. But the alacrity with which state legislatures have customarily acceded to the wishes of lobbyists for industry is not an encouraging omen. ("The states have no ability to regulate the insurance industry and their track record proves it," Herbert Denenberg told a Senate committee not long ago. "To turn national health insurance over to the states would be disastrous.") Moreover, state regulation of public utilities has often been a dismal failure. Utility companies have packed regulatory commissions with their friends, and have used their influence with state legislators to deprive commissions of the professional staffs they would need in order to do a proper job of regulation. An investigator who looked into utility regulation in the states recently reported, "Four public service commissions have no attorney on their staff; seventeen, only one; another nine, only two. . . . Twenty commissions have only one or two accountants."

Federal agencies, too, can be co-opted or emasculated by the industries they are supposed to regulate. Just recently, a Senate committee heard testimony that drug experts employed by the Food and Drug Administration had been transferred or fired after declining to clear certain new drugs whose safety or efficacy had not, in their professional opinion, been clearly demonstrated by their drug-company sponsors. But federal regulatory agencies at least are scrutinized more sharply—by Congress, by the press, and by Ralph Nader—than their state counterparts, and therefore probably tend to do a better job. It is true that provision can be made, as in the insurance-industry bill, for the federal government to second-guess the states in the matter of hospital costs and the like. But quite apart from the awkwardness of such an arrangement from an administrative standpoint, a federal agency that sticks its nose into a state's business, even with statutory authority to do so, is almost certain to raise a furious political storm. In any case, if the states cannot be counted on to do a proper job of regulating the flow of public money to doctors, hospitals, nursing homes, and insurance companies, it would seem sensible to let the federal government do the regulating in the first place.

"For too long," Senator Edward Kennedy has complained, "we have accommodated the vested interests of the health-care industry—the special pleaders, the healer-dealers, and the health imperialists. They have had carte blanche for generations to develop the health system for their own private benefit, to the detriment of the public interest. . . . Rome is burning, and yet the American Medical Association doesn't even smell the smoke." The only way to put out the fire, Kennedy suggested on another occasion, was to pass the health insurance bill backed by organized labor—a bill whose enactment, he said, would guarantee high-quality and humane medical care for all Americans, and would result "not only in billions of dollars saved, but also in millions of lives preserved and untold human suffering averted."

This sort of talk is obviously not calculated to win the hearts and minds of America's doctors. Even those who cannot fairly be categorized as either healer-dealers or health imperialists, and who may themselves be critical of the way medical care is bought and sold in America, have tended to write Kennedy off as a political quack whose nostrums would do the patient more harm than good. Their suspicions of what had come to be known as the Kennedy Bill were doubtless strengthened when Kennedy himself backed away from it, noting sadly that the country wasn't ready yet for such a measure, and joined Mills in supporting a compromise bill less threatening to doctors and the insurance industry, and less alarming to fiscal conservatives.

But even though the remedy that Kennedy once so enthusiastically prescribed would be unlikely to act with the miraculous efficacy he claimed for it, the fault is with the label he put on the bottle, not with its ingredients. The old Kennedy Bill, as some congressmen have taken to calling it, is a carefully thought-out proposal, reflecting the views of a number of well-respected academic experts on public health and the economics of medical care. It is the only plan commanding serious Congressional support that contains all the elements I have listed as essential to a proper health insurance system. And while the odds are against its enactment into law in the next few years, it is indispensable as a yardstick against which to measure the merits and demerits of competing schemes.

The aims of the old Kennedy, or Health Security, bill have sometimes been misrepresented by its opponents. President Nixon, in his 1974 State of the Union address, warned darkly of politicians who would "put our whole health-care system under the heavy hand of government." He went on to say, "This is the wrong approach that has been tried abroad and it's failed. It is not the way we do things here in America. . . . Government has a great role to play, but we must always make sure that our doctors will be working for their patients and not for the federal government."

Nixon's comments were misleading in two respects. If he was alluding to England's National Health Service when he spoke of a wrong approach, his claim that it has failed would certainly be disputed by most Englishmen. Moreover, the English variety of socialized medicine is not at all what the drafters of the Health Security bill had in mind for the United States. In England, hospitals are almost all run by local governments. Fee-for-service medicine exists only for a relatively few people who are willing to pay their doctors' bills themselves; with few exceptions, general practitioners must rely for their livelihood on fixed annual retainers—so many pounds a year for each patient on their lists—while specialists must have salaried hospital jobs. And while an Englishman can choose his own GP, he can not ordinarily choose his surgeon or psychiatrist. Under the Health Security bill, by contrast, most Americans would still be taken care of, when seriously ill, in independent, not-for-profit hospitals run by their own autonomous boards of directors. Doctors would be free to decide for themselves how they would be paid, and in what sort of setting they would work. A surgeon or a family physician or a radiologist might choose to work as a salaried member of a hospital staff. Or he might become a partner in, or an employee of, a group of doctors affiliated with a prepaid group practice plan. Or he might elect, as most doctors do now, to go into private practice, charging by the visit or by the operation, and deciding for himself what hours he would keep, how many patients he would see, and what kinds of diseases he would treat. Patients, for their part, unless they had contracted with a plan like Kaiser for all their medical care, would be free to consult, at government expense, any doctor they liked—

provided only that the doctor was not one of those, presumably few in number, choosing to stay outside the health insurance system.

But if the Health Security bill were to become law, medical care in America would become, far more than it is now, a social, if not a socialist, enterprise. Hospitals, HMOs, and doctors in private fee-for-service practice who agreed to participate in the new insurance scheme would be paid exclusively and directly by the federal government. Medical care would be available to everybody on the same terms as the privilege of walking in a city park or driving on an interstate highway. No American would have to pay to have a baby delivered or an appendix removed, to go to a doctor for a shot or a checkup, or to get regular psychiatric help. Eye examinations, eyeglasses, and hearing aids would be free, and so would most prescription drugs. Children under fifteen at the time the plan went into effect would be entitled to free dental care (orthodontia excepted) for the rest of their lives. Eventually, when enough dentists and technicians had been trained to satisfy the demand for their services, free dental care would be available to everybody. To help pay for all this, there would be a new 3.5 per cent payroll tax (to be paid by employers); a 1 per cent tax on employees' paychecks; a 1 per cent tax on dividends and other unearned income; and a 2.5 per cent tax on the earnings of people who work for themselves. Each dollar raised in this fashion would be matched by a dollar taken from general tax revenues and earmarked for medical care.

If the Health Security bill had been in effect in 1973 it would have cost around $80 billion, and opponents have thrown up their hands in dismay at the thought of putting so huge a load on the back of the suffering American taxpayer. But such criticism is rather disingenuous. Almost all the money that would be raised in new taxes would be used to pay for the same goods and services that Americans would otherwise be paying for through private insurance plans, through taxes to support Medicaid and Medicare, and by shelling out money directly to doctors and hospitals. Some money, perhaps $5 billion a year, would be spent on drugs, hearing aids, dental care, routine checkups, and other medical goods and services that people need but are not getting now because they can't afford them. But the main effect of financing medical care in the manner proposed by the backers of the Health Security bill would be to make each person's contribution roughly proportional to his ability to pay. People earning, say, $10,000 to $15,000 a year would pay a lot less for medical care than they do now, and less than they would have to pay under any of the other plans that Congress has been considering. People in higher brackets would, of course, generally pay more—which no doubt explains much of the violent opposition to the bill.

There is also fierce opposition to the bill because it would largely do away with private health insurance and make the federal government, in Kennedy's words, "the insurance agent for all Americans." Thus President Nixon, noting that his own scheme for national health insurance would rely extensively on private insurers, told Congress early in 1974, "I firmly believe we should capitalize on the skills and facilities already in place, not replace them and start from scratch with a huge federal bureaucracy to add to the ones we already have." This attitude is widely shared in Congress.

But the choice is not really between a vast new federal bureaucracy and no bureaucracy. Rather it is between a new federal bureaucracy and the old private bureaucracy we already have. Under present arrangements a doctor already has to fill out and sign, in the course of a month, a bewildering variety of claim forms: one for Medicare, another for Medicaid, another for Blue Shield, and still others for private insurance companies. Not long ago, when I visited the offices of a medical group affiliated with a small hospital in Monterey County, California, the director told me that the group does business with more than two hundred insurance companies. "We have as many girls working on insurance claims as we have doctors," he said gloomily. A Congressional expert on the economics of medical care, who had a hand in drafting the Health Security bill, recently observed, "If you took the administrative bureaucracy that we've tucked away in individual hospitals all over the country, and in doctors' offices, and in insurance companies—if you take all the hospital people handling insurance claims, there's a bureaucracy out there that's incredibly complex. The only difference is that it's not visible—it's all spread out."

Actually, a health insurance scheme that covers everyone automatically, and is financed by federal taxes, should be much easier and cheaper to administer than our existing mixture of public and private insurance. With no need to sell people health insurance policies, there would be no need to lay out money for advertising or for commissions to agents or salesmen. Hospitals and doctors would have one set of claim forms to fill out, and one set of rules to follow. (Under the Health Security bill, bookkeeping would be further simplified because there would be no need to deal with co-payments and deductibles.) Finally, when everyone is entitled to the same benefits, there is no need to spend tens of millions of man-hours each year, as would be necessary under many of the plans Congress has been looking into, to determine who is eligible for government subsidies, and in what amounts. (Anyone who thinks this would not be a serious problem is invited to consider the following passage from the Nixon Administration's 1974 insurance bill: "An assisted health care insurance plan," it begins, "must, subject to paragraph [4], impose, with respect to all items and services other than outpatient drugs and biologicals, and other blood and blood products, a per individual per calendar year deductible equal to the following percentages of the deductible base. . . .")

The question remains whether, under a system in which medical care is financed by tax money, that money can be distributed to doctors and hospitals more efficiently by private organizations or by the government. George Meany of the AFL-CIO, who is convinced the government can do a better job, has cited the low overhead costs of government-run health insurance plans in Canada. In one recent year, he pointed out to the House Ways and Means Committee, the province of Saskatchewan reported administrative costs amounting to only 2.1 per cent of total payments to hospitals, and 4.94 per cent of the total sum paid out to doctors. In neighboring Manitoba the corresponding figures were 1.5 per cent and 4.08 per cent. In the United States, by comparison, administrative costs absorb 4 to 5 per cent of the money that Blue Cross collects from subscribers to its hospitalization plans, and around 11 per cent of the money that Blue Shield subscribers pay for medical coverage. The figures of course are not exactly comparable (Saskatchewan and Manitoba don't have to solicit subscribers) but they do suggest that government bureaucrats can do an efficient job of handling payments under a national health insurance plan. Furthermore, as I have indicated, the insurance companies and Blue Cross and Blue Shield have not been notably efficient in taking care of the government's Medicaid and Medicare business.

Elaborate data-processing systems have been set up by private insurers to handle the huge volume of business that they do, and obviously it would be foolish for the government to replace these with systems of its own. This is not what the authors of the Health Security bill had in mind. "Actually, there's nothing in the bill that says the government won't contract for a great deal of what needs to be done," one of Kennedy's assistants points out. "If you think about it, you are almost obliged to do this. There's a tremendous technology out there in the sheer claims-processing machinery. And very likely the government would try to sign contracts with some of the major carriers to do that on a cost-plus arrangement." With proper government supervision, such arrangements—which would have been mandatory under the Mills-Kennedy compromise bill—would make good sense. But there is no reason why the insurance industry should be granted the privilege it has been vigorously claiming, which is to be allowed to go on operating pretty much as it does now, but with the government underwriting a greatly stepped-up demand for its services. To put the industry in this cozy situation, as the AMA and the Nixon Administration were both proposing in 1974, makes little more sense than if we were to relieve the Internal Revenue Service of the responsibility for collecting the income tax, and to farm the job out to private firms.

Supporters of the Health Security bill can derive some comfort from the fact that the AMA is past its political prime. One clear sign is that it was unable to prevent the passage, in 1972, of the law under which Professional Standards Review Organizations are being set up to watch over the quality and cost of hospital care paid for by Medicare and Medicaid—a law that the AMA's president-elect described, shortly after its enactment, as "the greatest threat to the private practice of medicine of any piece of legislation ever passed by Congress."

If politicians have grown more skeptical of the AMA's apocalyptic pronouncements it is partly because the AMA's stubborn opposition to Medicare convinced many people that, in political and social matters, the doctor does not necessarily know best. The AMA's authority has also been sapped by the enormous expansion of medical-school faculties, and by the entry of more and more hospitals into arrangements under which their medical staffs are selected and supervised by medical-school professors. This has given great power and prestige to a class of physicians who often do not bother to join the AMA, and whose main business is teaching and research, or directing the work of teachers and researchers.

These bishops and archbishops of scientific medicine, having thrived on federal subsidies and in the administrative jungles of academic medical centers, do not, as a rule, share the morbid fear of government, and the fierce attachment to entrepreneurial medicine, that are so commonly displayed by doctors in private practice. They tend, therefore, to look with favor on schemes for national health insurance that include provisions intended to jack up the quality of medical practice and to hold down doctors' fees. A few have even had harsh words to say about the idea of fee-for-service medicine. Dr. Martin Cherkasky, an accomplished federal grantsman who is the director of Montefiore Hospital in the Bronx, has called the fee-for-service system "professionally undignified" and "a mechanism of payment almost calculated to seduce the doctor into placing cash before care." The views expressed by people like Cherkasky are treated respectfully by Congress and the media, and they have made it much harder for the AMA to present its opinions as revelations whose truth is necessarily accepted by everyone with a license to practice medicine. At the same time, the private practitioner's ability to set his patients straight on the economics of medical practice has been impaired as his encounters with them have become briefer and more impersonal. A doctor seeing forty patients a day doesn't have time to explain why limitations on doctors' fees would destroy American medicine.

But even though the AMA's views have come to strike a great many Americans as archaic and self-serving, they still carry a lot of weight in Washington. In 1972 and 1973, for instance, the AMA was able to cool down, to a point only a few degrees above absolute zero, the Nixon Administration's earlier enthusiasm for Kaiser-style HMOs. One reason its lobbyists are so successful is that they are prepared to put their money where their mouths are. Between the Presidential election in 1972 and September, 1974, the AMA's political arm, the American Medical Political Action Committee, together with its state affiliates, contributed a total of more than $600,000 to the campaign funds of twenty-one senators and 205 members of the House of Representatives. The beneficiaries included Representative Omar Burleson of Texas, a leading supporter of the AMA's Medicredit plan, who got $4000 even though he was unopposed in both the 1974 Democratic primary and in the general election that followed. Moreover, senators and congressmen are convinced that the doctors who count in their communities generally take their cue from the AMA's leaders, and that a politician who gets on the AMA's list of enemies can be badly hurt at the polls. "The AMA is still very, very potent," a member of the staff of Senator Kennedy's Subcommittee on Health said recently, with mingled awe and resignation. "They're well financed, their organization is incredible, and the average physician trusts them. He may have problems with the AMA, he may disagree with it because he's to the right or left of where it is. But if it really comes to the crunch, he'll trust that what they're saying is the best way to defend his interests."

In opposing the Health Security bill—and in opposing any compulsory insurance scheme financed by taxes—the AMA is in a much stronger position than when it fought the PSROs. In that battle, the AMA had few allies, and it was under fire not only from liberals, but from conservative senators and congressmen who were tired of watching the way money spent on Medicaid and Medicare was being wasted. By contrast, the AMA now has powerful allies, namely the drug manufacturers and the insurance companies, who can also find campaign funds for their friends even when their friends are not campaigning, and who are no less determined than the AMA to keep the federal government from interfering in any serious fashion with established ways of doing business in the health-care industry.

The AMA's cause has also been favored by the political climate of the past two or three years. Even before nerves were numbed by Watergate, enthusiasm for complex and expensive social legislation had been dampened by a conviction that the animating principle of the Great Society—namely, Lyndon Johnson's belief that there was nothing much wrong with America that couldn't be fixed up by passing a law—was rather naive. Even liberals had grown wary of laws that would make government more complicated and cost the taxpayers more money. "Let's face it," an assistant to a senator who had been an early supporter of the Health Security bill observed in 1973, "the 1972 campaign, with its repudiation of McGovern's economics, has put the fear of God into many people in Congress about espousing big spending plans." As for the voters, when it came to health insurance their voice was muted and tentative. Poll after poll indicated that most Americans wanted national health insurance. But it was not clear how far they wanted Congress to go in remodeling the medical-care system, and by 1973 the polls were showing that while people might be concerned about medical care, they were more concerned about education and welfare and race relations—and, of course, inflation. "Now and then someone writes," Senator Russell Long, the chairman of the Senate Finance Committee, which handles health insurance legislation, told a reporter. "But frankly, there's no spontaneous march on Washington or letter writing for anybody's health program unless it's a put-up job."

It was presumably with all this in mind that Senator Kennedy abandoned, at least for a time, his efforts to get the Health Security bill passed, and joined with Mills in backing a bill that turned out to be acceptable neither to labor, nor to the new Ford Administration, nor to the AMA's conservative sympathizers on Mills's own committee, who refused to go along with any insurance scheme financed and controlled by the federal government. A conviction that the country was not yet ready for the Health Security bill also helped persuade another of its supporters, Senator Abraham Ribicoff of Connecticut, to throw in the towel. In 1973, Ribicoff joined with Senator Long, a leading conservative, in introducing a bill that would replace Medicaid with a much better program of medical benefits for the poor and the near-poor, and that would provide catastrophic insurance for just about everybody, but that would otherwise leave things as they are. "Just because we cannot pass the Kennedy bill does not mean we should sit back and do nothing," Ribicoff told the Senate. "We cannot wait for the 'climate to be right' for full national health insurance. I am not such a purist that I am going to wait for the whole loaf when thousands of families are being financially wiped out by huge medical bills."

Enactment of a free-standing catastrophic insurance bill would constitute a kind of surrender to the AMA and its allies, putting off for many years the passage of a comprehensive and universal insurance plan. But unless Watergate, inflation, and recession are harbingers of a great wave of Populism and reform, such as surged through Congress in the 1930s, the chances are slim that Congress will soon enact, or the President sign, any measure written along the lines of the Health Security bill. That does not, however, make its passage any the less desirable.

14

Getting a Better Run for Our Money

While universal health insurance will alleviate some of the symptoms of distress that afflict American medicine, and will make it easier to alleviate others, it will not in itself make medical care better or cheaper. Nor will it steer more young doctors into family practice, or persuade those who are so steered to open up offices in Roxbury or Watts or rural Arkansas. If these aims are to be realized, other kinds of therapy are indicated, and in this chapter, and the next, I propose to examine some measures that may prove helpful.

Let us look, to begin with, at some of the schemes that have been put forward for holding down the cost of medical care. I use the term "holding down" because none of these proposals—and no combination of proposals—stands any chance of reducing our annual bill for medical goods and services. That bill, whether it is stated in constant dollars or as a percentage of the gross national product, is bound to go on rising. One reason is that, when national health insurance goes into effect, Americans will demand more medical care. And in the long run they will almost surely get it. Beyond this, the history of medicine in this century strongly suggests that, as the art of medicine advances, medical care tends to become more, not less, expensive. Clearly there are exceptions. The discovery of Isoniazid, by helping to make possible the closing down of most of the world's tuberculosis hospitals, has saved not only lives, but a great deal of money as well. But such savings have been more than offset by the high cost of so many of the techniques that have been developed for treating diseases that were previously untreatable, diseases from which the patient ordinarily died before he had a chance to run up a huge medical bill. Kidney dialysis is a particularly striking example. By hooking themselves up to a machine for a few hours two or three times each week, some 18,000 Americans who would otherwise have died are alive—working, mowing lawns, and, in a few cases, even playing golf. Once the value of this lifesaving treatment had been clearly established, it was out of the question to limit it to those patients who could afford its enormous cost, amounting to $10,000 to $20,000 a year. And there seemed to be no other ethically defensible way to ration the use of kidney machines. In 1972, as a result, Congress voted to have the government pay for kidney dialysis for anyone requiring it, even though this may, in time, cost the taxpayers half a billion dollars a year or more. Other forms of treatment are almost certain to be developed that will be just as valuable as kidney dialysis, just as expensive, and just as unrationable.

But there are many things we can do to avoid paying for medical goods and services that we don't need, and to avoid paying too much for those we must have. One useful step, as I have said, would be to establish a fee schedule for all doctors undertaking to treat patients under national health insurance, and to forbid them to charge anything extra for their services. It should also be possible, even without doing away with fee-for-service medicine, to cut down on the number of unnecessary operations. It is clear that a lot of unnecessary surgery—and a lot of bungled surgery—is performed by doctors with little formal training as surgeons, and the authors of the Health Security bill have therefore proposed that the government should pay for major operations only if they are performed by a certified specialist. The bill would also require surgeons wishing to undertake certain operations to get a second opinion from another specialist, a precaution that, as I have said, has proved quite effective in saving members of some union health insurance plans from unnecessary surgery. Finally, if the Health Security bill were enacted, a surgeon performing certain kinds of operations would be required, in each case, if he wished to be paid by the government for his work, to submit a summary (taken from the patient's medical chart) of what he had done to the patient, and why, plus the hospital pathologist's postoperative report. This would obviously mean a fair amount of paperwork, but the requirement could be waived—subject to periodic spot-checking—in the case of hospitals with effective procedures of their own for restraining the enthusiasm of over-eager operators.

A lot can be done, too, to save some of the money that is now spent for prescription drugs. Senator Gaylord Nelson, who succeeded the late Senator Kefauver as the chief congressional critic of the big drug companies (Senator Kennedy has lately been running a strong second) has made the reasonable proposal that the government should publish a formulary containing information about all drugs judged to be "necessary for good medical practice." A doctor would be free to prescribe a drug not listed in the formulary, but the government would not pay for it. The formulary would be compiled by a committee made up mainly of nongovernmental experts on pharmacology, and it would contain comparative information. That is, it would list the relative merits and demerits of all drugs commonly used for treating a particular condition—a seemingly useful service, but one that the drug companies see as a dangerous threat to the American way of merchandising. The main purpose of the formulary would be, of course, to help doctors use drugs more intelligently. But since its compilers would almost surely exclude a great many high-priced drugs of the me-too and fixed combination variety it would tend to encourage doctors to prescribe more economically as well as more effectively.

Nelson has suggested other ways of undermining the influence of drug-company detail men. In the late 1960s four out of five of some 9000 doctors surveyed by the AMA agreed that they had "difficulty in obtaining reliable, unbiased information on drugs." To ease this difficulty Nelson would have the government publish, in addition to the more exclusive formulary, a compendium of information about *all* drugs on the American market. The compendium would include prices, which big drug companies do not ordinarily like to talk about in the presence of doctors, and Nelson would further require manufacturers to list prices in their advertisements. Nelson would also encourage doctors to prescribe generically by requiring manufacturers of nonpatented drugs to show that they are not only chemically identical to the patented drugs on which they are modeled, but that they are absorbed into the bloodstream at the same rate, and can therefore be assumed to have the same therapeutic effect. This would make it harder for detail men to dismiss generic products as "junk" and "schlock drugs."

It would also be helpful to modify the patent law as it applies to drugs. Nelson has introduced a bill that would, under certain circumstances, compel the holder of a drug patent to license the drug's manufacture by other companies willing to pay a reasonable royalty for the privilege. The patent-holder would also have to furnish all technical data in its possession that would help the licensee to manufacture the drug economically and to get it on the market quickly. Under Nelson's plan, the government could require licensing if there was a moderately brisk demand for a drug (sales of a million dollars a year or more for at least three years); and if its price was unreasonably high—that is, if it was being sold for more than five times the cost of its manufacture, or if it was available at a lower price in another country. Nelson has estimated that this might cut the total cost of prescription drugs by as much as 18 per cent, or $2 billion a year. However that might be, compulsory licensing would have the further merit of forcing the big companies, by reducing their profit margins, to cut back on detailing. This, coupled with more and better instruction in the use of drugs in medical schools and in graduate-training programs, would tend in itself to make it harder to sell high-priced products that offer no advantage over cheaper drugs.

Doctors have recently put forward a number of schemes intended to lower the cost of malpractice insurance by changing the rules under which malpractice suits are brought and tried. The most sweeping of these proposals would not simply change the rules, but would abolish the game, replacing malpractice litigation with no-fault compensation. Under a no-fault system, a patient confined to a hospital bed for six weeks because an operation on his hip had gone wrong would be entitled to compensation without his having to prove that the surgeon had been incompetent or careless.

The advantages to both doctors and patients from such an arrangement are obvious, though it is hardly a sure-fire remedy for what has been bothering the doctors. Even with fixed ceilings on how much would be paid for specified injuries—so much for the loss of a leg, so much for each week spent in the hospital or convalescing—the total amount of money paid out to victims of medical accidents, and the insurance premiums required to cover the payments, would almost surely be a lot bigger than they are now. One basis for this prediction is to be found in the long and meaty report published in 1973 by the federal government's Commission on Medical Malpractice. Under the commission's sponsorship, a panel of doctors and lawyers examined the medical records of a representative sample of more than eight hundred hospital patients and concluded that sixty-two of them had been injured—eight of them fatally—as a result of the treatment they had received. The panel further concluded that in eighteen of the sixty-two cases there was evidence of negligence on the part of the doctor or hospital. Yet, judging by historical statistics, the commission pointed out, it was unlikely that more than one or two of the injured patients would ever file a malpractice claim. Under a no-fault system, by contrast, all sixty-two patients in the sample would be entitled to compensation, and most could be expected to claim it.

Another reason why a no-fault system would cost a good deal more than is often supposed is that deciding whether a claimant had a right to compensation—and, if so, how much he should get—could be a complicated and expensive business. If a factory worker's hand is mashed in a drill press, and he loses two fingers, he has no difficulty in showing that he was injured on the job and is therefore entitled to workmen's compensation. But if a skier breaks a leg and winds up with a permanent limp, it will not be so easy for a compensation board to determine whether the limp is a result of the original tumble or the subsequent treatment. Difficult questions would also arise as to whether, for example, a patient who has agreed to undergo a risky operation should be compensated if the operation happens to go wrong.

Despite its high cost, and the hard administrative problems it would pose, no-fault compensation is worth a try. However, to the extent that malpractice litigation tends to make doctors and hospitals careful, and to turn a spotlight on incompetence, patients would lose if malpractice suits were outlawed. A no-fault system should therefore not be seriously considered until the quality of American medical care has been made subject to much stricter legal and professional controls.

Some current ideas for revising the rules of malpractice litigation, rather than doing away with it entirely, have little merit. One such notion that particularly appeals to doctors, most of whom believe the boom in malpractice suits is largely the work of unscrupulous and aggressive lawyers, is to abolish the contingent fee in malpractice cases. This is the arrangement whereby a plaintiff's lawyer gets nothing if his client loses, but ordinarily pockets one third to one half of any out-of-court settlement or jury award. Doing away with contingent fees might save insurance companies money in some cases, since a lawyer working for a fixed fee, and therefore having no financial stake in the outcome of a suit, might be less insistent on a big settlement or award. But it is illogical to suppose, as many doctors do, that contingent fees encourage frivolous litigation. On the contrary, a lawyer who knows he is going to be paid whether his client wins or loses may be more willing to take on a shaky case than one who stands to get nothing for his time and trouble if his client loses. Abolishing contingent fees would, to be sure, save money by reducing the number of malpractice suits. But the savings would be achieved, to a large extent, at the expense of people who had, in fact, been injured by careless or incompetent treatment. Bringing a malpractice suit is an expensive business—securing the opinions and testimony of medical experts can cost thousands of dollars—and many people with legitimate grounds would be unable to sue if they had to pay the full cost regardless of how their suit might turn out.

Another proposal of doubtful value that many doctors favor is to limit the size of malpractice awards. The trouble with this plan, apart from its dubious constitutionality, is that million-dollar settlements and awards are not nearly so common as many doctors suppose. Unless the ceiling on awards were fixed at a level that most people, including most doctors, would consider much too low, the cost of malpractice insurance would hardly be lowered at all. In 1972 through 1974, for example, insurance companies settled some 6500 malpractice claims against members of the New York State Medical Society. Only six of these were settled for $300,000 or more. If a $300,000 ceiling had been in force, the saving to the companies would have amounted to only $635,000, or just 1.4 per cent of the $46 million they paid out over the three years. A $500,000 ceiling, such as New York doctors have recently been calling for, would have resulted in an even smaller saving.

Some other reforms that doctors have been urging make more sense. Compulsory arbitration of relatively small claims—for, say, $20,000 or less—might cut legal costs for both parties, while enabling plaintiffs to get their cases settled faster than if they had to go to court. Compulsory mediation may be an even better idea. In New York, anyone who brings a malpractice suit is now required, before his case can go to trial, to submit it informally to a mediation panel. The panel ordinarily consists of a physician active in the medical speciality involved in the suit; a trial lawyer; and the judge to whose court the suit has been assigned. If the panelists conclude that the plaintiff has a case, they so inform the two sides, and suggest what they think would be a fair settlement. Neither party is bound to accept the panel's recommendation, but in Manhattan, where the system went into operation in 1971—it was extended to the entire state in 1974—the proportion of suits settled at the mediation stage has risen from one quarter to one third.

Many doctors have suggested that this proportion would be much larger if the parties to a suit were not barred, as they are now, from making the panel's recommendations known to the jury if the suit goes to trial. Their theory is that allowing a panel's findings to be introduced in evidence would discourage plaintiffs' lawyers from pressing suits that the panel had concluded were without merit. There is a danger, of course, that a plaintiff will not get a fair trial if the jury is told that a panel of experts, including the judge presiding at the trial, has already, in effect, decided in favor of the defendants. This objection might be overcome, however, by specifying that the judge who takes part in mediating a suit must not also be on the bench if the suit goes to trial. Attorneys for both sides might also be permitted, in some circumstances, to bring members of the mediation panel into court and question them about their findings—in an attempt to show, for example, that certain facts were not known to the panel when it made its recommendations.

Some other changes in the rules governing malpractice litigation are probably in order. Limits might be placed on the size of contingent fees, which are already regulated in some localities. In New Jersey, for instance, a lawyer may charge a plaintiff in a malpractice suit 50 per cent of the first $1000 his client recovers, and 40 per cent of the next $2000. But in the case of larger awards, the lawyer's maximum share is much smaller, dropping off to 10 per cent of any sum recovered in excess of $100,000. Such a fee schedule not only protects clients from greedy lawyers but may help to hold down the cost of malpractice insurance, since a jury may be less generous in awarding money to a plaintiff if the jurors know he is not going to have to split it fifty-fifty with his lawyer. Another useful reform would permit a judge, if he concludes that a malpractice suit has been instituted or pressed in bad faith, to order the plaintiff—or his lawyer—to pay all or part of the defendants' court costs and legal fees.

Finally, it may be that the legal definition of medical malpractice should be slightly narrowed. Ordinarily a plaintiff can collect damages only if he can show exactly how his doctor deviated from standard medical practice and exactly how that deviation resulted in injury. But in cases where the deviation is gross and inarguable—when, for example, a pair of scissors has been sewed up in the patient—the legal doctrine of *res ipsa loquitur* ("the thing speaks for itself") may permit a patient to collect from a surgeon without having to demonstrate a specific act of negligence on the surgeon's part. This outrages doctors, and while the number of *res ipsa* cases won by plaintiffs is very small, changing the rule would make doctors feel better. A patient who discovered that his stomachaches were due to scissors in his abdomen could still sue the hospital for damages on the ground that it had failed to properly train or supervise its operating-room staff.

One of the merits of a national insurance plan under which all hospital bills are paid by the government is that it puts the government in a position to do something about hospital costs. The five-member board that would administer the Health Security Act could refuse to reimburse a hospital for the cost of building or operating a new wing, or for equipping and staffing a new surgical suite, the need for which had not been certified by the appropriate state planning agency. The board could also order a hospital, on pain of losing its government business, to close down a largely unused maternity wing, or arrange with another hospital for joint staffing of a single emergency room; in some circumstances, it could even cut off all payments to a hospital or nursing home whose services had been found no longer to be required by the community. Such decisions would, and should, be made only after public proceedings during which everybody concerned would have ample opportunity to mobilize and deploy the political forces at their command. Even so, the prospect can hardly be pleasing to trustees and administrators of voluntary hospitals, who would have to adapt themselves as best they could to the noisy and abrasive process of political bargaining. But this is the only alternative to a system in which the public is, in effect, taxed, at rates that go up year after year, to support hospitals over whose expenditures it has no control.

Another way to hold down hospital costs is to keep people out of hospital beds who don't need to be there. This is one of the jobs that has been assigned to the new Professional Standards Review Organizations, or PSROs. PSROs will employ a coordinator (typically, a registered nurse) to make a daily check of patients' hospital charts. If the coordinator suspects that a patient shouldn't have been hospitalized in the first place, or is being kept in the hospital longer than is necessary, she will notify a PSRO physician, who, if he agrees, can put pressure on the hospital, and on the attending physician, to have the patient discharged. PSROs now have nothing to say about the hospitalization of patients other than those whose bills are paid for by Medicare or Medicaid, or by certain other government programs. But most health insurance bills Congress has been looking at would place just about all hospital care under their jurisdiction.

PSROs are meant to operate along much the same lines as medical care foundations, and these, as I have pointed out, have had some success in keeping down the use of hospitals. Certainly PSROs are likely to be more effective than the conventional utilization committee, on which doctors serving on the staff of a hospital take turns in policing one another. (Doctors taking their turn as PSRO utilization-control officers will not be expected—or permitted—to monitor any hospital with which they themselves are connected.) Yet even granting for the moment that doctors can be counted on to do a good job of policing themselves (a tricky question that I will get to presently) it is unlikely that the PSROs will make much headway against the phenomenon of over-hospitalization. The trouble is that, in general, they can deal only with its symptoms. They cannot rescue a patient from the financial difficulty posed by the fact that his insurance will pay for the treatment he needs only if he is confined to a hospital bed when he gets it. And even if this sort of absurdity is eliminated by national health insurance that pays for out-of-hospital care, a PSRO will still be unable to build the nursing homes or the self-help convalescent units, or to organize the home-care services, that would enable doctors to get their patients out of the hospital promptly without endangering their health. Nor will a PSRO be in a position to build, equip, and staff clinical centers, such as those established by Group Health Cooperative of Puget Sound, that make it both safe and convenient for doctors to diagnose and treat even fairly complicated diseases without putting patients into a hospital bed.

Recently there have been attempts to make hospitals more efficient, and less extravagant, by doing away with the cost-pass-through method of reimbursement—the system under which hospitals are paid by Blue Cross and other third parties on the basis of how much money they have spent in the course of a year. These efforts have mostly taken the form of what is called prospective reimbursement, or rate-setting. In New York and some other states, Blue Cross and Medicaid reimbursement rates (the sum that a hospital is entitled to collect for each day of hospital care) are determined at the beginning of the year, instead of the end; the hospital must, in effect, live within a fixed budget. A common variant is for the hospital's chief customers—Blue Cross and Medicare, for instance—to negotiate a target cost-per-patient-day figure for the coming year. If actual costs exceed that figure, the hospital has to absorb all or most of the loss; if costs are less than had been allowed for, the hospital keeps a portion of the money it has saved by its efficiency.

But for all their plausibility, such schemes have serious weaknesses. For one thing, hospitals differ in the services they offer, and in the kinds of patients they care for. A small community hospital obviously has lower costs than the university medical center to which it refers patients who have complicated diseases, or who require complicated testing or surgery. There is no single standard of fiscal performance to which all hospitals, even all hospitals of roughly the same class, can be expected to conform. In the circumstances, rate-setting becomes a game in which the hospital administrator has the advantage of being able to cast his adversaries—the officials with whom he must bargain over his budget—as heartless villains trying to save a few dollars at the expense of suffering patients. The record suggests that the administrator usually comes out ahead in contests of this kind. In Canada, for example, where almost all hospital bills are paid for in full by the government, each hospital must have its annual budget approved in advance by a government agency empowered to withhold funds if a hospital's proposed expenditures are seriously out of line with those of other hospitals of its size and type. Yet during the ten years after this system went into effect hospital costs in Canada actually rose faster than in the United States, and two American researchers reported, after taking a close look, that they had been able to find "no evidence that the National Hospital Act and the budget review process have had any appreciable effect in slowing down cost increases in Canada."

It is doubtful, too, whether it helps much to offer incentive bonuses to hospitals that come in under their budgets. Hospitals—to be precise, hospital administrators—have little control over many of a hospital's expenses. It is the doctors on the staff of a hospital, not its administrator, who determine how many x-rays are taken, and how many laboratory tests are performed. Moreover, the administrator himself has nothing to gain by cost-cutting even if it will yield a modest bonus for his institution. This point has been emphasized by two Harvard experts on hospital economics who studied a number of experiments that have been made with incentive awards in the United States. "The prestige of a hospital does not stem from its ability to operate with the highest of economy," they note, "but from its reputation as the source of effective medical care. It attracts better physicians by offering them better facilities and training opportunities. The physicians attract patients. The larger and more complex the institution and the larger its budget, the higher is the salary of its administrator. These are the facts of life . . . and we delude ourselves if we think that essential priorities are going to be changed by the offering of some financial reward that is insignificant in size, two years late in coming, and rarely directed to the people within the institution who are making the cost consequential decisions."

Several of the cost-saving schemes I have described, and hospital rate-setting in particular, would work better if money for medical care were rationed—that is, if there were a ceiling on how much money could be paid out each year to the country's doctors, hospitals, and nursing homes. One of the merits of the

Health Security bill is that its authors have provided for such a ceiling. Government spending for medical care—and there would be little medical spending of any other kind—would be limited each year to a sum equal to the number of dollars generated by the new Social Security taxes, plus the same number of dollars taken from general tax revenues. Over the years, if employment grew and wages went up, tax yields would rise proportionately, and more money would be available. But unless Congress voted to change the rules by, for example, raising the payroll-tax rate, total expenditures for medical care, figured as a percentage of the gross national product, would remain more or less at their present level.

One obvious result of such an arrangement would be to force doctors and hospitals to compete politically with one another for money. Under the Health Security bill the country would be divided into more than a hundred health-service areas, and, at first, each of these areas would be allocated a sum roughly equal to the amount of money people in that area had been spending for medical care before passage of the bill. As time went on, however, this formula would be modified. The board charged with administering the act would be required to give extra-large slices of the budgetary pie to areas where per capita expenditures for medical care had been relatively low. This could, in time, mean more doctors and better hospitals for states like Mississippi and West Virginia, which everybody would agree is a good idea. It could also mean fewer doctors and smaller hospital budgets for New York and Massachusetts, which will not command the same universal enthusiasm.

It is plainly impossible to work out a mathematical formula for determining exactly how much money should go to Vermont and how much to Iowa, or for determining how Vermont and Iowa should divide up the money they get. If the Health Security bill were to become law, each state and each community—and each hospital within each community—would be compelled to clamor for more money than it was, in strict fairness, entitled to. For a hospital that was honest and modest in its demands would, of course, end up with less than it deserved. But if we want to keep the yearly rise in the country's medical bill within reasonable limits we will have to reconcile ourselves to the kind of budgetary medicine prescribed by the authors of the Health Security bill, with all the political tugging and hauling that remedy implies. What we must do is to contrive matters so that the business of parcelling out funds for medical care is decentralized—Washington should not tell Rutland or Des Moines how to spend its money—and so that the bargaining takes place in full public view, and with full opportunity for the public to take part in the process.

As some critics have pointed out, enactment of the Health Security bill could lead to our spending too little on medical care rather than too much. As medical technology became more elaborate, and therefore more expensive, Congress might balk at levying the new taxes needed to pay the cost, and more and more prosperous, middle-class Americans might find themselves in hospitals that were overcrowded, understaffed, and dilapidated—the sort of hospitals for which the poor have usually had to settle. In these circumstances, some people would choose to buy their way out of the national health insurance plan, paying doctors out of their own pockets and patronizing private hospitals that provided the amenities and personal attention no longer to be had at the typical community hospital. If enough people were to do this we could end up with another two-class system of care, in which lawyers, stockbrokers, bankers, and business executives would have cornered for themselves a disproportionate share of the country's medical services and facilities and, having done so, would be most reluctant to have their taxes hiked to improve things for the rest of the population.

But things are unlikely to get to such a pass, for the reason that the disadvantaged class of patients would be made up not only of migrant workers and domestics and welfare mothers, but of factory workers, shoe clerks, auto mechanics, and teachers. It would, in fact, include most Americans. And this majority, having no real choice but to avail themselves of the publicly-financed medical-care system, would be fairly certain to insist on whatever steps were necessary to prevent its deterioration. In any case, this is what has happened in England, where the National Health Service was at one time badly underfinanced, but where new funds were pumped into the system before the rich had begun to abandon it in significant numbers. This point has been made by, among others, Dr. Paul B. Beeson, an American physician who was for many years a leading member of the Yale Medical School faculty, and who left Yale in 1965 to become Nuffield Professor of Clinical Medicine at Oxford. Speaking of the National Health Service, Beeson recently noted that "people belonging to all social classes use it. We see some of Oxford's most distinguished citizens on our ward services, and they accept this quite naturally."

There are two fundamentally different ways of dealing with the excessive cost of medical care in the United States. The first way—the one discussed so far in this chapter—is to accept the medical-care system pretty much as it is, but to subject it to various controls. The purpose of these controls would be to keep doctors and hospitals and drug manufacturers from drawing checks on the public in whatever amounts seemed right to them. The other approach to holding down costs is to modify the system so as to get rid of certain built-in incentives to extravagance, inefficiency, and excessive treatment. Probably the most useful thing that can be done along these lines is for the government to offer strong inducements to both doctors and patients to sign up with prepaid group practice plans.

The Health Security bill includes several such inducements. Sponsors of Health Maintenance Organizations, or HMOs (the bill defines the term so as to include medical care foundations as well as plans like Group Health Cooperative of Puget Sound) would be eligible for generous grants and loans to cover planning and start-up costs. Patients enrolled in HMOs would get certain drugs free that they would otherwise have to pay for. To further stimulate the growth of HMOs, and to encourage them to keep a tight rein on costs, bonuses would be given out to any HMO whose enrollees spent less time in the hospital than a comparable group of people being cared for under conventional fee-for-service arrangements. These bonuses, which could be quite large, would differ in two important ways from the incentive payments to hospitals that I have described. For one thing, an HMO's doctors would ordinarily share in the bonus, and would therefore have a personal stake in keeping patients out of the hospital if at all possible. For another, an HMO's directors and administrators would also stand to gain by keeping hospitalization low, since whatever part of the year-end bonus was not passed along to the doctors would be available to them to expand and improve services, and thereby to attract more enrollees. The government's budget-reviewers, for their part, would be spared the necessity of checking on doctors' fees, and of determining whether Mrs. Jones really needed to be kept in the hospital for seventeen days after her gall-bladder operation. One reason they wouldn't have to worry about her is that the managers of a prepaid group practice would be impelled by self-interest to develop a good home-care service, and to build and operate self-care units, in which convalescing patients could be accommodated at a much lower cost than in a hospital. These are not the sort of projects that fire up the enthusiasm of a hospital administrator who is losing sleep over the number of empty beds he sees on his daily rounds.

Obviously there is a danger, as I have said, that doctors in prepaid group practice plans would try to fatten their bonuses by under-treating and under-hospitalizing their patients—or that an HMO's managers would not take on enough doctors to care adequately for the plan's members. But this is not likely to happen if, as the Health Security bill provides, the government is prepared to do business with an HMO only if it is organized as a not-for-profit enterprise, and only if its members have a voice in formulating policy. Anyway, skimping on services to patients would be self-defeating: it would tend to drive members out of an HMO and into the offices of fee-for-service doctors—a switch that a dissatisfied patient could make at the relatively small cost of having to pay for more of the drugs that he might need.

When the new Professional Standards Review Organizations were voted into being in 1972, Congress was mainly, but not exclusively, impelled by a desire to save money for the taxpayers. The PSROs were also given the job of checking up on—and, if possible, improving—the technical competence of doctors who treat the elderly and the poor. Congress has also been considering a number of other measures aimed at doing something about those doctors who habitually dose patients with the wrong drugs, misdiagnose their ailments, and subject them to unnecessary operations or to forms of therapy that have been shown to be useless or even harmful. Even the AMA's leaders seem inclined to concede that the question is not whether the government should take steps to protect people against incompetent or careless doctors, but what those steps should be.

One approach is to lean hard on doctors to police themselves more effectively than they have in the past. Such policing, or peer review, as it is called in the trade, is quite effective in university hospitals, where doctors must routinely defend their diagnoses to their associates, and justify the treatments they have ordered. It also works well in prepaid group practice plans, whose doctors don't want their own professional reputations compromised by bungling colleagues. To be sure, when a Kaiser medical group fires a bungler and, as often happens, he rents an office of his own and builds up a thriving private practice, nothing has really changed except that his incompetence is being visited on a different set of patients.

But incompetence is a condition that can, in many cases, be prevented and cured. "It is doubtful that the average physician knowingly employs questionable practices," the sociologist Eliot Freidson has written. "Isolated from others, he simply comes to believe that his poor records, shortcuts, and readiness to prescribe are all harmless and insignificant practices." A corollary of this proposition is that a doctor who might fall into sloppy habits if practicing by himself may do an adequate, if not brilliant, job in the setting of a group practice, where he sees how other doctors handle problems, and where his own performance is subject to frequent review, not only by the plan's medical audit committee, but also informally by colleagues who have occasion to see his patients and therefore to consult the charts that he keeps.

But at a great many hospitals, for reasons I have set forth in Chapter Seven, peer review is a meaningless exercise. It was with this in mind that Congress charged the PSROs with setting guidelines for the treatment of Medicaid and Medicare patients sick enough to be confined to hospitals or skilled nursing homes. These guidelines may specify, for instance, what tests should ordinarily be performed before a patient's tonsils or gall bladder are removed, or what drugs, in what dosages, are generally appropriate in treating a seventy-five-year-old man with lobar pneumonia. A doctor who deviates from these standards may be questioned by a doctor, or by a committee of doctors, practicing in the same area (but not at the same hospital). If his explanation is considered unsatisfactory, the government may refuse to pay him for his work. In time, PSROs may be given the further task of monitoring the care patients get in doctors' offices and in the outpatient clinics of hospitals.

Although PSROs are probably a good idea, they have two serious weaknesses. One is that there is no provision for consumers—that is, the public—to take a hand in the reviewing process. Obviously a tax lawyer or a housewife or a union shop steward is in a poor position to make a firsthand judgment as to whether Doctor X was justified in taking out Mrs. Y's uterus, or whether Doctor Z regularly overdoses patients with antibiotics. But with the help of their own medical expert, a sort of minority counsel, consumers sitting on a review committee could at least put a damper on any tendency toward professional log-rolling, and they could demand answers to questions which, in their absence, might never have been raised. Unfortunately, most practicing physicians explode at any suggestion that they be evaluated by nonphysicians, and getting consumers into the reviewing act, however desirable, may have to wait a while.

The other weakness of PSROs—at any rate, a potential weakness—is that they will deprive doctors of the freedom they need to do a good job. "The tendency," a committee of public health experts reported recently to the National Academy of Sciences, "will be . . . to institutionalize a laundry list of processes for given disease conditions, deviation from which may result in the imposition of a sanction. If this happens . . . the flexibility and 'room' for innovation and experimentation will be sacrificed." A similar warning has been sounded by, among others, Dr. Saul B. Gilson, a New York kidney specialist. In a recent letter to the *New England Journal of Medicine,* Gilson observed that the standards a PSRO draws up may simply reflect what most doctors in the area do in their own practices, and he went on to suggest that "consensus medicine" may call for the use of procedures that were once popular but that have proven to be worthless or even dangerous. "Ultimately," he writes, "medicine by the norm enforces medicine by authority, by majority, and bans the more eccentric. Must I now send coronary patients to the surgeon for a popular but invalidated operation?"

It may be, as the proponents of the PSRO law hope, that PSROs will have the opposite effect from that feared by Gilson. Under the right kind of pressure from the government, they may in turn put pressure on doctors to drop forms of treatment that they might otherwise have clung to out of habit, laziness, or ignorance. But rigidity in the enforcement of treatment standards will be hard to avoid. In the circumstances, hospital boards would do well to take advantage of a provision of the law that permits a PSRO to loosen the regulatory reins if a hospital shows that it is doing a good job of policing and upgrading the work of its own medical staff. It may turn out, in fact, that one of the best things about the PSRO bill is that it will nudge hospital trustees and medical staffs, in the interest of maintaining their own autonomy, into taking a much harder line with medical bunglers and incompetents.

Another way to set about improving the quality of medical practice in the United States is to stiffen the educational standards that doctors must meet. Thus under the Health Security bill, as I have already pointed out, the government would, as a general rule, pay for major surgery only if done by a doctor who had gone through a five-year surgical residency, and whose competence had been certified by the American Board of Surgery or a similar professional body. This would almost certainly result in better surgery as well as fewer operations. It is less clear, though, how much good would be done by a related provision of the bill aimed at making doctors keep up with new developments. A doctor wishing to be paid by the government for his services would have to show that he was putting in a specified number of hours each year attending postgraduate courses. This makes sense for neurosurgeons and cardiologists and other specialists, who ordinarily have no difficulty keeping up with their fields if they are willing to take the time. But, as I have said earlier, seminars and lectures laid on for family doctors very often have little or no relevance to the problems they face in their daily work, and therefore have little or no effect on the way they practice.

Postgraduate courses for family physicians seem to be most effective when they are given by a hospital for members of its own medical staff; and when they are aimed at correcting specific deficiencies uncovered by the hospital's own internal audits. A number of hospitals now run educational programs designed along these lines. For example, if a study of patient charts has shown that antibiotics are being much too freely dispensed, the doctors on the staff may be asked to take part in drawing up general guidelines for their use. When they have done this, they may be given a pencil-and-paper quiz testing their ability to apply the new standards in a variety of circumstances. The hospital's director of medical education may then plan a conference, or a series of conferences, focused on problems having to do with the administration of antibiotics that had given the doctors on the staff the most trouble. It was mainly by such methods that Chestnut Hill Hospital in Philadelphia reduced the number of complications resulting from hysterectomies, and brought about the other improvements in the work of its medical staff that I have described in Chapter Three. The educational provisions of the Health Security bill would be more effective if all hospitals were required to conduct educational programs based, like Chestnut Hill's, on regular and close analysis of the performance of their own doctors.

A further and logical step, as Senator Kennedy and some reformers within the medical profession have suggested, would be to stop issuing unrestricted lifetime licenses to practice medicine. Every doctor might be required from time to time—every ten years, let us say—to re-establish his competence by passing a stiff examination either in general medicine, or else in surgery, or radiology, or pediatrics, or any other branch of medicine in which he wishes to keep his standing as a specialist. The examination might be coupled with a look at how a doctor actually treats his patients: the examiners might rely on the evidence of the charts he has kept, or they might have an observer sit in with him and accompany him on his hospital rounds for a day or two.

A doctor scoring poorly on this combined test and performance check might be required to spend three months in a full-time training program, run by a teaching hospital or a prepaid group practice plan, designed to help him remedy the weaknesses the examiners had found. After this he would be examined again. If he still did poorly, his unrestricted license would be taken away, and until such time as he could pass muster with the examiners he would be allowed to practice medicine only under the close supervision of another physician, who would be held legally responsible for the quality of his work. All this examining and reviewing and retraining would obviously cost a lot of time and money, but probably not nearly as much as is now consumed by the malpractice suits that could thereby be avoided.

Besides the schemes I have described for raising the level of American medical practice, there are, finally, some specific measures that can be taken to increase the effectiveness with which doctors make use of drugs. For one thing, it should be made easier for doctors to obtain accurate information about drugs. The publication of a national drug formulary, along the lines proposed by Senator Nelson, would help, and so would the establishment of a National Center for Clinical Pharmacology, as called for in a bill introduced by Senator Kennedy and Senator Jacob Javits of New York. One of the center's responsibilities would be to see that medical students and young house officers got more and better instruction in pharmacology, a field that has generally been scanted in the curricula of medical schools and teaching hospitals. The center would also be charged with collecting, analyzing, and sending out information on adverse reactions to drugs; and with trying out plans such as the provision of free, expert telephone advice to doctors having specific questions about a drug, or class of drugs. Prescribing the right drug would also be easier if drug manufacturers were forbidden to make claims of safety and effectiveness that were not based on hard evidence—on controlled, double-blind tests. To this end, Senator Nelson has sensibly proposed that the testing and evaluation of new drugs be taken out of the hands of drug companies and assigned to an independent center for clinical testing.

The extent to which Americans benefit from the drugs that they swallow, or that are injected into their bodies, depends not only on the knowledge and judgment of their doctors, but on the intelligence with which the federal government regulates the flow of new drugs onto the market. As the government's regulator, the FDA has performed in a rather uneven fashion. At times it has been too easy on the drug companies. It has let them test potentially dangerous new drugs without keeping close track of how many people were getting the drug, and in what doses and for how long they were getting it. It has also allowed the industry to continue selling drugs of no proven effectiveness long after they should, by law, have been taken off the market. On the other hand, the agency has sometimes been too slow, partly because of bureaucratic timidity, to approve the marketing of genuinely useful new drugs. One important reason for the FDA's lapses, as the Brookings Institution pointed out in a 1971 study, is that policing drug manufacturers is not the sort of work that attracts first-rate chemists and pharmacologists. What the agency needs is to be deeply engaged in pharmacological research, both on its own and in collaboration with medical schools, the National Institutes of Health, and independent research institutes. Its efforts should not be limited to finding out what effects particular drugs have on mice or people; they should extend to the more interesting and basic questions of why drugs work the way they do. This would make it easier for the FDA to hire good people, and would have a tonic effect on the whole enterprise of drug regulation.

15

How to Deal with the Doctor Shortage

In 1974, spokesmen for the Nixon Administration, over the protests of some of its own manpower experts, suggested to Congress that the time had come to stop worrying about the doctor shortage. Noting that twenty-seven new medical schools had opened for business in the United States since 1963, and that enrollment in all American medical schools had gone up by 60 per cent over the same period, they argued that, by 1980 or soon thereafter, there would be plenty of doctors to go around. Consequently, they concluded, there was no reason for the government to spend its money subsidizing any further expansion of the country's medical schools.

In making this assessment, the Administration's spokesmen appeared to take for granted that the United States will, and should, continue to get a large proportion of its new doctors—perhaps as many as a third—from other countries. One trouble with this assumption is that in recent years tens of thousands of foreign medical graduates, or FMGs, as they are called in the trade, have been allowed to practice here even though, as I have noted, they do not measure up to the standards required of doctors educated in the United States. If this dispensation is withdrawn—and a number of influential people in Congress have been pressing for its withdrawal—the number of FMGs entering practice in the United States may fall off sharply. This effect could be partly offset if hospitals offering postgraduate training to FMGs were to stop treating them simply as a kind of stoop labor, as is now often the case, and were to try conscientiously to remedy the deficiencies, as seen from the American point of view, in the education they have had as undergraduates. But while this is the least we owe to young doctors coming here from abroad—and the least we owe to their patients—it is obviously absurd to expect countries like India, Thailand, and the Philippines to spend hundreds of millions of dollars over the next five or ten years training medical students who will end up taking care of patients in West Hartford or Kansas City or Seattle. The situation makes so little sense, indeed, that there is no reason to think that it will continue. China and Cuba do not export doctors to the United States, and it will not necessarily take a revolution to persuade our Asian suppliers to put their young doctors to work at home. In the circumstances, investing federal money to further boost the output of our own medical schools seems a reasonable thing to do.

What we mainly need, of course, are more family physicians, and expanding our medical schools will do little good if the great majority of their graduates choose to take up careers as surgeons or radiologists or heart specialists. It is true that the idea of going into family practice is more popular with medical students than it was a few years ago, and in 1974 one out of five graduating seniors applied for family-practice residencies. A smaller but substantial number, who elected to take their postgraduate training in pediatrics or internal medicine, did so with the intention of devoting themselves to first-line, or primary care rather than becoming specialists in the treatment of rare and complicated disorders. But we are still failing to produce nearly enough new family doctors even to replace those who retire or die each year, let alone enough to ease a shortage of family physicians that will be even more painfully felt when national health insurance steps up the demand for their services. The AMA has accordingly suggested that medical schools should steer fully half their graduates into family practice, and even that is probably too few. In England, nearly three quarters of all doctors are general practitioners, while prepaid group practice plans in the United States have found that the right mix for their medical staffs is two-thirds family doctors, one-third specialists. This would suggest that even after we have eliminated the existing shortage of family doctors, two out of every three medical-school graduates will have to go into family practice just to keep things in balance.

A shift of this magnitude in the career choices of young doctors is not going to occur without a lot of prodding. So long as medical-school faculties are made up almost entirely of scientists and super-specialists, who select as students those applicants who seem best qualified to follow in their footsteps, the job of looking after the general run of human aches and ailments is going to strike a great many students as unrewarding hackwork. Moreover, not all the young men and women now taking family-practice residencies are going to stay in family practice. Drawn by the lure of easier hours, higher prestige, and greater intellectual challenge, a fair number are likely to decide at some point to take a year or so of additional hospital training in, say, endocrinology or cardiology, and so to become specialists after all. This is much easier to do, of course, than it was before hospital residents were paid a living wage.

However, there are a number of things that can be done to draw doctors into family practice and to keep them there. One is to induce medical schools, by appropriate manipulation of the federal subsidies on which they increasingly depend, to establish a great many more family-practice residencies. (In 1974, there weren't nearly enough to accommodate all the students who put in for them.) Encouraging the growth of prepaid group practice will also help. Plans like Kaiser-Permanente can offer a family doctor many of the advantages of specialty practice: close association with a hospital, regular hours, long vacations, and time off for education. Also, as more and more medical schools set up prepaid group practice plans, as many of them are now doing, more and more medical students will be able to see for themselves that family practice need not mean drudgery, hackwork, and professional isolation.

Another way to steer more young doctors into family practice is to make it harder for them to take up careers in the already overcrowded field of surgery. Dr. Francis D. Moore, a professor of surgery at Harvard who has been directing a five-year study of surgical manpower in the United States, estimates that no fewer than 92,000 of the roughly 300,000 doctors practicing here are either full-time surgeons, or designate surgery as their major interest. This is a "remarkable imbalance," Dr. Moore notes, in that "about a third of the practitioners in the country do surgical procedures as a principal activity. This is much higher than any other country I know of. The comparable figures from Western Europe are 15 per cent to 20 per cent." Bills aimed at redressing this sort of imbalance were introduced in

Congress in 1974 by Senator Kennedy, and by Representative William Roy, a Topeka, Kansas, gynecologist then serving in Congress. Both bills would have established a national council, and a group of regional subcouncils, authorized to set limits on the number of residencies in general surgery, and in other specialties. Nurses, medical students, and laymen would serve on these councils, as well as doctors, and their decisions would be enforced by the federal government. Similarly, the Health Security bill provides that a doctor can be licensed only if he has received his graduate training in a program certified by the Secretary of Health, Education and Welfare on the recommendation of a regional council. This would perhaps put too much power in the Secretary's hands, however, and much the same result could be achieved by reducing government payments to hospitals having uncertified training programs. The public indirectly foots a good part of the bill for the training of hospital residents, and there is no reason why it should not get the kinds of doctors it needs.

Channeling more doctors into family practice is an easier job than persuading them, once channeled, to practice where their services are most needed. Getting doctors to take care of residents of Bedford-Stuyvesant or Watts or the Kenwood-Oakland district of Chicago is not the main problem. A doctor does not have to live in a slum to practice there. Nor need he feel driven, once Medicaid is replaced by a plan that pays doctors just as well for treating the poor as for treating anyone else, to see fifty or sixty patients a day. Arrangements can also be made, as they have been by the Harvard Community Health Plan, that will permit a doctor who spends most of his time seeing patients in, say, an East Harlem clinic to spend some of his time working in a teaching hospital, and some of his time seeing patients who are not desperately poor.

It is much harder to make it attractive for a doctor to settle in a community like Slaterville, the old Pennsylvania coal-mining town described in Chapter Three. Young physicians do not see the small-town or country doctor as a heroic figure, but as an exile condemned to a lifetime of drudgery beyond the boundaries of scientific medicine. Even when a young doctor is willing to take a shot at rural practice, at least for two or three years, his wife may find the prospect—and the actuality—depressing. This was brought home to me by a doctor who recalled, in a talk we had not long ago, his determination, at the time he was finishing his residency in pediatrics at Bellevue Hospital in New York, to do something more useful to society than just settling into a comfortable suburban practice. After some exploring he found what he was looking for. It was a chance to join a group practice connected with a small hospital in the Kentucky coalfields that had been built by the United Mine Workers. "After talking things over with the people there, I went down to the cafeteria to meet my wife," he said. "I was very excited. I said, 'Honey, this is *it!*' She burst into tears." As it turned out, he worked in Kentucky for two and a half years, and then moved to New York, where he is now a mover and shaker on the staff of a neighborhood health center, and his wife is working on a Ph.D. in art history.

Attempts have been made to lure doctors into small-town and rural practice by offering them guaranteed incomes, free office space, and other financial incentives. But in a time when a doctor can make a good living almost anywhere he chooses to go, these efforts have largely failed. For the last ten years, for instance, medical students borrowing money under a special federal program have been offered partial forgiveness of their loans in return for practicing for two or three years in an area where doctors are in critically short supply. Between 1965 and 1972, one third of all students graduating from medical or dental schools (some 30,000 students in all) had borrowed money on these terms. Yet as of October, 1973, only 86 doctors and 133 dentists had actually spent some time in one of the specified areas, and four out of five of these said they would have done so without any special incentive.

In 1974, discouraged by these and other similar statistics, the Senate (though not the House) passed a bill, sponsored by Senator J. Glenn Beall of Maryland, that would have sent more than three thousand doctors a year into big-city ghettos and sparsely settled rural counties. It would have accomplished this by requiring all medical schools, on pain of losing their federal subsidies, to reserve one quarter of the places in each entering class for students volunteering to spend at least two years delivering primary care in an area with a serious doctor shortage. The volunteers would have been eligible for generous federal scholarships, and any student going back on his promise would have had to pay over to the government twice as much money as he had received in scholarship aid, plus interest—a sum that could have amounted to more than $50,000. The Senate adopted Beall's proposal after voting down a stiffer measure, sponsored by Senators Kennedy and Javits, that would have allowed the Secretary of Health, Education and Welfare to draft young doctors, by lottery, for two years of practice in areas where more doctors were most badly needed. As the supporters of both proposals pointed out, the taxpayers are now paying more than half of the cost of putting students through medical school, and they have a right to ask some return on the investment in the form of national service.

Drafting doctors for rural service, or compelling them to volunteer for it, may be the quickest way to improve matters in towns like Slaterville, but in the long-run a less coercive sort of remedy might be better. Under the right kind of national health insurance plan, state or federal agencies could contract with a hospital or an HMO—or with a consortium of hospitals and HMOs—to provide complete medical care, at so many dollars per head, for everyone living in a particular rural county or cluster of counties. The government would lay down certain requirements. It might specify, for example, that 95 per cent of the area's residents should be able to get to an emergency room in forty minutes or less, and that there should be the equivalent of five full-time primary care physicians for every 10,000 persons. It would be up to the hospital or HMO to meet the government's specifications in whatever way it thought best. It would decide to what extent it would rely on circuit-riding doctors and nurses, and to what extent it would rely on a special bus service to bring patients to the doctors. It would decide whether to try to attract more independent practitioners into the area, or whether to establish clinics staffed by doctors working on salary, or whether to do both. When a contractor did decide to open clinics, it could choose to staff them with fully-trained doctors, with doctors taking family-practice residencies, or, in part, with medical students. A large hospital or a prepaid group practice undertaking to furnish care on these terms would be in a position to modify some of the features of rural practice that put young doctors off. It could, for instance, arrange for a doctor working in an outlying clinic or office to swap places from time to time with a hospital resident. It could also provide him with the part-time help of medical students and visiting specialists, with a closed-circuit television link (for diagnostic purposes) to the nearest medical center, and with sensible—that is, relevant—postgraduate training.

For some years many medical educators and government planners have contended that one of the best ways to alleviate the doctor shortage is to train people other than doctors to take on some of the tasks that doctors have traditionally performed. The idea first gained currency during the Vietnam War, when the armed forces each year were discharging thousands upon thousands of military corpsmen, or medics, who had been highly effective in treating battle casualties. For a fraction of what it costs to train a doctor, it was argued, these ex-medics could be trained to take medical histories, give physical examinations, sew up cuts, treat sprained ankles and poison ivy, monitor the progress of diabetics, and handle other more or less routine jobs that may take up half or more of the time of the average pediatrician or family physician. Seizing the opportunity to beat swords into ploughshares, a number of medical schools began enrolling ex-corpsmen and turning them into a new kind of medical worker—the physician's assistant, or P.A.—whose arrival on the medical scene in the late 1960s was hailed by the Surgeon General of the United States as "the hottest thing in health care delivery." At the same time medical and nursing schools began turning out nurse practitioners: registered nurses who had been trained, for example, to examine and advise pregnant women, and to deliver babies—that is, to work as midwives; or to deal with most of the problems that mothers are concerned about when they bring their children into a pediatrician's office for their periodic checkups.

Since doctors in family practice often feel over-trained and over-qualified for many things they are called on to do for their patients, they should be delighted to hand over some of their work to nondoctors. Yet many doctors have strongly resisted any such transfer. In part, no doubt, this is because they are unwilling to concede that so much of what they do (and what they are so highly paid for doing) can be done by an ex-medic or a nurse who has had a year or two of special training. As for nurse practitioners, resistance may be fortified by a lingering conviction that nurses are all right in their places, but should not be encouraged to get uppity. Even when doctors accept in principle the validity of sharing their work with nondoctors, they may find the reality hard to take. "Probably the biggest problem is that we physicians are so stubborn about accepting the idea of using others to help us," a California physician, Dr. Len Hughes Andrus, has written. "When faced with change, they feel that their authority and control are threatened. We have to face these feelings in our own group. We have learned that these fears are unfounded but they nevertheless exist."

Mainly because of such fears, the new health practitioners, or NHPs, as they are sometimes called, have not proliferated as their advocates had hoped. In 1974, according to the best available estimates, fewer than 1800 men and women completed training programs leading to their certification as physician's assistants or nurse practitioners. Since a doctor who adds an NHP to his office staff can not count on being able to increase the size of his practice by much more than a third, these 1600 NHPs are, in terms of productivity, the equivalent of no more than perhaps 600 doctors, whereas some authorities have estimated that the United States needs to enlarge its stock of primary-care physicians (or their equivalents) by more than 100,000. Moreover, most NHPs have found work in city hospitals, in group-practice plans like Kaiser, and in neighborhood health centers, rather than in rural areas where their services may be most needed. One reason for this is that, in many states, the law allows an NHP to practice only under the direct orders and supervision of a physician; this means that a nurse practitioner, for example, can go to work in a rural community only if there is already a doctor there, and only if that doctor is willing to hire her.

The question naturally arises as to the quality of the care patients get when a PA or a nurse practitioner and a physician are working in collaboration. The evidence is very clear that the care is usually excellent—at least as good as when patients are seen by a doctor alone. In one recent test, for example, two family physicians practicing in partnership in Burlington, Ontario, a middle-class suburb of Toronto, hired two nurse practitioners and turned over to them some five-hundred families who had agreed to take their medical problems, in the first instance, to one of the nurses instead of to the doctor who had previously been seeing them. The nurses were told to call in one of the doctors if they had any doubt as to what should be done. As it turned out, however, they handled two out of three office visits entirely on their own.

Over a two-year period, the patients assigned to the two nurses were judged by outside reviewers to have been treated with the same degree of technical competence as those patients seen only by one of the doctors. Judging by such measures as the number of days they had spent in bed, they seemed, moreover, to enjoy just as good health. In another experiment, a group of patients attending a hospital clinic for treatment of chronic diseases such as hypertension and arthritis were assigned to nurses rather than doctors for their care. At the end of a year they had fewer complaints about the way they felt, and were much more likely to be holding down a job, than a closely matched group of clinic patients who had been seen regularly by a doctor. Patients getting much or all of their medical care from nurse practitioners are usually quite happy with the arrangement. In Colorado, for example, a survey of mothers whose children were under the joint care of a pediatrician and a nurse indicated that three out of five mothers believed that their children were getting better care than they had previously gotten from a pediatrician alone.

Although patients may not be the best judges of the quality of care, the mothers in this case were probably right. Nurse practitioners, and physician's assistants as well, usually see fewer than half as many patients in the course of a day as the doctors they work with, and therefore spend proportionately more time with those they see. The resulting benefits to the patient have been pointed out by the authors of a report, published in *Pediatrics,* on the work of a pediatric nurse practitioner employed by a medical group in a suburb of Denver. "Mothers frequently will discuss things with the nurse which they may have considered too trivial to bring to the attention of the physician," they observe. "When the nurse spends a long and uninterrupted period of time with the mother, the latter will frequently become quite communicative and participate in a much more meaningful discussion. This, in turn, has resulted in earlier recognition and more effective management of behavior problems that are already present or, in other instances, in the initiation of measures to prevent their development."

Because they have more time to give to patients, NHPs can

sometimes also be effective in helping adult patients cope with emotional problems. A physician's assistant, a large, deep-voiced man who had recently been hired by two doctors practicing in partnership in a small New England town, told me that while he was mainly occupied with strictly medical tasks—doing physicals, treating scrapes and bruises, ordering laboratory tests and bringing the results to the doctors' attention, explaining to patients the regimen they should follow when they get home from the hospital—he also puts in a fair amount of time just listening to patients. "When people come in, and seem troubled, I make myself a fairly good sounding board," he said. "Quite often I can help ward off a deep depression by asking the right questions at the right time—but mainly by *listening*."

As all this would suggest, the new health practitioners should not be thought of simply as cheap substitutes for real doctors. Rather, they tend to offset, or dilute, the harsh impersonality and the impatience with trivial disorders—or those judged to be imaginary—that are so often encountered in doctors' offices. This is not to say, of course, that physicians' assistants and nurse practitioners are invariably sympathetic and understanding in their transactions with patients. "A transformation occurs as the nurses learn the practitioner role," Dr. Harold Wise, the former project director of the Dr. Martin Luther King, Jr., Health Center in New York, has written. "They develop some of the physician's chutzpah. They stop wearing the nurse's uniform and begin to wear a doctor's white coat. They walk more assertively, and lose interest in making home visits. They love the practitioner's role, perhaps too much." But while some of the new health practitioners are bound to prove to be as brusque and condescending as any doctor, their faults will be attributable to their personalities, not their training. Unlike doctors, they will not have been conditioned to find professional fulfillment mainly in the diagnosis and treatment of complex organic disorders—an attitude which, whatever may be said in its favor, may incapacitate a doctor for dealing patiently and imaginatively with the common run of physical and emotional problems that people bring to their family physician.

16

Making Medicine More Human

Nothing Congress or anyone else can do will bring back the kind of medical care that most Americans could count on seventy-five years ago. The family doctor who is a close family friend, who is always on call, who is ready to sit through the night at the bedside of a dying patient, who treats patients regardless of whether or not they can pay him—no matter how we tinker with the system, this exemplar of the Samaritan strain in medicine will not be restored to life.

But the powerful new technologies that have turned medicine into a social and bureaucratic enterprise need not rule out compassion in ministering to people who are worried and in pain. Nor does the physician's new power over disease justify a disdain for those disorders that are rooted in human existence, and that cannot be made to yield to surgery or drugs. ("The haughty physician," Dr. Edward H. Reinhard, Professor of Medicine at the Washington University School of Medicine, has written, "finds it so easy to dismiss the patient as a crock. It is so much more trouble, indeed it may be considered unmanly, to listen to the patient, to hear, to understand, to experience the terror. God forgive us for our arrogance.") Indeed, the healing potential of scientific medicine cannot be fully realized if the patient is afraid to tell the doctor how he lives and how he feels, or if the doctor ignores what he says or shuts him off. In this last chapter, I propose to suggest some things that might be done about the inhumanity, the narrowness of outlook, and the condescension that too often characterize the care we get when we are sick, or are afraid we might be.

One remedy might be to change the standards that medical-school admissions committees apply in deciding who shall, and who shall not, have a chance to become a doctor. I have described how American medical schools have come to think of biomedical research as their principal mission or, at any rate, their most exciting one. Not surprisingly, they have tended to favor applicants who have spent at least half their time as undergraduates taking courses in physics and chemistry and biology, and who have gotten As in all of them. Such students are less likely to flunk out during the first two years of medical school, during which they will be occupied mainly with courses in biochemistry, anatomy, and other so-called preclinical subjects. They are also more likely to get high scores on the examination that all medical students must take at the end of these two years, and thereby to reflect credit on their teachers.

But while the standard-model premedical student may well develop into a competent radiologist, pathologist, or anesthesiologist, he is less likely, perhaps, to turn out to be the kind of doctor we want as a medical adviser. He is likely to have arrived at medical school already inclined to the belief that the true business of medicine is to develop and apply the kind of chemical and surgical techniques that have permitted doctors to prevent polio, cure tuberculosis, and prolong the lives of cancer victims. This belief can lead, in the words of a student speaker at a recent medical-school commencement, to "the idea that good management of emotional problems is easier to master than the more strictly organic aspects of our art; that 'real doctors' shouldn't bother with patients' feelings because nonphysicians can easily handle them, people like nurses, social workers, volunteers, and freshman medical students—people of 'lower status.' "

As these remarks suggest, the schools' preference for hard scientists has not gone entirely unchallenged. In the late 1960s, under heavy pressure to make medical education less baroque and more "relevant," some admissions committees began accepting students whose grounding in mathematics, chemistry, and physics did not look too solid, but who had shown an interest in, and an aptitude for, the softer, behavioral sciences such as anthropology, psychology, and sociology. The idea was that such students would be more likely to manifest, as doctors, a strong interest in the psychological and social setting in which their patients' symptoms were embedded. Dr. H. Jack Geiger, one of the founders of the Mound Bayou health center in Mississippi, who is now Professor of Community Medicine at the State University of New York at Stony Brook, recently recalled the fate of this experiment: "With the whole shutdown of space engineering, and this enormous glut of kids coming into pre-med now and wanting to be doctors, the medical schools have deliriously abandoned all other criteria and have gone back to trying as hard as they can to pick the kid with a Medical College Admissions Test score of 998." What the schools are getting, Geiger added, are "the straight, square, very competitive, highly motivated kids" who have straight-A science records. "Medical schools were always very comfortable with these students," he said sardonically. "We're done with the crazy years now."

Geiger has said that probably the best way to open up the profession to more young anthropologists and sociologists—and, for that matter, to more young history and English majors—is to put other people as well as medical-school deans and professors on the schools' admissions committees. The demand is legitimate; since we, as taxpayers, are putting up several hundred million dollars a year to train medical students, we have a right to some say about who is chosen for this training. It is not clear what criteria should be used in picking medical students (though obviously *some* knowledge of, and aptitude for, science is necessary). But some clues might be found by looking into the background and personalities of practicing physicians who are judged by their peers to be technically competent, and whose patients consider them to be sympathetic and understanding. It might turn out that a high proportion had, in their teens, been more interested in music and poetry than in science, and had decided to become doctors only late in their college years. In any case, enlarging admissions committees to include union officials, health-center administrators, family physicians, nurses, and patients seems more likely to produce the kinds of doctors the rest of us want than leaving the task of selection wholly in the hands of medical-school professors who may have little respect for the kind of physician who merely takes care of people.

A doctor's attitude toward his work not only reflects the kind of person he was when he was admitted to medical school, but it is shaped by the institutions in which he learns his trade. One trouble with the training of doctors in America is that it takes place almost entirely in university hospitals, or in big teaching hospitals that are closely affiliated with medical schools. Such a setting affords the prospective pediatrician or internist or family physician no more than a glimpse of the real world of family practice, in which he will probably spend most of his time treating people who are not really very sick, and in which, to do a good job, he will have to concern himself with the messy emotional and social problems of his patients. Moreover, the men responsible for his training as a medical student, and later as an intern and resident, may make little effort to hide their conviction that family practice is tedious and depressing work, and he may well end up agreeing with them. Some schools have tried sending students out for brief periods to work with old-style general practitioners, the idea being to give them a notion of what family practice is like. But the students have often been so put off by what struck them as the slipshod work habits of their preceptors that they have abandoned any notion they might have had of going into family practice.

This is changing, however. The University of Illinois's new medical school at Rockford has been opening up two-to-six-man offices, or health centers, to provide comprehensive (and presumably nonslipshod) care to residents of a number of nearby communities that have had to get along for years without a doctor of their own. Throughout his years at the school, each student spends two half-days a week working at one of these centers. A few medical schools have made similar arrangements for students to work in clinics run by prepaid group practice plans.

More importantly, some medical school graduates (those who are taking family-practice residencies) are getting much of their postgraduate training in settings where the main business is the provision of primary care. In Santa Monica, California, for example, the Santa Monica Community Hospital operates a clinic that is intended to furnish several thousand low-income families with the services they would get from a good family doctor. When I visited the clinic in 1972, there were six young residents taking care of patients there. The director of the program, Dr. Thomas L. Stern, a former family physician, told me that during a resident's first year he spends most of his time in the hospital, learning how to deliver babies, for example, and how an intensive-care unit functions. But by the beginning of his third year he will be putting in half of his time at the clinic where he will be responsible (together with a social worker and a public health nurse trained to provide home care) for two hundred families. In this last year of his residency it will be up to him how he spends the other half of his time. Each resident thus has a chance, Dr. Stern explained, to get training in those specialties that will be most useful to him in the particular kind of practice he expects to go into. "We will highly recommend four months of psychiatry," he said. Both of the residents with whom I spoke said they would probably follow this advice. "It's already obvious that being able to spot psychological strains, and hopefully to deal with them, is an important part of family practice," one of them told me. "You can't just poke a pill down somebody."

The Medical University of South Carolina has a similar program. Family-practice residents work in a medical center furnishing primary care to a large clientele that includes prosperous as well as poor people. The physician in charge of their training, Dr. Hiram Curry, has said that he wants to turn out doctors who are more than skilled medical engineers. A patient's "personal ecology," he told an interviewer, "includes not only the physical condition of his body, but also such factors as the impact of relationships within which he lives—especially his family—the beliefs and values which give meaning to his life, the mechanism for coping with problems and expressing feelings, and the particular social and economic situation in which he finds himself." Prepaid group practice plans also are offering residencies in family practice, giving young doctors a chance to be trained in a setting where technical standards are high, but where the main emphasis is on out-of-hospital care, and where—at any rate in the clinics of well-run plans like Group Health Cooperative of Puget Sound—doctors are to some extent accountable to their patients.

This last point is important: the attitudes toward patients and their diseases that pervade the university hospital should not be allowed to dominate the training of family doctors, even though the prospective family doctor needs to learn much of what academic medicine has to teach him. One way to prevent this domination is to make someone other than a medical school responsible for postgraduate training. This is what has been done in Rockford, Illinois. In Rockford, the training of family practitioners (and, for that matter, all postgraduate training in which the new medical school is involved) has been put under the auspices of an independent foundation. The foundation, which contracts with the medical school to run the training programs that it sponsors, is governed by a board whose members include lawyers, labor leaders, businessmen, educators, politicians, and clergymen, as well as representatives of the medical school and of the community hospitals where much of the training actually takes place.

As medical care comes more and more to be furnished by institutions rather than individuals, it becomes more and more important to devise arrangements that will shield people from perhaps the worst offense of bureaucratic enterprise, namely, the assumption that clients exist for the bureaucracy's convenience instead of the other way around. With this in mind, the American Hospital Association has drafted a bill of rights for patients, which it has urged its members to adopt and abide by. The proposed bill specifies that a patient is entitled to be told, in plain English, what the doctors think is wrong with him, what they propose to do about it, what are the risks of the proposed course of treatment, and what alternatives are open to him. The association also believes a patient should have the right "to know, by name, the physician responsible for coordinating his care," the right to refuse to be experimented on, and the right to privacy—"Case discussion, consultation, examination, and treatment are confidential and should be conducted discreetly."

The adoption by a hospital of such a bill of rights is plainly a move in the right direction. A patient who believes he has been experimented on without being told what the experimenters were up to is in a better position to sue the hospital if he can show that it was violating its own rules. Indeed, one reason commonly given by administrators of hospitals that have not adopted the proposed bill of rights is that to do so would encourage unhappy patients to sue. But for a hospital's trustees simply to hand out printed copies of a bill of rights is not enough. Unless a patient has some way of enforcing those rights at the time they are violated—or are about to be violated—the fact that they have been listed on a piece of paper is not likely to do much good. In the words of Dr. Willard Gaylin, a psychiatrist who teaches at the Columbia University Law School, and who is a leading student of medical ethics, "It is the thief lecturing his victim on self-protection—i.e., the hospital instructs the patient to make sure the hospital treats him according to the rules of decency and law to which he is entitled."

What the patient needs is access to an ombudsman, or patient's advocate, who can act quickly and effectively on his behalf. A number of hospitals now have people whom they call patient's advocates. But as a rule they have little power, and are expected to spend most of their time soothing ruffled feelings. As George J. Annas, a law professor who is director of Boston University's Center for Law and Health Sciences, has pointed out, a patient's advocate cannot be what his title suggests if he is simply a wheel in the hospital's public-relations machinery. Annas argues that if an advocate is really to represent patients instead of the hospital, he must be appointed and paid by an independent public body; he must have automatic access to all medical records; he must have the authority to call in qualified consultants to give an opinion on the validity of a patient's complaints; and he must be an ex-officio member of all hospital committees that monitor medical care. A patient's advocate should also be in a position, if necessary, to take a patient's grievance to arbitration.

In most cases, of course, nothing like arbitration would be required. In a recent issue of the *Journal of Nursing Administration,* Annas and an associate, Joseph Healey, give an illustration of just how a patient's advocate might go about his job. They begin by quoting from an article, published in 1972 in the University of Pennsylvania's alumni magazine, titled "Notes of a Dying Professor." The author had been admitted to a hospital for a series of tests, and had been examined by a neurologist and three medical students. In his words, "I got a reinforcement of the sense of not only am I a patient who is supposed to behave in a certain way, but I'm almost an object to demonstrate to people that I'm not really people any more, I'm something else. I'm a body that has some very interesting characteristics about it. . . . I began to feel not only the fear of this unknown, dread thing that I have, that nobody knows anything about—and if they know, they're not going to tell me—but an anger and a resentment of 'Goddamn it, I'm a human being and I want to be treated like one!' And feeling that if I expressed anger, I could be retaliated against, because I'm in a very vulnerable position." In such a situation, Annas and Healey write, there are a number of things an advocate could do. "The advocate would be a person that the patient could talk to without fear of retaliation. A person who could pull out his medical records and tell him whether a diagnosis had been made. A person who, on behalf of a busy medical staff, could take the time to explain the reason for the tests, why medical students were present, that he could have them excluded if he wished, that no matter what his attitudes toward the medical staff or his expressions of fear and resentment, no retaliatory action would be taken against him in any manner."

If every hospital patient had a doctor of his own as counselor and guide—and as protector—there would be little need for ombudsmen or patient's advocates. But, as I have said, even a person who can perfectly well afford a doctor of his own is likely to find himself, when he is seriously ill, in the situation of the Dying Professor—cared for, that is, by an ad hoc and shifting coalition of interns, residents, and senior specialists of one variety or another, no one of whom is, in the traditional sense, "his" doctor. In the circumstances, while doctors may be less than enchanted by the prospect of patient's advocates poking into their affairs and calling them to account, they cannot reasonably object if the rest of us insist on appointing nondoctors to do a job that doctors too often are unwilling or unable to perform.

Another way to narrow the gap between what we want from doctors and hospitals, and what we often get, is to insist that nonprofessionals (consumers, as they are usually described) be put in charge of the country's medical-care system. Many congressmen and senators are already convinced that parceling out federal money for medical care is a job that should not be left entirely in the hands of doctors, hospital administrators, and federal bureaucrats. In 1974, for example, Congress passed, and President Ford later signed, a bill establishing a network of so-called Health Systems Agencies, or HSAs. The HSAs will have a lot to say about how certain kinds of federal funds for health care are allocated in their areas of jurisdiction, and the new law specifies that a majority of the people on the governing board of an HSA must be consumers—that is, not in any way involved in providing medical care.

This principle might well be applied to the governing boards of hospitals, HMOs, and health centers of all kinds. It is true that most hospital boards already are made up mainly of consumers. But as a rule they are extremely well-heeled consumers—tax lawyers, bankers, philanthropists, and corporate executives. This may be appropriate for the board of a hospital situated in a prosperous suburb. But the board of a hospital situated in or on the border of a low-income city neighborhood should include a large contingent of poor and working-class people who get most of their medical care in the hospital's clinics and emergency room. In the late 1960s some hospitals did set up advisory committees that included representatives of the poor and near-poor, but they have had little impact. "We had our first meeting several months after I got my letter of appointment," a "community member" of the Patient Care Committee of the Boston City Hospital told an interviewer. "The major topic was whether inpatients should be provided with toothpaste. I tried to steer the conversation toward broader issues but the professionals on the committee had command of the situation. . . . They dream up these committees as a means of perpetuating the system. I want to be a trustee because that's the only way to change things in the hospital—that's where the decisions are made. But when I called to submit my name for the opening on the Board they said they were looking for another businessman."

As voting members of a hospital board, representatives of low-income families would be in a position to press for more significant reforms than free toothpaste—to insist, for example, that the hospital's clinics be kept open in the evenings, that enough doctors be assigned to them to keep patients from having to wait for hours, that patient's advocates be stationed in the clinic area, and that arrangement be made for clinic patients to have their questions answered by telephone. Poor patients are not the only ones who stand to benefit by being represented on a hospital's governing board. A board member who owes his election to his union, or to some other group in the community, is more likely than the average banker or corporation president to be aware of—and to become angry about—the hospital's shortcomings in its treatment of the ordinary run of patients.

It is not easy for nonprofessionals to exert a strong influence on the operation of an institution as complicated as a hospital or an HMO. They may be frustrated by an inability to get at, and interpret, the information they need in order to challenge an administrator's proposal, or to draw up workable alternatives. For this reason, consumers sitting on a hospital board should have at their disposal the services of the equivalent of a minority counsel, an expert on hospital administration who has access to all hospital records, and who can help his clients arrive at informed judgments of the proposals they must vote on. Even without such help, however, there is evidence that medical care is better when patients have some say in how it is delivered. For all the weaknesses of the community boards that are involved in the operation of neighborhood health centers, the centers, by and large, seem to offer patients, as I have said, a warmer and less condescending brand of care than is available in the outpatient clinics of the average big-city teaching hospital. Moreover, Group Health Cooperative of Puget Sound appears to pay a good deal more attention to patients' complaints and suggestions than Kaiser-Permanente does, and the difference is almost surely due to the fact that Group Health Cooperative is run by an elected board, and Kaiser-Permanente is not. This conclusion is in line with the results of a study made some years ago, in which six cooperatively-run prepaid group practice plans were compared with six plans run entirely by doctors. The author of the study, Jerome L. Schwartz, reported that the cooperative plans generally offered more benefits and services to their members, and were much better about handling members' complaints. ("In several physician plans," Schwartz wrote, "the business manager saw his duty as shielding the physicians from the annoyance of complaints.")

All this is not to suggest that putting schoolteachers and plumbers and welfare mothers on the boards of hospitals and HMOs will work miracles. But there must be a forum in which the conflict between what patients want in the way of medical care, and what doctors and hospital administrators find it convenient to give them, can be compromised, if not resolved. Putting control of medical institutions into the hands of the people who use them is one way of restoring some of the bargaining power that patients enjoyed when there were plenty of doctors, and when a doctor who consistently failed to satisfy his patients was likely to end up not having any.

The bargaining power of the poor would, of course, be greatly enhanced by a health insurance system that guaranteed everybody free (or virtually free) medical care, and that paid doctors at the same rate for treating the poor as for treating anybody else. But even if such a system were in effect, some additional steps would still be in order to help the poor use their new leverage to best advantage. It is obviously important to avoid, insofar as we can, having one set of people and institutions that care for the middle class and rich, and another set that care mainly for the poor. To this end, federal grants and loans to HMOs should be contingent on their enrolling a specified number, or proportion, of people with low incomes. Furthermore, since the poor tend to be in poorer health, and to need more medical attention, than the rich, an HMO should be paid extra for each of its enrollees whose income falls below a certain level. (The bonus should be large enough to permit an HMO to run a minibus service for patients living in ghetto areas with poor public transportation.) This would encourage HMOs to compete for the patronage of the poor, and to incorporate into primarily middle-class practices a great many people who would otherwise be getting their medical care in hospital clinics or emergency rooms, or in the offices of doctors who rarely see a prosperous patient.

But it is obviously impractical to bus every ghetto resident out of the ghetto for his medical care. For many years to come, no matter what kind of health insurance is passed by Congress, hundreds of thousands of families living in vast slums like Watts and Bedford-Stuyvesant will still be treated by doctors working in parts of the city where few middle-class people venture except on business. Fortunately, national health insurance of the sort I would like to see enacted would put new life into existing neighborhood health centers, and would encourage the establishment of more of them. Since the centers would be guaranteed a monthly sum for each family coming to them regularly for care, they would no longer be dependent on fluctuating Congressional appropriations, or on the good will of budget officers in Washington. Their fiscal health would depend, rather, on their ability to attract and hold, as patients, the people in their neighborhoods. It is true, as I have pointed out, that the promoters of some California HMOs, organized as get-rich-quick schemes, have signed up large numbers of Medicaid patients by promising much more in the way of services than they intended to deliver. But fraud of this kind is unlikely if the government refuses to do business with a health center or HMO unless, once it has gotten under way, it is run by a board a majority of whose members are chosen by its enrollees.

Another way to improve the care meted out to the poor is to strengthen the bargaining power of inner-city health centers in their dealings with the hospitals to which they send their patients. This could be done by channeling payments to a hospital through the HMO, or neighborhood health center, in which a patient is enrolled, instead of handing the money directly to the hospital. A health center located in a low-income neighborhood would thereby be put in a position, as a major purchaser of hospital services for its members, to insist that the health center's doctors be given hospital staff privileges. It could also put pressure on a hospital to provide better care, in its specialty clinics, to health-center patients needing to be seen by an endocrinologist, a cardiologist, or some other variety of super-specialist whose services were not available at the health center itself.

It would be naive to suppose that changes of the kind I have suggested in the way that medical care in America is organized and paid for will do everything that reformers such as Senator Kennedy sometimes claim for them. Certainly they will bring about no dramatic improvement in the country's health as measured by life expectancy. Cancer and diseases of the arteries and heart have replaced infectious disorders like pneumonia and tuberculosis as the chief causes of death in the United States, and in the present state of knowledge none of these diseases is curable. As for prevention, doctors and nurses alone cannot be expected to persuade Americans to eat more wisely, exercise more, give up smoking, and stop poisoning the air they breathe. Nor will the reforms that I have proposed make all doctors humane, or secure for the poor the same medical care that the rich enjoy, or do away with all waste and extravagance.

It must be admitted, too, that changes in complicated economic and social systems, however carefully thought out, almost always have unpleasant side effects that have been foreseen only dimly, if at all, by the authors of the changes. Disagreeable consequences are bound to flow from a decision to make medical care available, at little or no out-of-pocket cost, to everybody who needs it; and disagreeable consequences will also flow from the decision—already taken—to hold doctors and hospitals to account for the quality, cost, and efficiency of their services. For one thing, it will be harder for people to get the prompt, personal attention from their doctors that some rich and middle-class patients can now command. For another, as medical care becomes more bureaucratic, doctors and patients both will have to learn to cope with a complex set of regulations dealing with such matters as whether a patient is entitled to another consultation, to home nursing care, or to an extra week or ten days in the hospital. In the new order, the ideal provider of medical care will not be the family doctor practicing on his own, but something more like one of the health centers operated by Group Health Cooperative of Puget Sound. The reformer's job then will be to find ways to preserve, insofar as possible, the intimacy and flexibility that is perhaps the chief merit of our present system of medical care, but that fewer and fewer people are fortunate enough to enjoy.

But there are good reasons why we should press very hard for the kinds of reforms I have been talking about. While it is true that medical care is a complicated business that we tamper with at our peril, improving medical care is a much easier job than bringing peace to the Middle East, stopping the deterioration of our cities, eliminating slums, or guaranteeing every black or Puerto Rican or Chicano child—or, for that matter, every *white* child—a first-rate education. As England's experience has shown, it is possible to do away with the worst faults of entrepreneurial, pay-as-you-go medicine without changing the larger political and economic system of which medicine is a part. And if we want to use the power inherent in popular government to change for the better the terms on which we live together—a power in whose reality many Americans have understandably lost faith—reshaping the enterprise of medical care is a good way to start. If we are reasonably successful in this endeavor, it may give us the confidence to set about changing in an orderly way, and without bloodshed, other powerful institutions that, like cancer, have recently seemed to be running completely out of control.

Notes

INTRODUCTION: What Crisis?

Page

xi Kennedy quotation: Address before New York Academy of Medicine Conference on National Health Programs, April 30, 1971.

xiii *"American medicine . . . brink of chaos . . ."*: *Fortune* 81, No. 1 (January 1970), p. 79.

xiii *"I ask you to picture . . ."*: *Bulletin of the New York Academy of Medicine* 46, No. 12 (December 1970), p. 1026.
Survey findings: Stephen P. Strickland, *U.S. Health Care: What's Wrong and What's Right* (a Potomac Associates Book; New York: Universe Books, 1972), p. 27.

xiv Citizens Board of Inquiry: Quotations are from *Heal Yourself, Report of the Citizens Board of Inquiry Into Health Services for Americans* (n.d.), pp. iii, iv.

xiv–xv Coles quotation: *Health Care in America, Part 1,* Hearings before the U.S. Senate Committee on Government Operations, Subcommittee on Executive Reorganization, 90th Congress, 2nd session (April 25, 1968), pp. 460–61.

xv *"Vandalia exhibits . . ."*: Joseph P. Lyford, *The Talk in Vandalia,* A Report to the Center for the Study of Democratic Institutions, 1962, p. 48.

xv National survey figures: Mac F. Cahal, "The Image," *Journal of the American Medical Association* 185, No. 3 (July 20, 1963), pp. 183–87.

CHAPTER ONE: Buying Health in a Sellers' Market

1 Hospital costs: Interview with Ruth Baine, American Hospital Association.

1 Doctors' fees: U.S. Department of Labor, *Monthly Labor Review.*

1 *In the year ending June 30, 1974, the country's medical bill . . .* : Nancy L. Worthington, "National Health Expenditures, 1929–74," *Social Security Bulletin* 38, No. 2 (February 1975), pp. 3–20.

1 Comparisons with other countries: In 1968 the United Kingdom and the Netherlands were each spending less than 5 per cent of their gross national product on medical care ("International Health Expenditures," *Social Security Bulletin*, December 1970). In 1970 Norway was spending 6.4 per cent (David M. Cleary, "Europe's Differing Health Plans," reprint of articles appearing in *The Philadelphia Bulletin* in the summer of 1970).

1-2 National Cancer Foundation study: Cancer Care, Inc., and the National Cancer Care Foundation, *The Impact, Costs and Consequences of Catastrophic Illness on Patients and Families* (New York, 1973).

2 De Lury testimony: Quoted in Godfrey Hodgson, "The Politics of American Health Care," *The Atlantic*, October 1973, p. 52.

2 David Halberstam: Quoted in A. J. Vogl, "See Yourself as V.I.P.s See You: David Halberstam," *Medical Economics*, January 21, 1974, p. 92.

2 Earnings of hospital workers: Local 1199, Drug and Hospital Union, *Fact Sheet*, December 8, 1970; interview with James Boykin of Local 1199, Drug and Hospital Union, New York City.

2-3 Henry K. DeWitt: Quoted in Harold B. Meyers, "The Medical Industrial Complex," *Fortune* 81, No. 1 (January 1970), p. 90.

3 Edwin L. Crosby: Crosby, "What Happened to Hospital Costs?" statement distributed by American Hospital Association.

4 Hospital costs in England: Theodore E. Chester, "United States Hospital Costs in International Perspective," *The Annals of the American Academy of Political and Social Science*, January 1972, p. 75.

4 Dr. Charles E. Lewis: Quoted in John H. Lavin and Linda C. Busek, "What Makes Americans So Operation-Happy?" *Medical Economics*, January 8, 1973, p. 69.

4-5 Dr. Sidney Wolfe: Pennsylvania Insurance Department, Public Hearings on Premium Request of Blue Shield of Pennsylvania and the Health Delivery System, Harrisburg, September 26, 1972 (transcript, pp. 282, 299).

5 John P. Bunker: Bunker, "Surgical Manpower: A Comparison of Operations and Surgeons in the United States and England and Wales," *New England Journal of Medicine* 282, No. 31 (January 15, 1970), pp. 135-44.

6 Lembcke-Johnson studies: Paul A. Lembcke and Olive G. Johnson, "A Medical Audit Report: Comparison of the Findings in a 200-Bed Suburban Hospital with Those in University Teaching Hospitals . . . ; also, "The Findings Before and After a Continuing Medical Audit was Established in a Large Community Hospital," School of Public Health, UCLA, 1963, pp. iv, vii, ix, 49, 56, 63.

7 *. . . the plan's members underwent 20 per cent fewer operations . . .* : W. A. MacColl, talk delivered at Insurance Finance Conference, Regina, Saskatchewan, June 30, 1971.

7 *Other comparisons have indicated . . .* : G. S. Perrott and J. C. Chase, "The Federal Employees' Health Benefits Program: Sixth Term Coverage and Utilization," *Group Health and Welfare News*, Special Supplement, October 1968, p. viii.

7 Mine Workers' program: Warren F. Draper, "The Medical Care Program of the UMWA Welfare and Retirement Fund," address to the New England Hospital Assembly, March 1958; quoted in Herman Miles Somers and Anne Ramsay Somers, *Doctors, Patients and Health Insurance* (Washington, D.C.: The Brookings Institution, 1961), pp. 409-10.

7 United Store Workers' program: Nancy Hicks, "A Second Opinion Reduces Surgery," *New York Times*, June 19, 1973.

8-9 All Bolande quotes are from Robert P. Bolande, "Ritualistic Surgery—Circumcision and Tonsillectomy," *New England Journal of Medicine* 280, No. 11 (March 13, 1969), pp. 591-96.

8 Tonsillectomies in Massachusetts: "Tonsillectomy and Adenoidectomy in Massachusetts," *New England Journal of Medicine* 285, No. 27 (December 30, 1971), p. 1537.

9 Williams estimates: *How to Avoid Unnecessary Surgery* (New York: Warner Paperback Library, 1972), p. 182.

9-10 Hospitalization in Russia: John Fry, *Medicine in Three Societies: A Comparison of Medical Care in the USSR, USA, and UK* (Aylesbury, Bucks: MTP Chiltern House, 1969).

10 Yale researchers: Raymond S. Duff, Charles D. Cook, Gary R. Wanerka, et al., "Use of Utilization Review to Assess the Quality of Pediatric Inpatient Care," *Pediatrics* 49, No. 2 (February 1972), pp. 169-76.

10 . . . surveys of federal employees . . . : For example, United States Civil Service Commission, *Reports of the Federal Employees Health Benefits Program and the Retired Federal Employees Health Benefits Program for the Fiscal Years 1961-62, 1962-63, 1963-64*. Comparisons for 1972 are in Marjorie Smith Mueller, "Private Health Insurance in 1972: Health Care Services, Enrollment, and Finances," *Social Security Bulletin*, March 1974, p. 26.

10-11 General Accounting Office estimate: GAO, *Study of Health Facilities Construction Costs*, Report to the Congress of the United States, December 1972, p. 98.

11 Pierre de Vise: De Vise, "Pressures for Change: The Social Pressures," *Hospitals* 45 (February 1, 1971), pp. 51-55.

11 Chicago Regional Hospital Study: Ibid.

11 Inter-Society Commission: Inter-Society Commission for Heart Disease Resources, Surgery Study Group, "Optimal Resources for Cardiac Surgery," *Circulation* 44 (September 1971), A-221-A-236.

12 Denenberg: Quoted in Rose De Wolf, "Fighting Spiraling Health Care Costs," *Chicago Tribune*, November 8, 1971.

12 President's Commission on Heart Disease, Cancer and Strokes: Cited by William Fullerton, "The Problem of Rising Hospital Costs, February 6, 1968: A Report by the Library of Congress Legislative Reference Service," printed in *Health Care in America, Part 1*, Hearings Before the U.S. Senate Committee on Government Operations, Subcommittee on Executive Reorganization, 90th Congress, 2nd Session (1968), p. 169.

12 James Brusstar: Quoted in Harry T. Paxton, "Whatever Happened to the Hospital Bed Shortage?" *Medical Economics*, February 28, 1972, p. 44.

13 *"misguided boom"*: Victor Cohn, "Unneeded Hospital Building Boom in Area," *Washington Post*, August 26, 1973, 96:1b.

13 . . . *the average occupancy rate* . . . : *Hospitals* 48, No. 8 (April 16, 1974), p. 23.

13 Cost of surplus beds: Cohn, in his *Washington Post* story, quotes the American Hospital Association as saying an empty bed costs two thirds as much as a full one; another source estimated the cost of an empty bed at only 15 to 20 per cent of the cost of a full one.

13–14 Lembcke study: Paul A. Lembcke, "Hospital Efficiency—A Lesson from Sweden," *Hospitals* 33, No. 7 (April 1, 1959), pp. 34–38, 92.

14 American Hospital Association study of costs: Cited in National Advisory Commission on Health Manpower, *Report*, Vol. I (Washington, D.C.: Government Printing Office, 1967), p. 55.

14 Rashi Fein: Quoted in de Vise, "Pressures for Change: the Social Pressures."

Chapter Two: Buying Health in a Sellers' Market (Continued)

15 Dr. John H. Knowles: "Dr. Knowles and the Foundations," *Intellectual Digest*, February 1972, pp. 28–31; Lawrence K. Altman, "Dr. Knowles Is Facing Censure over His Allegations on Medical Profits and Surgery," *New York Times*, June 5, 1972, p. 15.

15 Doctors' fees before and after Medicare: *Medical Care Costs and Prices: Background Book*, Department of Health, Education and Welfare, Social Security Administration, Office of Research and Statistics, January 1972, pp. 40–41.

15–16 Doctors' incomes, 1965–1970: Arthur Owens, "Physicians' Earnings: Leveling Off," *Medical Economics*, October 11, 1971, pp. 203–11.

16 . . . *in the six months after controls were taken off* . . . : *Social Security Bulletin* 38, No. 1 (January 1975), p. 72.

16 . . . *sketch of a Florida physician* . . . : James A. Reynolds, "My Retirement's Taken Care of—I Can Live It Up Now," *Medical Economics*, March 18, 1974, pp. 88–95.

16–17 Doctors' earnings in 1971: William N. Jeffers, "Self-employed M.D.s' Earnings and Expenses: How High the Bind?" *Medical Economics*, November 20, 1972, pp. 131–47.

17 Internal Revenue Service study: Cited in Henry Aubin, "Doctors' Incomes Soaring Above Rise in Cost of Living," *Washington Post*, June 21, 1971, 94:1c.

17 *Knowles has explained* . . . : Altman, "Dr. Knowles is Facing Censure. . . ."

17 . . . *physicians such as Dr. Vernon E. Martens* . . . : Ronald Kessler, "Pathologists: More Profits, More Pay," *Washington Post*, November 1, 1972, 95:1.

18 *Knowles has pointed out* . . . : Altman, "Dr. Knowles Is Facing Censure. . . ."

18 *A West Coast radiologist* . . . : James N. Kastal, "Something Is Rotten in Radiology!" *Medical Economics*, June 5, 1972, pp. 170–75.

18–19 *A California surgeon* . . . : Clifford L. Graves, "Are Surgeons Squeezing the System?" *Medical Economics*, March 18, 1974, pp. 222–26.

19 . . . *a survey of physicians in and around Hartford* . . . : Ray H. Elling and Joyce K. Bain, "The System of Medical Practice in the Hartford Capitol Region," mimeographed, August 1971, p. 44.

19 . . . *an analysis of 1960 census data* . . . : Cited in Nancy Hicks, "Doctors' Median Income ($40,550) Spurs Fee Debate," *New York Times*, September 13, 1971.

19–20 What interns and residents earn: Interview, Rosemarie Maune, executive secretary, National Association of Residents and Interns.

20 Medical school applications: In 1964–65, there were 19,168 applicants, of whom 9043 were accepted.

20 . . . *young graduates often grew so discouraged* . . . : Richard H. Shryock, *The Development of Modern Medicine* (New York: Alfred A. Knopf, 1947), p. 258. A survey of 100 young doctors graduating from medical schools around the turn of the century disclosed that seventy-five had quit medicine within five years, mainly to find a way to make a better living.

20 Flexner critique: Abraham Flexner, *Medical Education in the United States and Canada*, A Report to the Carnegie Foundation for the Advancement of Teaching, Carnegie Foundation Bulletin No. 4., New York, 1910.

21 Closing down of medical schools and new licensing requirements: Rosemary Stevens, *American Medicine and the Public Interest* (New Haven: Yale University Press, 1971), pp. 68–69.

21 Medical school enrollments: Shryock, *The Development of Modern Medicine*, p. 340; Stevens, *American Medicine and the Public Interest*, pp. 177, 354. Role of AMA: Reuben A. Kessel, "The AMA and the Supply of Physicians," *Law and Contemporary Problems* 35, No. 2 (Spring 1970), pp. 267–83.

21 AMA on need for more doctors: The Carnegie Commission on Higher Education, *Higher Education and the Nation's Health* (New York: McGraw-Hill, 1970), p. 101.

22 Surgeons' earnings: Arthur Owens, "Too Many General Surgeons? Then Why Aren't They Poor?" *Medical Economics*, April 15, 1974, pp. 137–42.

23 Cost of drug-company promotional efforts: The drug industry would deny spending more than a billion dollars a year on promotion. I am following T. Donald Rucker, "Economic Problems in Drug Distribution," *Inquiry* 9, No. 3 (September 1972), pp. 43–50. Rucker, now a professor at Ohio State University, was Chief of the Drug Studies Branch of the Social Security Administration's Office of Research and Statistics. His estimate squares with a study by the Department of Health, Education and Welfare, based on 1966 financial data, which showed that seventeen of the most successful pharmaceutical companies were spending 35 per cent of their gross revenues on "marketing and general expenses"; allowing 10 per cent for general expenses (not including manufacturing costs, or cost of materials, or the cost of research and development) this would mean that twenty-five cents of every dollar taken in by these seventeen companies was being spent on the marketing of their products.

23 Pierre Garai: Garai, "Advertising and Promotion of Drugs," in Paul Talalay, ed., *Drugs in Our Society* (Baltimore: The Johns Hopkins Press, 1964), p. 191.

24 *A survey of 86,000 hospital patients* . . . : Commission on Professional and Hospital Activities, "Therapeutic Use of Antibiotics," *The Record*, August 22, 1962; quoted in Robert S. McCleery et al. *One Life—One Physician*, A Report to the Center for Study of Responsive Law (Washington, D.C.: Public Affairs Press, 1971), p. 24.

24 Dr. Harry Dowling on antibiotics: Quoted in Calvin M. Kunin, Thelma Tupasi, and William A. Craig, "Use of Antibiotics: A Brief Exposition of the Problems and Some Tentative Solutions," *Annals of Internal Medicine* 79, No. 4 (October 1973), pp. 555–60.

24 *Yet two medical researchers* . . . : Paul D. Stolley and Louis Lasagna, "Prescribing Patterns of Physicians," *Journal of Chronic Diseases* 22 (1969), pp. 395–405.

24–25 . . . *another commentator on B_{12}'s popularity* . . . : Richard Burack, *The New Handbook of Prescription Drugs* (New York: Pantheon Books, 1970), p. 281.

25 Stolley on antihistamines: Paul D. Stolley, "Cultural Lags in Health Care," *Inquiry* 8, No. 3 (September 1971), pp. 71–76.

25 Prevalence of bad reactions to antibiotics: Henry E. Simmons and Paul D. Stolley, "This is Medical Progress? Trends and Consequences of Antibiotic Use in the U.S.," *Journal of the American Medical Association* 227, No. 9 (March 4, 1974), pp. 1023–28.

25–26 Rise of Gram-negative infections: Kunin et al., "Use of Antibiotics . . . ."

26 Dr. Martin Shargel: *Examination of the Pharmaceutical Industry, 1973–74, Part 4*, Hearings before the U.S. Senate Committee on Labor and Public Welfare, Subcommittee on Health, 93rd Congress, 1st and 2nd sessions (May 3, 1974), p. 1299.

26 Colonel Robert H. Moser: Cited in Burack, *The New Handbook of Prescription Drugs*, p. 5.

26–27 Kefauver and estrodiol: *Administered Prices, Part 14*, Hearings before the U.S. Senate Committee on the Judiciary, Subcommittee on Antitrust and Monopoly, 86th Congress, 1st Session (1959), p. 7881.

27 Cost of Valium: Senator Gaylord Nelson, "Public Health Price Protection Act," *Congressional Record*, September 29, 1972, p. S16336.

27 Nelson on drug prices in other countries: Ibid.

28 Price of Serpasil: *Competitive Problems in the Drug Industry: Summary and Analysis* (Committee Print), U.S. Senate Select Committee on Small Business, Subcommittee on Monopoly (November 2, 1972), p. 15.

28 ... *thirteen of the fifty most frequently prescribed drugs* ... : "National Prescription Audit," *Pharmacy Times*, April 1974, p. 38. Prices are those listed in the standard industry compilation, *Drug Topics Red Book*.

28 Dispensability of Butisol: Burack, *The New Handbook of Prescription Drugs*, p. 81.

28 Prices of butabarbital, Butisol, etc.: *Drug Topics Red Book* for 1974.

28–29 *As Richard Harris has written* ... : Harris, *The Real Voice* (New York: The Macmillan Co., 1964), p. 76.

29 Stetler quotation: *Competitive Problems in the Drug Industry: Summary and Analysis*, pp. 31–32.

29 1973 drug-company earnings: *Fortune*, May 1974.

29 Mueller on drug-industry profits: *Competitive Problems in the Drug Industry: Summary and Analysis*, p. 33.

30 ... *the Kefauver committee calculated* ... : *Study of Administered Prices in the Drug Industry (Senate Report No. 448)*, U.S. Senate Committee on the Judiciary, Subcommittee on Antitrust and Monopoly, 87th Congress, 1st session (1961), p. 39.

30 *A government study* ... : U.S. Department of Health, Education and Welfare, *The Drug Makers and the Drug Distributors*, Task Force on Prescription Drugs, Background Papers, December 1968.

30 Witness at Canadian inquiry: *Competitive Problems in the Drug Industry, Part 5*, Hearings before the U.S. Senate Select Committee on Small Business, Subcommittee on Monopoly, 90th Congress, 1st and 2nd sessions (1967–1968), p. 1917.

30 *Yet the Social Security Administration has estimated* ... : Marjorie Smith Mueller, "Private Health Insurance in 1973: A Review of Coverage, Enrollment, and Financial Experience," *Social Security Bulletin* 38, No. 2 (February 1974), pp. 21–40.

30–31 Metropolitan Life's uninsurables: *Commercial Health and Accident Insurance Industry, Part 1*, Hearings before the U.S. Senate Committee on the Judiciary, Subcommittee on Antitrust and Monopoly, 92nd Congress, 2nd session (1972), pp. 973–1013.

31 The case of Paul R: Committee for National Health Insurance, *Health Security News* 2, No. 4 (March 1973).

31–32 Woodcock quotation: *Commercial Health and Accident Insurance Industry, Part 1*, p. 13.

33 Kennedy-Smythe dialogue: Quoted in Edward M. Kennedy, *In Critical Condition: The Crisis in America's Health Care* (New York: Simon & Schuster, 1972), pp. 38–41.

CHAPTER THREE: The Question of Quality

34–35 *"The [American] general practitioner ...":* Milton I. Roemer, "The Impact of Hospitals on the Practice of Medicine in Europe and America," *Hospitals* 37 (November 1, 1963), pp. 61–64, 124.

35 Infant mortality statistics: *UN Demographic Yearbook for 1973* (New York: United Nations, 1974). The appearance of Malta on this list is probably a statistical or epidemiological accident. In 1969 through 1971, and again in 1973, infant deaths occurred with much greater frequency in Malta than in the U.S. On the other hand, New Zealand, which apparently failed to supply the UN with an infant-mortality figure for 1972, would almost certainly have made the list if it had done so. For many years before 1972 the infant-mortality rate was lower in New Zealand than in the U.S., and preliminary figures indicate that that was so in 1973 as well.

36 *. . . 120,000 fewer American babies would have died . . .* : Calculated from *UN Demographic Yearbook for 1973.*

36 *As the AMA has put it . . .* : Quoted in "International Health Statistics: Who's to Believe What?" *Perspective, the Blue Cross Magazine,* 3rd quarter, 1971, p. 7.

36 Infant mortality in Britain: In England and Wales, infant mortality in 1945 was 46 deaths per thousand births, as compared with 38.3 deaths per thousand in the U.S. *Report of the Ministry of Health for the Year Ended 31st March 1946* (London: H.M.'s Stationery Office, 1946); U.S. Department of Commerce, *Historical Statistics of the United States, Colonial Times to 1957,* and *UN Demographic Yearbook for 1973.*

37 Rutstein on Swedish midwives: David D. Rutstein, *The Coming Revolution in Medicine* (Cambridge, Mass.: The MIT Press, 1967), pp. 26–27.

37 De Vise quotation: Pierre de Vise, "Slum Medicine: Chicago Style," in Pierre de Vise et al., *Slum Medicine: Chicago's Apartheid Health System,* Report No. 6, University of Chicago Community and Family Study Center, January 1, 1969, p. 69.

38 Infant mortality in Denver: André Chabot, "Improved Mortality Rates in a Population Served by a Comprehensive Neighborhood Health Program," *Pediatrics* 47, No. 6 (June 1971), pp. 989–94.

38 Infant mortality in Holmes County: "A Dramatic Cut in Infant Mortality," *Medical World News,* October 27, 1972, pp. 80–84.

39–40 Fitzsimmons testimony: Quoted in Edward M. Kennedy, *In Critical Condition: The Crisis in America's Health Care* (New York: Simon & Schuster, 1972), pp. 155–56.

39 Kerr White quotation: *American Journal of Public Health* 59, No. 1 (January 1969), Supplement, p. 67.

40 *A second Teamsters' Union study . . .* : Columbia University School of Public Health and Administrative Medicine, *A Study of the Quality of Hospital Care Secured by a Sample of Teamster Family Members in New York City* (1964).

40 *Similar findings were reported by the Yale investigators . . .* : Raymond S. Duff, Charles D. Cook, et al., "Use of Utilization Review to Assess the Quality of Pediatric Inpatient Care," *Pediatrics* 43, No. 2 (February 1972).

40–41 Chestnut Hill Hospital: Clement R. Brown, Jr., "How to Evaluate: Models and Mechanisms," in James E. C. Walker et al., eds., *Evaluation of Care in the University and Community Hospital,* Proceedings of the University of Connecticut School of Medicine Conference, Hartford, Conn.,

Health Services Research Series, No. 2 (1970); also, Clement R. Brown, Jr., and H. S. M. Uhl, "Mandatory Continuing Education: Sense or Nonsense?" *Journal of the American Medical Association* 213, No. 10 (September 7, 1970), pp. 1660–68.

41–42 *A study recently reported . . .* : Robert H. Brook and Robert L. Stevenson, Jr., "Effectiveness of Patient Care in an Emergency Room," *New England Journal of Medicine* 283 (October 22, 1970), pp. 904–907.

42 *Investigators at Johns Hopkins . . .* : Cited in Richard A. Shaffer, "Grim Diagnosis," *Wall Street Journal*, October 5, 1971, 51:1.

42–43 Institute of Medicine study: National Academy of Sciences, Institute of Medicine, *Assessment of Medical Care for Children* (Washington, D.C., 1974), pp. 4, 6, 180, 188.

43–44 Peterson study: Osler L. Peterson et al., "An Analytical Study of North Carolina General Practice, 1953–1954," *Journal of Medical Education*, December 1956, Part 2. Also, Lois Hoffman, "How Do Good Doctors Get That Way?" in E. Gartly Jaco, ed., *Patients, Physicians and Illness* (New York: The Free Press, 1958).

44 Canadian study: Kenneth F. Clute, *The General Practitioner* (Toronto: University of Toronto Press, 1963), pp. 313–15.

45 *The United States has more doctors . . .* : *The American Almanac: The U.S. Book of Statistics and Information for 1972*, The Statistical Abstract of the United States, 92nd edition. (New York: Grosset & Dunlap), pp. 799–800.

46 *Weldon Barton . . . told: Physicians Training Facilities and Health Maintenance Organizations*, Hearings before the Subcommittee on Health of the Committee on Labor and Public Welfare, U.S. Senate, 92nd Congress, 2nd session (May 1, 1972), p. 2044.

46 Illinois Medical Society: Cited in Alex Gerber, *The Gerber Report* (New York: David McKay, 1971), p. 45.

46 Chelsea, Mass., figures: Howard H. Hiatt, "Medical Care for Northbridge: A Model for Teaching Hospital-Community Interaction," *New England Journal of Medicine* 284, No. 11 (March 18, 1971), pp. 593–602. Hiatt identifies the community he writes about only as "Northbridge," but it is clear from internal evidence, as well as from other sources, that Northbridge is Chelsea.

46 De Vise quotation: Pierre de Vise, "Persistence of Chicago's Dual Hospital System," in de Vise et al., *Slum Medicine: Chicago's Apartheid Health System*, Report No. 6, University of Chicago Community and Family Study Center, January 1, 1969, p. 20.

47 *When physicians at one hundred and fifty hospitals . . .* : H. Margulies, L. S. Bloch, and F. K. Cholko, "Random Survey of U.S. Hospitals with Approved Internships and Residencies: A Study of the Professional Qualities of Foreign Medical Graduates," *Journal of Medical Education* 43 (June 1968), pp. 706–16.

47–48 Foreign graduates who are unlicensed or have limited licenses: R. J. Weiss, J. C. Kleinman, and U. C. Brandt, "Foreign Medical Graduates and the Medical Underground," *New England Journal of Medicine* 290, No.

26 (June 27, 1974), pp. 1408–13. Also, Lawrence K. Altman, "Many Foreign Physicians in U.S. Found Unlicensed," *New York Times,* June 19, 1974, p. 1.

CHAPTER FOUR: The Bitter Taste of Charity

49 *"The hospital's physical plant . . ."*: De Vise, "We Spend Enough Money on Care for the Poor, But We Spend it Badly," *Modern Hospital* 114, No. 5 (May 1970), pp. 84–86, 148.

49 *"The family does not like the [hospital] clinics. . . ."*: Harold B. Wise, "Medicine and Poverty," in E. Fuller Torrey, ed., *Ethical Issues in Medicine* (Boston: Little, Brown, 1968), pp. 349–70.

49 *"I thought I was expecting a baby . . ."*: *Heal Yourself: Report of the Citizens Board of Inquiry Into Health Services for Americans,* p. 2.

50 Mississippi survey: Southern Regional Council, *Special Report: Hungry Children* (May 1967); printed in *Health Care in America, Part 1,* Hearings before the U.S. Senate Committee on Government Operations, Subcommittee on Executive Reorganization, 90th Congress, 2nd session (1968), pp. 476–79.

50–51 Head Start children: A. F. North, Jr., "Project Head Start and the Pediatrician," *Clinical Pediatrics* 6 (April 1967), pp. 191–94.

51 Children's health in Washington, D.C.: National Academy of Sciences, Institute of Medicine, *Assessment of Medical Care for Children* (Washington, D.C., 1974), pp. 51, 54, 183.

51–52 Eligibility for Medicaid: *Heal Yourself,* pp. 2–3, 35.

52 *. . . an angry Medicaid recipient . . .* : *Social Welfare in Vermont: Biennial Report to the Governor and General Assembly* (July 1966–June 1968), pp. 18–19.

52 *A federal task force found . . .* : U.S. Department of Health, Education and Welfare, Office of the Secretary, *Report of the Task Force on Medicaid and Related Programs,* June 1970, p. 2.

52 *"Once I called 20 different doctors . . ."*: *Heal Yourself,* p. 4.

53 *In Portland, Oregon . . .* : Ibid., p. 4.

53 *"I joined Medicaid . . ."*: Henry Aubin, "Some D.C. Doctors Like Medicaid, Others Shun Program," *Washington Post,* June 25, 1971, 94:1c.

53 *Dr. Kavaler wrote . . .* : Florence Kavaler, "People, Providers and Payment—Telling It How It Is," *American Journal of Public Health* 59, No. 5 (May 1969), pp. 825–29.

53 *Leon A. Katz . . . reported . . .* : Edward Ranzal, "Strict Bill in Council Aims to Curb Medicaid Abuses," *New York Times,* January 27, 1973.

53–54 Welfare physicians in Chicago: Pierre de Vise et al., *Slum Medicine: Chicago's Apartheid Health System,* Report No. 6, University of Chicago Community and Family Study Center, January 1, 1969, pp. 51, 53, 57, 58, 64.

54 . . . *two doctors practicing in one of the poorest sections* . . . : R. Kotulak and T. Powers, *Chicago Tribune*, June 12, 1969.

54–55 New York City emergency rooms: Eli Ginzberg and the Conservation of Human Resources Staff, *Urban Health Services: The Case of New York* (New York: Columbia University Press, 1971), p. 122; also, Max H. Seigel, "Emergency Rooms Found Misused by New York City Patients," *New York Times*, April 30, 1974.

55–56 Columbia student's report: Barry Siegel, "Inside the Booker," unpublished manuscript, 1972. (On file in the library of the Graduate School of Journalism, Columbia University.)

56 Roth quotations: Julius A. Roth, "The Treatment of the Sick," in John Kosa, Aaron Antonovsky, and Irving Kenneth Zola, eds., *Poverty and Health: A Sociological Analysis* (Cambridge, Mass.: Harvard University Press, 1969), p. 230.

57 *"Welfare cases . . ."*: Ibid., p. 232.

57–58 "*. . . welfare clients questioned recently in New York . . .*": Margaret C. Olendzki, Richard P. Grann, and Charles H. Goodrich, "The Impact of Medicaid on Private Care for the Urban Poor," *Medical Care* 10, No. 3 (May–June 1972), pp. 201–206.

58 *Brook and Stevenson* . . . : Robert H. Brook and Robert L. Stevenson, Jr., "Effectiveness of Patient Care in an Emergency Room," *New England Journal of Medicine* 283 (October 22, 1970), pp. 904–907.

59 *A young San Francisco woman* . . . : Quoted in Edward M. Kennedy, *In Critical Condition: The Crisis in America's Health Care* (New York: Simon & Schuster, 1972), p. 97.

60 Harvard medical student: Letter, February 27, 1975.

60 *As recently as 1968* . . . : M. A. Fredericks, J. Kosa, and L. S. Robertson, "The doctor and the poor: a study of physicians' attitudes toward treating the poor," paper presented at the annual meeting of the Eastern Sociological Society, New York, April 1969.

62 *Rose Lamb Coser* . . . : Coser, *Life in the Ward* (East Lansing, Michigan: Michigan State University Press, 1962).

63 *Health Law Newsletter:* August 1971.

63 *. . . according to Pierre de Vise* . . . : De Vise, "Cook County Hospital: Bulwark of Chicago's Apartheid Health System," *The New Physician*, June 1971, pp. 394–98.

63–64 *. . . staff physicians at the District of Columbia General Hospital* . . . : "Statement of the House Staff Association of the District of Columbia General Hospital Before the Survey Team of the Joint Commission on Accreditation of Hospitals," quoted in William Worthington and Laurens H. Silver, "Regulation of the Quality of Care in Hospitals: The Need for Change," *Law and Contemporary Problems* 35, No. 2 (Spring 1970), pp. 305–306.

64 *A resident physician at San Francisco General* . . . : *Physicians' Training Facilities and Health Maintenance Organizations*, Hearings before the

Subcommittee on Health of the Committee on Labor and Public Welfare, U.S. Senate, 92nd Congress, 2nd Session (1972), p. 1976 (testimony of Kenneth Barnes, M.D.).

64 Society of Urban Physicians report: Matthew Fine, Jeffrey Sacks, et al., "Nursing in New York City Municipal Hospitals," Society of Urban Physicians, p. 7.

64 *"At least fifteen cases . . ."*: Quoted in a press release from New York State Senator Roy M. Goodman, October 15, 1970.

64–65 *A year later, Edmond O. Rothschild . . .* : Rothschild, "The Level of Health Care in Municipal Hospitals is Shocking," *New York Times*, November 27, 1971.

65 *Thus David Sudnow . . .* : Sudnow, "Dying in a Public Hospital," in Orville G. Brim, Jr. et al., eds., *The Dying Patient* (New York: Russell Sage Foundation, 1970), p. 206.

65–66 *Sometimes, Sudnow suggests . . .* : Sudnow, "Dead on Arrival," in Anselm L. Strauss, ed., *Where Medicine Fails* (Chicago: Aldine, 1970), p. 123.

CHAPTER FIVE: The Price of Scientific Medicine

67 L. J. Henderson: Quoted in Alan Gregg, *Challenges to Contemporary Medicine* (New York: Columbia University Press, 1956), p. 13.

67 *. . . one historian has written . . .* : Erwin H. Ackernecht, *A Short History of Medicine* (New York: The Ronald Press, 1955), p. 178.

69 *Even in pediatrics . . .* : William N. Jeffers, "Self-employed M.D.s' Earnings and Expenses: How High the Bind?" *Medical Economics*, November 20, 1972, p. 133.

69 Atchley quotations: Dana W. Atchley, "Changing Patterns of Medical Education," *Journal of Medical Education* 41 (April 1966), pp. 325–31.

69–70 Student poll at Downstate: Samuel W. Bloom, "The Medical School as a Social System," *The Milbank Memorial Fund Quarterly* 59, No. 2 (April 1971), Part 2, pp. 100, 190–91.

70 Haggerty quotation: Robert J. Haggerty, "Etiology of Decline in General Practice," *Journal of the American Medical Association* 185, No. 3 (July 20, 1963), pp. 179–82.

70 Number of doctors beginning family-practice residencies: American Academy of Family Physicians, quoted in *Medical Economics,* July 8, 1974, p. 16.

70–71 *. . . the more than 16,000 men and women . . .* : *Directory of Approved Internships and Residencies, 1973–74* (Chicago: American Medical Association, 1973), p. 11.

71 Decline in number of GPs: "Can Washington Tell Doctors Where to Go?" *Medical World News*, September 13, 1974, pp. 46, 54.

71 *Medical Economics* poll: Howard Eisenberg, "What the Next Medical Generation Wants," *Medical Economics*, September 11, 1972, pp. 191–206.

71–72 *The poet Mark Van Doren* . . . : *The Autobiography of Mark Van Doren* (New York: Harcourt, Brace & Company, 1958), pp. 18, 19.

72–73 Duff and Hollingshead: *Sickness and Society* (New York: Harper & Row, 1968), p. 277.

73 Emily Mumford: Mumford, *Interns: From Students to Physicians* (Cambridge, Mass.: Harvard University Press, 1970), pp. 118, 169.

73–74 Deborah Josephs: Josephs, "The Right to Die With Dignity," *New York Times*, September 25, 1971, p. 31.

74 *David Sudnow . . . reports* . . . : Sudnow, "Dying in a Public Hospital," in Orville G. Brim, Jr. et al., eds., *The Dying Patient* (New York: Russell Sage Foundation, 1970), p. 204.

74 *. . . a young house officer* . . . : Duff and Hollingshead, *Sickness and Society*, p. 48.

74–75 *"It has always bothered me . . ."*: Ibid., p. 318.

75 Geiger: Interview, March 14, 1974.

76 Michael Crichton: Crichton, *Five Patients: The Hospital Explained* (New York, Alfred A. Knopf, 1970), p. 211.

76 Mrs. Helms: Duff and Hollingshead, *Sickness and Society*, pp. 162–63, 293–94.

77 ". . . *no tangible effort to diagnose mental illness* . . .": Ibid., p. 166.

77–78 The physician as Socratic teacher: Ibid., p. 380.

78 *. . . the young interns and residents in training* . . . : Ibid., p. 154.

79 John Knowles: Quoted in Crichton, *Five Patients: The Hospital Explained*, p. 200.

81 *The authors of a 1964 survey* . . . : R. P. Grant, C. P. Huttrer, C. G. Metzner, "Biomedical Science in Europe," *Science* 146 (October 23, 1964), pp. 493–501.

82 *. . . John H. Knowles has written* . . . : Knowles, "The Balanced Biology of the Teaching Hospital," in Knowles, ed., *Hospitals, Doctors and the Public Interest* (Cambridge, Mass.: Harvard University Press, 1965), p. 31.

82 *. . . a recent survey of medical-school faculties* . . . : James V. Maloney, "A Report on the Role of Economic Motivation in the Performance of Medical School Faculty," *Surgery* 68, No. 1 (July 1970), pp. 1–19.

82 Mumford: *Interns: From Students to Physicians*, p. 204.

83 *Emily Mumford reports* . . . : Ibid., pp. 206–207.

Chapter Six: Some Notes on the Sociology of Healing

85 *. . . in the words of one English commentator* . . . : Gilles Cremonesi in *New Society;* quoted in Michael Halberstam, "Patients Who Make the Doctor Feverish," *New York Times Magazine*, February 5, 1967.

86 *A recent poll* . . . : Cited in Alex Gerber, *The Gerber Report* (New York: David McKay, 1971), p. 108.

87–88 Ruth Brecher: Edward Brecher, "With a Life at Stake," *McCall's*, October 1967.

88 Czechoslovakia poll: "Poll Finds Czech Patients Satisfied with GPs; A Few Urge Improvements," *Hospital Tribune* 6, No. 2 (August 7, 1972).

89 *"The [clinic] physician . . ."*: Skrbkova and Vacek, "Some Problems of Health Care Organization in Czechoslovakia," *Medical Care* 9, No. 5 (September–October 1971), pp. 405–14.

89–90 *. . . a prepaid group practice studied by Eliot Freidson . . .* : Freidson, *Patients' Views of Medical Practice* (New York: Russell Sage Foundation, 1961), pp. 57–58, 228, 230.

90 *. . . a physician in Renton, Washington . . .* : Baird M. Bardarson, "Turn Away Welfare Patients? We Make It Unethical," *Medical Economics*, September 25, 1972, p. 171.

91 Verstandig: Ned Thomas, "Verstandig Sounds Warning," *New Haven Register*, March 28, 1969.

91 *Freidson reports . . .* : *Patients' Views of Medical Practice*, p. 51.

91–92 *When the American College of Surgeons first proposed . . .* : Beverly C. Payne, "Continued Evolution of a System of Medical Appraisal," *Journal of the American Medical Association*, August 14, 1967.

92 Beverly Hills doctor: Nancy Hicks, "Nation's Doctors Move to Police Medical Care," *New York Times*, October 28, 1973.

92 *. . . as Eliot Freidson points out . . .* : Freidson, *Profession of Medicine* (New York: Dodd, Mead, 1970), pp. 164–80.

93 *. . . a sociologist who looked into the reading habits . . .* : Theodore Caplow, "Market Attitudes: A Research Report from the Medical Field," *Harvard Business Review* 30, No. 6 (November–December 1952), pp. 105–12.

93 *Osler Peterson . . . found . . .* : Peterson et al., "An Analytical Study of North Carolina General Practice, 1953–1954," *Journal of Medical Educaton*, December 1956, Part 2.

93 *. . . a study of Kansas physicians . . .* : C. E. Lewis and R. S. Hassanein, "Continuing Medical Education: An Epidemiologic Evaluation," *New England Journal of Medicine* 282 (January 29, 1970), pp. 254–59.

94 *. . . as Peterson noted . . .* : Peterson, "An Analytical Study . . ." p. 82.

94 *"When I was a young faculty member . . ."*: Interview with Count Gibson, February 7, 1972.

94 *. . . a survey of members of the New Jersey Medical Association . . .* : Cited in "Prepayment for Medical Care in New York State, submitted by School of Public Health and Administrative Medicine, Columbia University, to Hon. Herman E. Hilleboe, Commissioner, Department of Health, and Hon. Thomas Thatcher, Superintendent of Insurance," October 1962.

95 *. . . studies in both the United States and Canada . . .* : See, e.g., Columbia University School of Public Health and Administrative Medicine, A

Study of the Quality of Hospital Care Secured by a Sample of Teamster Family Members in New York City, 1964; and Kenneth F. Clute, *The General Practitioner* (Toronto: University of Toronto Press, 1963).

95 *Malpractice claims . . . are running at a rate of more than 18,000 a year . . .* : Richard M. Markus, "You Doctors are Making Too Much of Malpractice," *Medical Economics,* May 28, 1973.

95 *. . . roughly half of all such claims . . .* : *Report of the Secretary's Commission on Medical Malpractice,* Washington, D.C., U.S. Department of Health, Education and Welfare Publication No. (OS) 73–88 (January 16, 1973), p. 10.

95–96 Robert C. Derbyshire: Quoted in Joann S. Lublin, "Do Doctors Need a Check-Up?" *Wall Street Journal,* February 25, 1974.

95 *. . . the story of a gynecologist . . .* : *Medical Times,* February 1972.

96 *. . . 214 doctors were asked . . .* : Joseph Kelny, "The Conspiracy of Silence," *Trial,* February-March 1970, p. 18.

96 *. . . Derbyshire pointed out . . .* : Quoted in John Carlova, "They're Going After Bad Apples as Never Before," *Medical Economics,* May 28, 1973, p. 145.

96 Dr. Ronald E. Clark: Anthony Ripley, "9 Deaths Studied in Doctor's Case," *New York Times,* December 3, 1967, p. 60; also, *New York Times,* June 30, 1968, and *Medical World News,* August 2, 1968, p. 25.

96–97 *Derbyshire has pointed out . . .* : Quoted in "Professional Standards: Enforcement Held Lax," *House Physician Reporter,* June 1973.

97 *AMA's code of ethics:* American Medical Association, *Opinions and Reports of the Judicial Council* (Chicago: AMA, 1969), p. vi.

97 *"This is a preposterous situation . . ."*: Quoted in Howard R. Lewis and Martha E. Lewis, *The Medical Offenders* (New York: Simon & Schuster, 1970), pp. 54–55.

97 *Derbyshire told an international conference . . .* : "Professional Standards: Enforcement Held Lax."

97 Holman: "Hard Cases Make Bad Law," *Journal of the American Medical Association,* October 29, 1973.

98 *. . . in one of the investigations . . .* : R. E. Trussell, M. A. Morehead, et al., *The Quantity, Quality, and Costs of Medical and Hospital Care Secured by a Sample of Teamster Families in the New York Area* (New York: Columbia University School of Public Health and Administrative Medicine, 1962).

98 Number of unaccredited hospitals and beds: *Guide to the Health Care Field* (Chicago: American Hospital Association, 1973). At the end of 1972 there were 5843 nonfederal short-term, general and special hospitals, with 884,000 beds. Of these, 4217, with 803,945 beds, were accredited.

99 Nader study-group report: Robert McCleery, *One Life-One Physician* (Washington, D.C.: Public Affairs Press, 1971), pp. 98–106, 149–50.

99 *Senator Kennedy has complained . . .* : *Physicians Training Facilities and Health Maintenance Organizations,* Hearings Before the U.S. Senate

Committee on Labor and Public Welfare, Subcommittee on Health, 92nd Congress, 2nd session (1972), pp. 1907–1908.

99 Porterfield: Quoted in "Hospital Accreditation," *Medical World News*, May 15, 1970.

100 *But as two legal scholars . . . have pointed out . . .* : Worthington and Silver, "Regulation of Quality of Care in Hospitals: The Need for Change," *Law and Contemporary Problems* 35, No. 2 (Spring 1970), pp. 306–33. (Quotation is on p. 312.)

100 *. . . Dr. Porterfield came back . . .* : "News," *Modern Hospital*, July 1970, p. 30.

101 *. . . the surveyor sensed something odd . . .* : McCleery, *One Life–One Physician*, pp. 103–104.

101–102 *"Is Peer Review a Force or a Farce . . . ?"*: *Hospital Physician*, January 1970, pp. 111–17.

102 *A team of physicians . . .* : Paul A. Lembcke and Olive G. Johnson, "A Medical Audit Report," School of Public Health, University of California at Los Angeles, 1963.

102 *. . . a study of appendectomies . . .* : Cited in *Health and Welfare Report*, published by the California Council for Health Plan Alternatives, April 6, 1972.

102–103 *In proprietary hospitals . . .* : For example, Mary E. W. Goss, "Organizational Goals and the Quality of Medical Care: Evidence from Comparative Research on Hospitals," *Journal of Health and Social Behavior* 11, No. 4 (December 1970), pp. 255–68, cites three studies suggesting that care is poorer in proprietary hospitals.

103 Illinois decision: *Darling v. Charleston Memorial Hospital*, 33 Ill. 2nd 326, 211 NE 2nd 253 (1965).

104 *. . . Robert Derbyshire has pointed out . . .* : "Professional Standards: Enforcement Held Lax."

104 *. . . a surgeon who was recently convicted of malpractice . . .* : "Doctor and Hospital Are Fined $3-Million for Needless Surgery," *New York Times*, November 28, 1973.

105 *Not long ago, . . . an official . . . told a Senate committee . . .* : *Medical Malpractice: The Patient vs. the Physician* (Committee Print), U.S. Senate Committee on Government Operations, Staff of the Subcommittee on Executive Reorganization, 91st Congress, 1st session (1969), p. 6.

106 *"You wind up ostracized . . ."*: Quoted in August Gribbin, "Senseless Surgery," *The National Observer*, July 29, 1972.

107 Bernzweig: *Medical Malpractice: The Patient vs. the Physician*, p. 18.

107 Rubsamen: Donald, McDonald ed., *Medical Malpractice*, Center for the Study of Democratic Institutions, Santa Barbara, California, 1971, p. 4.

108 *When the American College of Surgeons queried its members . . .* : U.S. Department of Health, Education and Welfare, Hearings before the Secretary's Commission on Medical Malpractice, Los Angeles, California, October 22, 1971, pp. 177–201.

108 Duke University study: "The Malpractice Threat: A Study of Defensive Medicine," *Duke Law Journal* (Durham, North Carolina). No. 5 (1971), pp. 939-93.

108 Blumberg: McDonald, ed., *Medical Malpractice*, p. 3.

CHAPTER SEVEN: The Lingering Odor of Snake Oil

110 Console: *Competitive Problems in the Drug Industry, Part 11*, Hearings before the U.S. Senate Select Committee on Small Business, Subcommittee on Monopoly, 91st Congress, 1st session (1969), p. 4496.

110 Kennedy: Quoted in Daniel S. Greenberg, "Medicine and Public Affairs," *New England Journal of Medicine* 290, No. 21 (May 23, 1974), p. 1211.

112 Console on asafetida: *Administered Prices, Part 18*, Hearings before the U.S. Senate Committee on the Judiciary, Subcommittee on Antitrust and Monopoly, 86th Congress, 2nd session (1960), p. 10373.

112 Console on research expenditures: *Competitive Problems in the Drug Industry, Part 11*, p. 4493.

112-13 Number of combination drugs on the market: *Competitive Problems in the Drug Industry, Part 20*, 92nd Congress, 1st session (1971), p. 7976.

113-14 Study of drug effectiveness: *Drug Efficacy Study: Final Report to the Commissioner of Food and Drugs* (Washington, D.C.: National Academy of Sciences, 1969); also, *Economic Priorities Report* 4, Nos. 4-5 (August-November 1973), pp. 15-17; and *Competitive Problems in the Drug Industry, Part 20*, p. 7972.

114 Zactirin: *Competitive Problems in the Drug Industry, Part 18*, 91st Congress, 2nd session (1970), p. 7451.

115 . . . a recent analysis of 490 separate studies . . . : A. Smith, E. Traganza, G. Harrison, "Studies on the Effectiveness of Antidepressant Drugs," *Psychopharmacology Bulletin*, March 1969, pp. 1-53.

115-16 Overprescribing of Chloromycetin: *Competitive Problems in the Drug Industry, Part 6*, 90th Congress, 1st and 2nd sessions (1967-1968), pp. 2167-2752; letter quoted is on p. 2576.

116 Decline in Chloromycetin sales: Richard Burack, *The New Handbook of Prescription Drugs* (New York: Pantheon Books, 1970), p. 85.

116 Gordon's estimate: Interview, October 17, 1973.

116 Stethoscopes, golf balls, etc.: Rick Barnhart, "The Medical Profession—Drug Industry Alliance," *The New Physician*, March 1971, pp. 164-71.

116-17 A Maryland physician . . . : *Examination of the Pharmaceutical Industry, Part 4*, Hearings before the U.S. Senate Committee on Labor and Public Welfare, Subcommittee on Health, 93rd Congress, 1st and 2nd sessions, May 3, 1974, p. 1296.

117 Sinequan promotion: Peter Frishauf, "Prescription Promotion: Selling The Doctor Drugs," unpublished ms. (on file in the library of the Graduate School of Journalism, Columbia University), pp. 1, 7, 9.

117 *Drug companies have on occasion . . .* : Testimony before U.S. Senate Committee on Labor and Public Welfare, Subcommittee on Health, reported in Morton Mintz, "Drug Industry 'Payola' Told," *Washington Post*, March 9, 1974; and Mintz, "Drug Promotions Defended," *Washington Post*, March 13, 1974.

117 *. . . a Tennessee physician . . .* : *Competitive Problems in the Drug Industry, Part 1*, 90th Congress, 1st session (1967), p. 326.

118 *"Tropical beaches . . ."*: *The New Physician*, March 1971, p. 137.

119 Eli Lilly and C-Quens: *Competitive Problems in the Drug Industry, Part 1*, p. 315.

119 Wallace Laboratories' "Dear Doctor" letter: Ibid., p. 313; also, Morton Mintz, "Misleading Drug Ads Conceded—Firm Informs Doctors on FDA Request," *Washington Post*, April 6, 1967.

120 Pillard testimony: *Competitive Problems in the Drug Industry, Part 13*, 91st Congress, 1st session (1969), pp. 5407–5409, 5416.

120–21 Serentil ad: Frishauf, "Prescription Promotion: Selling The Doctor Drugs," pp. 21–22.

121 Stelazine and Ritalin ads: See, e.g., *Medical Economics*, June 11, 1973, pp. 180–81, 222–23.

122 Directives to detail men, etc.: *Examination of the Pharmaceutical Industry, 1973–74, Part 3*, pp. 975, 1245–46.

122 Detail men instructed not to mention critical articles: Ibid., pp. 868–69.

122 Serino testimony: Ibid., pp. 782–83.

122–23 *. . . studies cited by witnesses . . .* : *Competitive Problems in the Drug Industry, Part 11*, p. 4346.

123 *"I have personally been very chagrined . . ."*: *Competitive Problems in the Drug Industry, Part 19*, 91st Congress, 2nd session (1970), p. 7749.

124 AMA's income from drug industry: *Examination of the Pharmaceutical Industry, 1973–74, Part 4*, p. 1340 (testimony of Dr. William R. Barclay, assistant executive vice-president of the AMA).

124–25 AMA and its Council on Drugs: *Competitive Problems in the Drug Industry, Part 23*, 93rd Congress, 1st session (1973), pp. 9608–42. For Adriani quotations see p. 9609.

125–27 Are Americans being deprived of important new drugs?: Ibid. Figures on decline in new drugs are on p. 9559; Warren quote is on p. 9669; Dripps' admission is cited on p. 9106; figures on "important new advances" are on p. 9559; Simmons quote is on pp. 9418–19.

127 Winstrol: *The Medical Letter* 15, No. 6 (March 16, 1973).

128 *In every other important drug-producing country . . .* : U.S. Department of Health, Education and Welfare, *The Drug Makers and the Drug Distributors*, Task Force on Prescription Drugs, Background Papers, December 1968, p. 38.

129 *. . . the FDA ordered the recall of nine batches . . .* : Burack, *The New Handbook of Prescription Drugs*, p. 16.

Notes 295

130 *Burack . . . recently wrote . . .* : "Massachusetts 'Generic Drug Law,' " letter, *New England Journal of Medicine* 285, No. 23 (December 2, 1971), pp. 1327-28.

130 Schmidt's views: *Examination of the Pharmaceutical Industry, 1973-74, Part 2*, pp. 441-42.

130 Feldmann's qualifications and statement: *Competitive Problems in the Drug Industry, Part 1*, 90th Congress, 1st session (1967), pp. 397-98, 412.

CHAPTER EIGHT: The Economics of Extravagance

132-33 Exploiting proprietary-hospital patients: Roger Rapoport, "The Patient Aution Block," *New Times*, January 11, 1974, pp. 18-22.

135 *"Your typical administrator . . ."*: Quoted by Herbert S. Denenberg, Pennsylvania Commissioner of Insurance, on opening day of public hearings on a request for a premium increase by Blue Shield of Pennsylvania, September 25-27, 1972.

137 *In a recent survey of doctors . . .* : Ray H. Elling and Joyce K. Bain, "The System of Medical Practice in the Hartford Capitol Regiðn," mimeographed, August 1971.

138 *. . . Blue Shield's 1970 fee schedule . . .* : *High Cost of Hospitalization, Part 1*, Hearings before the U.S. Senate Committee on the Judiciary, Subcommittee on Antitrust and Monopoly, 91st Congress, 2nd session (1970), pp. 362, 376.

138 *The General Accounting Office has estimated . . .* : GAO, *Study of Health Facilities Construction Costs*, Report to the Congress, December 1972, pp. 769-76; also, Nancy Hicks, "Cost of Health Care: A Case in Point," *New York Times*, February 2, 1974.

139 Gordon Chase: *High Cost of Hospitalization, Part 2*, 91st Congress, 2nd session (1970), p. 239.

139 Sander Kelman: Kelman, review of *Hospital Costs in Massachusetts: An Econometric Study, Inquiry* 6, No. 4 (December 1969), p. 57.

140 *. . . a series of well-documented articles . . .* : By Ronald Kessler, *Washington Post*, October 29, 30, and 31, and November 1, 1972.

141 *. . . The Western Voice of Motorola . . .* : Nicholas von Hoffman, "In the Pink of Health (and in the Black) in Phoenix," *Washington Post*, October 6, 1972.

142 Denenberg: Remarks on opening day of public hearings on request for premium increase by Blue Shield of Pennsylvania, September 25-27, 1972.

142-43 Kaitz study: Edward M. Kaitz, *Pricing Policy and Cost Behavior* (New York: Frederick A. Praeger, 1968), pp. 77, 79-80.

144-45 Denenberg vs. Blue Cross: Donald C. Drake, "Blue Cross, 80 Hospitals Ordered to Reduce Costs," *Philadelphia Inquirer*, March 18, 1971.

145 Results of new Blue Cross contract: Blue Cross of Greater Philadelphia, *Annual Report*, 1972.

145 *Denenberg, modestly describing . . .* : Press release, Commonwealth of Pennsylvania Insurance Department, February 27, 1973.

146–47 *. . . the* Los Angeles Times *reported . . .* : March 26, 29, 1972.

147 Children's Hospital: Ronald Kessler, "Too Many Empty Beds Cause Children's Hospital Deficit," *Washington Post*, November 2, 1972.

147 *In Philadelphia, the local Blue Cross plan . . .* : Blue Cross of Greater Philadelphia, *Annual Report*, 1972.

147–48 Competition in Oakland: Nancy Martin, "Will Practice Suffer If These Hospitals Don't Merge?" *Medical Economics*, February 5, 1973, pp. 94–107.

CHAPTER NINE: The Business of Insurance

149 Woodcock: *National Health Insurance*, Hearings before the U.S. Senate Committee on Finance, 92nd Congress, 1st session (1971), p. 114.

150 Origin of Blue Cross: Louis S. Reed, "Private Health Insurance in the United States: An Overview," *Social Security Bulletin*, December 1965.

151 California Blue Shield: Donald DuBois, "California Blue Shield," in Milton I. Roemer et al., eds., *Health Insurance Plans: Studies in Organizational Diversity* (University of California at Los Angeles, 1970).

151–52 Health insurance coverage: Marjorie Smith Mueller, "Private Health Insurance in 1973: A Review of Coverage, Enrollment, and Financial Experience," *Social Security Bulletin* 38, No. 2 (February 1974), pp. 21–40.

152 Metropolitan Life policy: Vincent Murphy, Metropolitan Life, interview, December 1974.

153 History of experience rating: Herman Miles Somers and Anne Ramsay Somers, *Doctors, Patients and Health Insurance* (Washington, D.C.: The Brookings Institution, 1961), pp. 309–12.

154 *In recent years, advertising [etc.] . . . have eaten up 45 cents of every dollar . . .* : In 1969–73, insurance companies collected $11.5 billion in premiums from individual policyholders, and paid out only $6.3 billion in benefits. Mueller, "Private Health Insurance in 1973 . . . ," p. 36.

154 National Liberty Corporation: *Commercial Health and Accident Insurance Industry, Part 1*, Hearings before the U.S. Senate Committee on the Judiciary, Subcommittee on Antitrust and Monopoly, 92nd Congress, 2nd Session (1972), pp. 598, 603.

154 *Another leading mail-order house . . .* : Ibid., p. 398.

154 *. . . at a hearing before Herbert Denenberg . . .* : *New York Times*, February 27, 1972.

156 *Two out of every three Americans . . .* : Mueller, "Private Health Insurance in 1973 . . . ," p. 22.

157 Aetna vs. the AMA: "AMA Takes Stand on Third-Party Payers," *American Medical News*, July 3, 1972; also, Barry Kramer and Priscilla Meyer, "Doctors Gain More Control from Aetna Life Over Disputed Payments on Medical Claims," *Wall Street Journal*, August 24, 1972.

158 Virginia Blue Cross: *High Cost of Hospitalization, Part 2: Blue Cross*, Hearings before the U.S. Senate Committee on the Judiciary, Subcommittee on Antitrust and Monopoly, 91st Congress, 2nd session (1970), pp. 32–40; also, Godfrey Hodgson, "The Politics of American Health Care," *The Atlantic*, October 1973, p. 54.

158 Louisiana Blue Cross and Utah Blue Shield: Social Security Administration audits, as summarized by the Washington office of the AFL-CIO.

158 *In 1970 the Senate Finance Committee dug into . . .* : *Medicare and Medicaid: Problems, Issues, and Alternatives*, Staff Report, U.S. Senate Committee on Finance, 91st Congress, 2nd Session (1970).

159 *. . . Ribicoff said angrily . . .* : *Medicare and Medicaid, Part 2*, Hearings before the U.S. Senate Committee on Finance, Subcommittee on Medicare-Medicaid, 91st Congress, 2nd session (1970), p. 211.

159 Denenberg on Blue Shield: Pennsylvania Insurance Department, public hearings on request for premium increase by Blue Shield of Pennsylvania, September 25–27, 1972 (transcript, p. 22).

159–60 McNerney: *Private Health Insurance and Medical Care*, Conference Papers, National Conference on Private Health Insurance, Washington, D.C., 1967.

160 *Its administrative and marketing expenses . . . absorb only about 6 per cent . . .* : Based on 1969–73 figures. Mueller, "Private Health Insurance in 1973 . . . ," p. 36.

160 *"We were very critical of Blue Cross . . ."*: *Commercial Health and Accident Insurance Industry, Part 1*, p. 415.

160–61 *As of 1973, only about one third of the plans . . .* : press release, Blue Cross Association, February 27, 1973, pp. 8–9.

161 *. . . the president of one plan . . .* : *High Cost of Hospitalization, Part 2: Blue Cross*, p. 26.

CHAPTER TEN: The Case for Health Maintenance Organizations

163 *Insurance companies, uneasily aware . . .* : Michael B. Rothfeld, "Sensible Surgery for Swelling Medical Costs," *Fortune*, April 1973, p. 110.

163 *. . . 1700 new HMOs by 1976 . . .* : U.S. Department of Health, Education and Welfare, "Toward a Comprehensive Health Policy for the 1970s—A White Paper," cited by Senator Edward Kennedy, "Health Maintenance Organizations," *Congressional Record*, April 10, 1973, p. S6934.

165 *In 1973, the cost of medical care provided by Group Health Cooperative . . .* : Letter from Richard Handschin, Research Director, Group Health Cooperative of Puget Sound, August 20, 1974.

166 Roemer study: Milton I. Roemer et al., *Health Insurance Effects: Services, Expenditures, and Attitudes Under Three Types of Plan*, Bureau of Public Health Economics, Research Series No. 16, School of Public Health, University of Michigan, Ann Arbor, 1972.

166 Comparative costs of medical care: Ibid., p. 46.

167 Incidence of chronic disease: Ibid., p. 16.

167 Insurance company estimates: Rothfeld, "Sensible Surgery for Swelling Medical Costs," pp. 114, 116.

167 Time spent in hospitals: Roemer, *Health Insurance Effects*, p. 21.

167 More preventive care for group-plan members: Ibid., p. 41.

169 *. . . doctors . . . were expelled from their local medical societies . . .* : Caldwell Blakeman Esselstyn, "The Professions Respond to Challenge," paper presented to the Southern District Branch Meeting, American Public Health Association, Roanoke, Virginia, May 3, 1962.

169 Larson Commission: Leonard W. Larson et al., "Report of the Commission on Medical Care," *Journal of the American Medical Association*, Special Edition, January 17, 1959.

169 *In accepting this report . . .* : "The President's Page," *Journal of the American Medical Association* 170 (1959), p. 1554.

170 *. . . Medical Economics reported . . .* : June 5, 1972, p. 17.

170 *The AMA itself has formally declared . . .* : Resolution of AMA House of Delegates, 1971, quoted in "Further Testing of HMOs Urged," *American Medical News*, July 5, 1971.

170 *Officers of the AMA have further warned . . .* : Health Maintenance Organizations, Part 1, Hearings before the U.S. House of Representatives Committee on Interstate and Foreign Commerce, Subcommittee on Public Health and Environment, 92nd Congress, 2nd session (1972), pp. 336 ff. (testimony of John R. Kernodle, M.D., vice chairman, board of trustees, AMA; and Dr. Russell B. Roth, Speaker of the AMA House of Delegates).

170 *Some newly organized plans in California . . .* : Robert Fairbanks, "New Gold Rush—Prepaid Medi-Cal Franchises Sought," *Los Angeles Times*, December 10, 1972; Harry Nelson, "Investigation of Prepaid Health Programs Asked," *Los Angeles Times*, February 24, 1973; "Prepaid California Health Plans Criticized on Care and Profits," *New York Times*, May 5, 1974; Bart Sheridan, "Will an H.M.O. Grab Your Pateints?" *Medical Economics*, September 17, 1973, pp. 220–43.

170–71 *. . . a recent advertisement . . .* : *Los Angeles Times*, September 17, 1972.

171 Kaiser plan in Portland: *Heal Yourself, Report of the Citizens Board of Inquiry into Health Services for Americans*, p. 52.

172 Kaiser drop-in clinics and complaint of Kaiser subscriber: Sheila K. Johnson, "Health Maintenance: It Works," *New York Times Magazine*, April 28, 1974, pp. 44, 50.

172 Harold Newman: Interview, February 1, 1972.

172 *Forty-three per cent of the people . . . , etc.*: Roemer, *Health Insurance Effects*, pp. 29, 31.

173 *"The Kaiser-Portland 'grievance procedure' . . ."*: *Heal Yourself*, p. 51.

173 Dr. Richard Handschin *. . . concedes . . .* : Interview, January 31, 1972.

173–74 Dr. Richard Weinerman *. . .* : Weinerman, "Problems and Perspectives of Group Practice," *Bulletin, New York Academy of Medicine* 44, No. 11 (November 1968), p. 30.

174 "Rational" care: Roemer, *Health Insurance Effects*, p. 42.

174 *. . . a study, made in the 1950s . . .* : Sam Shapiro, "End Result Measurements of Quality Medical Care," *Milbank Memorial Fund Quarterly* 45 (April 1967), pp. 7–30.

175 *When members of HIP were surveyed . . .* : Odin W. Anderson and P. B. Sheatsley, *Comprehensive Medical Insurance: A Study of Costs, Use, and Attitudes Under Two Plans*, Research Series No. 9, New York, Health Information Foundation, 1959.

175–76 Roemer findings on satisfaction, etc.: Roemer, *Health Insurance Effects*, pp. 51, 57–58.

176–77 Medical care foundations, and the San Joaquin foundation: "The Vanguard of the Rearguard," *Health/PAC Bulletin*, published by the Health Policy Advisory Center, New York, No. 49 (February 1973); Richard Sasuly and Carl E. Hopkins, "A Medical Society-Sponsored Medical Care Plan," *Medical Care*, July–August 1967, pp. 234–48; Richard Egdahl, "Foundations for Medical Care," *New England Journal of Medicine* 288, No. 10 (March 8, 1973), pp. 491–98.

177 CHAP scheme: Earl Brian, "Foundation for Medical Care Control of Hospital Utilization: CHAP—A PSRO Prototype," *New England Journal of Medicine* 288, No. 17 (April 26, 1973), pp. 878–82.

178 *In Phoenix, Arizona . . .* : *Health Maintenance Organizations, Part 3*, Hearings before the U.S. House of Representatives Committee on Interstate and Foreign Commerce, Subcommittee on Public Health and Environment, 92nd Congress, 2nd session (1972), pp. 1039–40.

178 *There is also persuasive testimony . . .* : See, e.g., *Physicians Training Facilities and Health Maintenance Organizations*, Hearings before the U.S. Senate Committee on Labor and Public Welfare, Subcommittee on Health, 92nd Congress, 2nd session (1972), p. 2029 (testimony of Dr. John Babich, treasurer of the Sacramento Medical Society Foundation).

178 *But foundations have not shown . . .* : Donald Harrington, president of the American Association of Foundations for Medical Care, has testified that three foundations doing pilot studies on Medicare reported that the average monthly cost per Medicare recipient was 11 to 17 per cent lower than under conventional arrangements (*Physicians Training Facilities and Health Maintenance Organizations*, Hearings, May 1, 1972). The San Joaquin Foundation estimates that it saves 12 to 15 per cent on premiums by controlling overutilization. By contrast, prepaid group-practice plans have reduced the use of hospitals by one third to one half, while members of the plans surveyed by Roemer and his associates were shown to be getting their medical care at a total cost 27 per cent lower than the cost of care for people covered by Blue Cross–Blue Shield. When plan members were compared with people covered by commercial health insurance, the saving was much less: 11 per cent. But plan members, as I have pointed out, were (a) getting more preventive treatment; and (b) presumably required more care of all kinds because so many more of them had chronic disorders.

178 Texas medical foundation: Austin Scott, "Doctors' Power Hit in Texas," *Washington Post*, December 26, 1972.

178 *. . . a young family doctor . . .* : At Kaiser, doctors start at around $25,000, and the average doctor's salary is about $45,000, plus a bonus that in recent years has ranged from $7000 to $9000. A hard-to-get specialist such as a neurosurgeon may make $100,000 (Johnson, "Health Maintenance: It Works," p. 35).

179 *. . . a 1970 poll of medical students . . .* : *Health Maintenance Organizations, Part 2*, Hearings, p. 391.

CHAPTER ELEVEN: The Trouble with Medicare and Medicaid

181 Federal spending for health: Interview, Barbara Cooper, Office of Research and Statistics, Social Security Administration, U.S. Department of Health, Education and Welfare, Washington, D.C.

182–83 Annis remarks: *New York Times*, October 14, 1971.

183 AMA poster: Richard Harris, *A Sacred Trust* (Baltimore: Penguin Books, 1969), p. 124.

184 *In 1968, according to a tabulation by the Senate Finance Committee . . .* : *Medicare and Medicaid: Problems, Issues and Alternatives*, staff report, U.S. Senate Committee on Finance, 91st Congress, 1st session (1970).

184 Rise in family doctors' fees: *Medical Care Costs and Prices: Background Book*, U.S. Department of Health, Education and Welfare, Social Security Administration, Office of Research and Statistics, January 1972, pp. 40–41; also, Arthur Owens, "Physicians' Earnings: Leveling Off," *Medical Economics*, October 11, 1971, pp. 203–11.

185 *"Medicare is the computer manufacturer's friend . . ."*: Quoted in Barbara and John Ehrenreich, *The American Health Empire* (New York: Random House, 1970), p. 106.

185 Rising cost of hospital care: Interview, Ruth Baine, American Hospital Association, Chicago.

185 *. . . a report by the staff of the Senate Finance Committee . . .* : *Medicare and Medicaid*, p. 18.

186 *. . . Medicare actually pays only 43 per cent . . .* : Walter C. Newburgher, 2nd vice-president, National Council of Senior Citizens, quoted in "The Problems Created by Medical Progress," *Medical World News*, April 7, 1972.

186 *But the National Council of Senior Citizens has complained . . .* : *Barriers to Health Care for Older Americans*, Hearings before the U.S. Senate Special Committee on Aging, 93rd Congress, 1st session (1973), p. 85.

186 *. . . in New York City doctors' bills . . .* : Max H. Seigel, "A Medicare Shortfall of Up to $70-Million Is Reported Here," *New York Times*, March 24, 1974.

187 *In New York City . . . nearly one third . . .* : *Barriers to Health Care for Older Americans*, p. 10.

188 *The essence of the new law* . . . : Rosemary Stevens and Robert Stevens, "Medicaid: Anatomy of a Dilemma," *Law and Contemporary Problems* 35, No. 2 (Spring 1970), pp. 348–425. (Except where otherwise noted, all facts about Medicaid coverage, history, eligibility rules, etc. are taken from this article.)

191 *Doctors have accepted kickbacks. . . . In New York City, the Health Department* . . . : Edward Ranzal, "Kickbacks Found On Medical Tests," *New York Times*, January 10, 1973.

191 *Pharmacists have kited* . . . : L. E. Bellin and F. Kavaler, "Policing Publicly Funded Health Care for Poor Quality, Overutilization, and Fraud: The New York City Medicaid Experience," *American Journal of Public Health* 60, No. 5 (May 1970), pp. 811–20.

191–92 Senator Moss: *Congressional Record*, September 17, 1971, p. S14518.

192 *Dr. Lowell Bellin . . . recently estimated* . . . : Edward Ranzal, "Medicaid Hearing Is Told of Abuses," *New York Times*, July 17, 1974.

192 *. . . sharp rise in the number of pregnant women. . . . Poor people are seeing doctors more often* . . . : *Health Service Use: National Trends and Variations*, Center for Health Administration Studies, University of Chicago, and National Center for Health Services Research and Development; U.S. Department of Health, Education and Welfare Publication No. (HSM) 73-7004, October 1972.

192 Pierre de Vise: De Vise, "We Spend Enough Money On Care for the Poor, But We Spend It Badly," *Modern Hospital* 114, No. 5 (May 1970), p. 86.

193–94 *And as Dr. Mildred Morehead* . . . : Mildred A. Morehead, Rose S. Donaldson, and Mary R. Seravalli, "Comparisons Between OEO Neighborhood Health Centers and Other Health Care Providers of Ratings of the Quality of Health Care," *American Journal of Public Health* 61 (July 1971), pp. 1294–1306.

194 *. . . a New York City public health officer* . . . : Interview with Dr. Anthony Mustalish, October 12, 1973.

CHAPTER TWELVE: Killing Rats in Mound Bayou: New Styles in Missionary Medicine

198 *Public transportation . . . was so poor* . . . : H. Jack Geiger, "Health in the Troubled City," in *Regional Medical Programs and Their Relationship to the Urban Community and the Poor*, U.S. Department of Health, Education and Welfare, Public Health Service, November 1968.

198 Conrad Herr: Statement to University Seminar on Social and Preventive Medicine, Columbia University, School of Public Health and Administrative Medicine, December 4, 1970.

198 *According to a door-to-door survey* . . . : Seymour S. Bellin and H. Jack Geiger, "Actual Public Acceptance of the Neighborhood Health Center by the Urban Poor," *Journal of the American Medical Association* 214, No. 12 (December 21, 1970), pp. 2147–53.

198 *The survey also turned up* . . . : Geiger, "Health in the Troubled City."

302 Notes

198–99 Mound Bayou center: H. Jack Geiger, "A Health Center in Mississippi—A Case Study in Social Medicine," in Lawrence Corey, Steven E. Saltman, and Michael F. Epstein, eds., *Medicine in a Changing Society* (St. Louis: C. V. Mosby, 1972), pp. 157–67; Richard Hall, "A Stir of Hope in Mound Bayou," *Life* 66, No. 12 (March 28, 1969), pp. 66–81; Lisbeth Bamberger Schorr, "The Neighborhood Health Center—Background and Current Issues," in *Medicine in a Changing Society*, p. 145.

199 *But there is persuasive evidence . . .¯*: Gerald Sparer and Joyce Johnson, "Evaluation of OEO Neighborhood Health Centers," *American Journal of Public Health* 61 (May 1971), pp. 931–42.

200 *"A family of eleven . . ."*: Harold B. Wise et al., "The Family Health Worker: A Multipurpose Health Worker with Nursing and Social Advocacy Skills," *American Journal of Public Health* 58 (October 1968), p. 1831.

201 *"The 'half-life' of the subprofessional . . ."*: Harold B. Wise, "Montefiore Hospital Neighborhood Medical Care Demonstration: A Case Study," *The Milbank Memorial Fund Quarterly* 46, No. 3 (July 1968), Part 1.

205 Dr. Samuel Standard: Standard, "Comment on the Neighborhood Health Center and the General Hospital," *Medical Care* 8, No. 4 (May–June 1970), pp. 252–53.

205–206 *The doctor working in a ghetto clinic . . .*: Eva J. Salber, "Community Participation in Neighborhood Health Centers," *New England Journal of Medicine* 283, No. 10 (September 3, 1970), p. 516.

206 *The professional . . . finds it "painful and stressful . . ."*: H. Jack Geiger, "Of the Poor, By the Poor, or For the Poor: The Mental Health Implications of Social Control of Poverty Programs," *Psychiatric Research Report* 21(April, 1967), p. 64.

206 *. . . Dr. Eva J. Salber, has written . . .*: "Community Participation in Neighborhood Health Centers," p. 516.

CHAPTER THIRTEEN: National Health Insurance: The Need for Heroic Therapy

210 *"City and state governments are terrified . . ."*: George A. Silver, "Is National Health Insurance the Question?" *American Journal of Public Health* 60, No. 10 (October 1970), pp. 1887–90.

210 *. . . George Meany . . . observed . . .*: Meany, "The Case for National Health Insurance," *American Federationist*, January 1970.

214–16 Effects of free medical care in Montreal: Philip E. Enterline, J. Corbett McDonald, et al., "Effects of 'Free' Medical Care on Medical Practice—the Quebec Experience," *New England Journal of Medicine* 288, No. 22 (May 31, 1972), pp. 1152–56; Enterline, Vera Salter, et al., "The Distribution of Medical Services Before and After 'Free' Medical Care—the Quebec Experience," *New England Journal of Medicine* 289, No. 22 (November 29, 1973), pp. 1174–78; Alison D. McDonald, J. Corbett McDonald, et al., "Effects of Quebec Medicare on Physician Consultation for Selected Symptoms," *New England Journal of Medicine* 291, No. 13 (September 26, 1974), pp. 649–52.

220 *An investigator . . .* : Cited in Jerry W. Finefrock, "Ma Bell: The Money Machine," *The Nation*, February 16, 1974, p. 199.

220 Harassment of drug experts: Anthony Ripley, "11 on Staff Accuse F.D.A. of Harassment on Studies," *New York Times*, August 16, 1974.

221 *. . . Kennedy suggested on another occasion . . .* : Address before New York Academy of Medicine Conference on National Health Programs, April 30, 1971.

224 *A Congressional expert . . .* : Interview, 1974.

225 Meany testimony: *National Health Insurance Proposals*, Hearings before the U.S. House of Representatives Committee on Ways and Means, 92nd Congress, 1st session (1971), p. 273.

226 *. . . one of Kennedy's assistants . . .* : Interview, 1973.

226 *. . . "the greatest threat to the private practice of medicine . . ."*: Richard D. Lyons, "Doctors Revolt Over A.M.A. Stand," *New York Times*, December 3, 1973.

227-28 AMA political contributions: Morton Mintz, "Gift List by AMA Revealed," *Washington Post*, September 15, 1974.

228-29 *"Let's face it . . ."*: Interview.

229 *"Now and then someone writes . . ."*: "Washington Front-Runner: Catastrophic Coverage," *Medical Economics*, April 16, 1973, p. 41.

229 *. . . Ribicoff told the Senate . . .* : *Congressional Record*, October 2, 1973, p. S18313.

CHAPTER FOURTEEN: Getting a Better Run for Our Money

233 Nelson's proposed formulary: S. 966, 93rd Congress, 1st session (1973). Other proposals by Senator Nelson having to do with drugs that are discussed in this chapter are also contained in this bill.

233 AMA survey: Cited in Art Douville, "The Drug Industry," *The New Physician*, March 1971, p. 143.

234 *Nelson has estimated . . .* : *Congressional Quarterly*, December 22, 1973, p. 3367.

241 *. . . two American researchers reported . . .* : Ronald Andersen and John T. Hull, "Hospital Utilization and Cost Trends in Canada and the United States," *Health Services Research* 4 (Fall 1969), pp. 198-222.

241 *. . . two Harvard experts . . .* : Katharine G. Bauer and Paul M. Densen, "Some Issues in the Incentive Reimbursement Approach to Cost Containment: An Overview," *Medical Care Review* 31, No. 1 (January 1974), pp. 61-100. The passage I have quoted is on p. 87.

244 *. . . Beeson recently noted . . .* : Paul B. Beeson, "Some Good Features of the British National Health Service," *Journal of Medical Education* 49, No. 1 (January 1974), pp. 43-49.

246 *. . . Eliot Freidson has written . . .* : Freidson, *Professional Dominance: The Social Structure of Medical Care* (New York: Atherton Press, 1970), p. 71.

246–47 PSROs: The law establishing PSROs (PL 92-603) is summarized, and its implications are thoughtfully considered, in Claude E. Welch, "Professional Standards Review Organizations—Problems and Prospects," *New England Journal of Medicine* 289, No. 6 (August 9, 1973), pp. 291–95.

247 *. . . a committee of public health experts . . .* : Quoted in Jay Winsten, "Imposing Controls on Doctors," *Resident and Staff Physician*, February 1974, pp. 45–47 (reprinted from *Wall Street Journal*).

247 Gilson letter: *New England Journal of Medicine* 289, No. 19 (November 8, 1973), p. 1045.

250 Kennedy-Javits bill: S. 3441, 93rd Congress, 2nd session (1974).

250 *At times it has been too easy . . .* : See Chapter 13, p. 220; also, Jonathan Spivak, "FDA Policies and Practices for Clearing Drugs Are Criticized Before Senate Units," *Wall Street Journal*, August 26, 1974.

250 *It has let them test potentially dangerous new drugs . . .* : Senator Abraham Ribicoff, "Experimental Use of Drugs on Human Subjects," *Congressional Record*, September 19, 1973, p. S16965. (Ribicoff cited a General Accounting Office study of the FDA's monitoring of tests on ten experimental drugs; in the case of eight of these drugs, Ribicoff told the Senate, the GAO had found that "FDA failed to halt human tests after receiving indications that the drugs were not safe.") See also Morton Mintz, "The Pill: Press and Public at Experts' Mercy," *Columbia Journalism Review*, Winter 1968–69, pp. 4–10.

250–51 *It has also allowed the industry to continue selling drugs of no proven effectiveness . . .* : Jim Mann, "FDA Ordered to Ban Drugs if Ineffective," *Washington Post*, August 24, 1972. In ruling against the FDA in a suit brought by the American Public Health Association, U.S. District Court Judge William B. Bryant wrote, "It seems inappropriate for an agency to adopt procedures . . . which effectively stay implementation of the Congressional mandate that drugs in the marketplace be both safe and effective."

251 *. . . the agency has sometimes been too slow . . .* : John Carlova, "Are Useful New Drugs Being Bottled Up by Bureaucracy?" *Medical Economics*, August 6, 1973, pp. 94–106.

251 Brookings Institution study: Ibid., p. 97.

CHAPTER FIFTEEN: How to Deal with the Doctor Shortage

252 Nixon Administration and the doctor shortage: *Congressional Quarterly*, May 25, 1974, p. 1390; Richard M. Schmeck, Jr., "Kennedy, Javits Say Nixon Risks Doctor Shortage," *New York Times*, June 24, 1974; "To Solve Primary Care Lacks—The Carrot and/or the Stick?" *Hospital Practice*, September 1974, pp. 54, 59.

253 *. . . one out of five graduating seniors . . .* : *Congressional Record*, September 23, 1974, p. S17281.

253 Proportion of family doctors in England and in U.S. prepaid group practice plans: U.S. Representative William Roy, quoted in "To Solve Primary Care Lacks," p. 48H.

254 *Dr. Francis D. Moore . . . estimates . . .* : Quoted in "Can Washington Tell Doctors Where to Go?" *Medical World News,* September 13, 1974, p. 48.

256 Results of loan forgiveness programs: *Congressional Record,* September 24, 1974, p. S17438.

256–57 Beall bill: actually, a substitute for S. 3585, the Kennedy-Javits bill.

258 Training of PAs and nurse practitioners: Alfred M. Sadler, Jr., Blair L. Sadler, and Ann A. Bliss, *The Physician's Assistant—Today and Tomorrow* (New Haven: Yale University School of Medicine, 1972); Susan Reverby, "The Sorcerer's Apprentice," *Health/PAC Bulletin,* No. 46 (November 1972), pp. 10–16.

259 *. . . Dr. Len Hughes Andrus has written . . .* : Andrus, "The Private Physician—Overcoming the Health Manpower Shortage," *The Bulletin of the American College of Physicians,* August 1969, pp. 381–84.

259 *In 1974 . . . fewer than 1800 men and women . . .* : According to the Association of Physician Assistant Programs, Washington, D.C., in the year ended June 30, 1974, 781 men and women completed courses leading to certification as physicians' assistants. Estimates of the number of nurse practitioners trained during this same period range from 750 to 1000.

259 Productivity of NHPs: See, e.g., D. W. Schiff, C. H. Fraser, and H. L. Walters, "The Pediatric Nurse Practitioner in the Office of Pediatricians in Private Practice," *Pediatrics* 44 (July 1969), pp. 62–68; Walter O. Spitzer, David L. Sackett, et al., "The Burlington Randomized Trial of the Nurse Practitioner," *New England Journal of Medicine* 290, No. 5 (January 31, 1974), pp. 251–56; Reverby, "The Sorcerer's Apprentice," p. 14.

259–60 *In one recent test . . .* : Spitzer, "The Burlington Randomized Trial."

260 *In another experiment . . .* : Charles E. Lewis, Barbara A. Resnik, et al., "Activities, Events and Outcomes in Ambulatory Patient Care," *New England Journal of Medicine* 280, No. 12 (March 20, 1969), pp. 645–49.

260 Colorado survey: Henry K. Silver and James A. Hecker, "The Pediatric Nurse Practitioner and the Child Health Associate: New Types of Health Professionals," *Journal of Medical Education* 45, No. 3 (March 1970), pp. 171–76.

260 *. . . a report, published in* Pediatrics *. . .* : Schiff et al., "The Pediatric Nurse Practitioner."

261 *"A transformation occurs . . ."*: The Martin Luther King, Jr., Health Center, *Fourth Annual Report* (1970), p. 15.

CHAPTER SIXTEEN: Making Medicine More Human

262 *. . . Dr. Edward H. Reinhard . . . has written . . .* : Reinhard, "Medicine and the Crisis in Confidence," *The Pharos,* October 1974, pp. 118–23.

263 *. . . a student speaker . . .* : David E. Reiser, "Struggling to Stay Human in Medicine," *The New Physician,* May 1973, pp. 294–99.

264 *. . . Geiger . . . recently recalled . . .* : Interview, March 14, 1974.

265 . . . *new medical school at Rockford* . . . : Robert L. Evans, Joseph G. Pittman, and Richard C. Peters, "The Community-Based Medical School—Reactions at the Interface Between Medical Education and Medical Care," *New England Journal of Medicine* 288, No. 14 (April 5, 1973), pp. 713–18.

266 . . . *Dr. Hiram Curry . . . told an interviewer* . . . : Peter Frishauf, "A Renaissance Man and His Residents," *The New Physician*, December 1973, pp. 770–75.

267 *In Rockford* . . . : Evans et al., "The Community-Based Medical School."

267 . . . *one reason commonly given* . . . : "Hospitals Scored for Ignoring Rights Bill," *Hospital Tribune*, December 10, 1973.

268 *In the words of Dr. Willard Gaylin* . . . : Gaylin, "The Patient's Bill of Rights," *Saturday Review of Science*, March 1973.

268 *Annas argues* . . . : Annas, "Patients Have Rights: How Can They Be Protected?" *Hastings Center Report*, September 1973.

268–69 Annas and Healey on patient advocates: "The Patient Rights Advocate," *Journal of Nursing Administration*, May-June 1974, pp. 25–31.

270 *But as a rule they are extremely well-heeled* . . . : See, e.g., Theodore Goldberg and Ronald Hemmelgarn, "Who Governs Hospitals?" *Hospitals* 45, No. 15 (August 1, 1971), pp. 72–79.

270 . . . *a "community member" of the Patient Care Committee* . . . : *Heal Yourself, Report of the Citizens Board of Inquiry Into Health Services for Americans*, pp. 61–62.

271 . . . *a study made some years ago* . . . : Schwartz, "Participation of Consumers in Prepaid Health Plans," *Journal of Health and Human Behavior* 5 (Summer-Fall 1964), pp. 74–84.

Index

Abortion, 36
Accreditation, hospital, 98–104
Adriani, John, 125
Advertising, drug-industry, 26–30, 117–22
Advocate, patients', 88, 268–69
Aetna Life and Casualty, 157
Albert Einstein Medical Center, 3
Ambulatory surgery, 138
American Academy of Family Physicians, 93
American Academy of General Practice, 69
American College of Surgeons, 91, 108
American Hospital Association, 14, 98; patients' rights and, 267–69
American Journal of Public Health, 210
American Medical Association (AMA): code of ethics, 97; doctor shortage and, 253; doctors' fees and, 16; drug industry and, 122–25; health insurance and, 149; HMOs and, 168–71; medical schools and, 21; Medicare and, 181–84; national health insurance and, 209–10, 217–18, 226–30; peer review and, 92, 104
American Medical Political Action Committee, 227–28
Analgesics, 114
Andrus, Len Hughes, 259

Annals of Internal Medicine, 25
Annas, George J., 268
Annis, Edward R., 182–83
Antibiotics, 23–26; adverse reactions to, 25–26, 115–16; testing of, 129
Antidepressants, 120
Antihistamines, 25
Appendectomies, 6, 7, 9, 41, 102
Arbitration, compulsory, 236–37
Argonaut Insurance Company, 106
Arrowsmith (Lewis), 90–91
Atchley, Dana W., 69
Atromid-S, 118–19

Baltimore City Hospital, 41–42, 58
Barton, Weldon, 46
Baylor University Hospital, 150
Beall, J. Glenn, 256–57
Beeson, Paul B., 243–44
Bellin, Lowell, 192
Bennett, Wallace F., 92
Bernzweig, Eli P., 107
Beth Israel Hospital, 205
Biomedical research, 81–83, 263
Birth control, 36
Black people, 50, 192, 198–99, 201
Blue Cross, 149–61; cost of, 152–53; extent of coverage of, 152; history of, 150–51; vs. HMOs, 166–67; hospital costs and, 135–46; limitations on, 155; national health insurance and,

Blue Cross (cont.)
158–61; public accountability of, 161; reimbursement methods of, 240–41
Blue Cross of Greater Philadelphia, 144–45
Blue Shield, 149–61; cost of, 152–53; doctors' fees and, 156–67; extent of coverage of, 152; fee schedule, 138; history of, 151; vs. HMOs, 166–67, 169; limitations on, 155; national health insurance and, 158–61
Blumberg, Mark, 108
Bolande, Robert P., 8–9
Bolivar County, Mississippi, 198
Boston City Hospital, 198
Brecher, Edward L., 87–88
Brecher, Ruth, 87–88
Brook, Robert H., 41–42, 58
Brookings Institution, 251
Brown, Clement, 41
Brusstar, James, 12
Bunker, John P., 5–6
Burack, Richard, 28, 130
Burleson, Omar, 228
Butisol, 28
Buzard, James A., 122

California Medical Association, 151
Canada, 44; national health insurance in, 214–17, 225, 241
Carnegie Foundation, 20
Center for Study of Responsive Law, 99
Certified Hospital Admissions Program (CHAP), 177
Charity care, 49–66; advantages of, 61–62; bargaining power and, 270–73; children's health and, 50–51; doctor shortage and, 46; emergency-room, 54–57; health centers and, 50–52, 197–208; infant mortality and, 37–38; Medicaid and, 51–54, 187–96; in outpatient clinics, 57–61; in public hospitals, 63–66; quality of, 37–38; in university hospitals, 62–63; in voluntary hospitals, 63
Chase, Gordon, 139
Check-ups, general, 43–44
Chestnut Hill Hospital, Philadelphia, 40–41, 101
Chicago Board of Health, 54
Children, health problems of, 42–43; black, 50
Children's Hospital, Washington, D.C., 147
Chloromycetin, 115–16, 123
Chronic disease, 78–79
CIBA, 28
Citizens Board of Inquiry Into Health Services for Americans, xiv, 51–52, 171
Clark, Ronald E., 96
Clinical medicine, standards of, 43–44
Clinic patients. *See* Outpatient clinics
Cold, common, 24–25
Coles, Robert, xiv
Columbia Point, Massachusetts, 198–99
Columbia Presbyterian Medical Center, 57–58
Commercialism, 91
Commission on Medical Malpractice, 107, 235
Community rating, 152–53
Coney Island Hospital, 64
Connecticut General, 167n
Console, Dale, 110, 112
Cook County Hospital, 63
Cordice, John W. V., Jr., xiii
Coser, Rose Lamb, 62
Cost-saving proposals, 231–51
Cost-sharing, 214
C-Quens, 119
Crechner, Harry D., 101–102
Crichton, Michael, 76
Crosby, Edwin L., 3
Curry, Hiram, 266
Czechoslovakia, 88–89

Death, physicians' attitude toward, 73–75
De Lury, John, 2
Denenberg, Herbert S., 12, 142–45, 154–55, 159–60, 220
Denver Department of Health and Hospitals, 38
Department of Health, Education, and Welfare (HEW), 203, 219
Deprol, 119
Derbyshire, Robert C., 95–97, 104
Detail men, drug-industry, 122–24
De Vise, Pierre, 11, 37, 46, 49, 63, 192
DeWitt, Henry K., 2
District of Columbia General Hospital, 63
Doctors: attitudes toward patients, 71–78, 262–67; autonomy of, 84–90; drug industry and, 23–30, 116–24; educational standards of, 248–50; emotional illness and, 75–78; fees, 15–23, 156–57, 183–84, 193; foreign-born, 47–48, 252–53; health centers and, 202–203, 205–206; health insurance and, 151, 156–57; HMOs and, 169–73; 176–80; hours, 19–20; incomes, 16–20; malpractice claims and, 95–109, 234–38; Medicaid and, 53–54, 193; medical schools and, 20–23, 253–55; Medicare and, 183–84; office visits to, 43–44; opposition to peer review of, 91–95; poor patients of, 37–38, 60–61; relocating, 255–58; shortage, 44–48, 252–61; standards of performance of, 39–41. *See also* Family physicians, Specialists
Doctor's Dilemma, The (Shaw), 4
Dowling, Harry, 24
Downstate Medical Center, Brooklyn, 69–70
Dripps, Robert D., 126
Drug Efficacy Study Group, 113–14

Drug Formulary Commission, 130
Drug industry, 23–30, 110–31; advertising, 30, 117–22; AMA and, 124–25; detail men for, 122–24; earnings, 29–30; FDA restrictions on, 125–28; gifts to doctors by, 116–18; pricing practices of, 26–28; promotions, 117–28; regulating, 233–34; trade names and, 128–31
Drugs. *See* Prescription drugs
Duff, Raymond S., 72, 74, 76–77
Duke University School of Law, 108

East Harlem Committee on Aging, 187
Economic Stabilization Program, 145
Electronic News, 185
Emergency rooms, 41–42; poor and, 54–57
Emotional illness, 48, 75–78, 193
England, 4–5, 35, 46, 85–87, 134; national health insurance in, 5, 36, 88, 222, 243
Ethics, code of, 97
Experimentation on dying, 74
Extravagance in hospitals, 132–48

Family health workers, 199–201
Family physicians, 22, 262; clinical standards of, 43–44; fee-for-service medicine and, 85–90; low status of, 69–71; relocating, 255–58; shortage of, 44–48, 252–61; training methods for, 265–67. *See also* Family practice
Family practice, 70–71, 253–55
Fee-for-service medicine, 85–90
Fees, doctors', 15–23, 156–57, 183–84, 193
Fein, Rashi, 14
Feldmann, Edward G., 130
Fitzsimmons, Frank, 39
Fleming, Alexander, 111
Flexner, Abraham, 20–21

Food and Drug Administration (FDA), 113–14, 220; antibiotics and, 24–25; drug advertising and, 118–19; restrictions on drug industry by, 125–28
Foreign-born doctors, 47–48, 252–53
Fortune, 167n
Foundation plans, medical care, 176–78
Freidson, Eliot, 89, 92, 173, 246
Funkenstein, Daniel, 60

Garai, Pierre, 23
Gaylin, Willard, 268
Geiger, H. Jack, 75, 198, 264
General practitioners. *See* Family physicians
Generic names, 28, 128–31
Ghettos, 46, 256
Gilson, Saul B., 247
Goldwater, Barry, 182
Gordon, Benjamin, 116
Government workers, 10
Gram, Hans, 25n
Gram-negative bacteria, 25–26
Graves, Clifford L., 18–19
Group Health Cooperative of Puget Sound, 7, 164–80, 240; cost of, 164–67; patients' complaints under, 271; waiting times under, 172
Group practice plans, 153, 162–80; advantages of, 173–74; AMA and, 168–71; charges against, 170–73; cost of, 164–67; doctors' incomes under, 178–79; federal subsidies to, 163; foundation plans and, 176–78; government workers and, 10; history of, 162–63; impersonality of, 89–90, 175; inducements to join, 244–45; reluctance of patients to accept, 168–69; undertreatment in, 170–71; unnecessary surgery and, 7. *See also* Health insurance, private; National health insurance

Haggerty, Robert J., 70
Halberstam, David, 2
Handschin, Richard, 173
Harlem Hospital, 55
Harris, Elma, 187–88, 191
Harris, Richard, 28
Harvard Community Health Plan, 255
Healey, Joseph, 268
Health centers, 38, 197–208; background of, 197–98; budgetary problems of, 202; doctors and, 202–203, 205–206; family health workers and, 199–201; infant mortality and, 199; Medicaid and, 197, 207–208; national health insurance and, 272–73; quality of care in, 50
Health insurance, private, 30–33, 149–61; cost of, 152; cut-rate hospital, 154–55; doctors' fees and, 156–57; extent of coverage under, 151–52; history of, 149–51; hospital care and, 137–46, 156; limitations on, 155, 157; national health insurance and, 157–59; poor and, 152–53. *See also* Group practice plans, National health insurance
Health Insurance Plan of New York (HIP), 89–91, 162, 174–75
Health Law Newsletter, 63
Health Maintenance Organizations (HMOs), 162–80; advantages of, 173–74; AMA and, 168–71; charges against, 170–73; cost of, 164–67; doctors' incomes under, 178–79; federal subsidies to, 163; foundation plans and, 176–78; history of, 162–63; impersonality of, 175; inducements to join, 244–45; nonprofessionals in, 270–73; reluctance of patients to accept, 168–69
Health Security bill, 211, 219, 221–30; allocating funds for, 242–43; educational standards of doctors and, 248–50; group prac-

tice plans and, 244–45; licensing of doctors and, 255; unnecessary surgery and, 232
Health Systems Agencies (HSAs), 269–70
Henderson, L. J., 67
Herr, Conrad, 198
Hoffmann-La Roche, 23, 27, 111–12, 128–29
Hollingshead, August B., 72, 74, 76–77
Holman, Edwin J., 97
Holmes County, Mississippi, 38
Hospitalization, unnecessary, 9–11, 137
Hospital Physician, 101
Hospitals, 1–14, 132–48; accreditation of, 98–104; charity care in, 49–66; cost of care in, 1–3, 238–40; denial of funds to, 145–46; duplication of services in, 147–48; health insurance and, 137–46, 154–56; inefficiency of, 13–14, 132–48; Medicaid and, 62–63; Medicare and, 185–86; national health insurance and, 238–40; nonsurgical use of, 9–11; occupancy rate in, 12–13, 137; PSROs and, 239–40; public, 63–66, 79–81; university, 62–63, 79–83; unnecessary surgery in, 4–9; voluntary, 63, 133–48
How to Avoid Unnecessary Surgery (Williams), 9
Hysterectomies, 5–7, 9, 41

Income, doctors', 16–20, 178–79
Incurable diseases, 78–79
Inefficiency, hospital, 13–14, 132–48
Infant mortality, 35–37, 199
Institute of Medicine, 42–43, 51
Insurance. *See* Group practice plans; Health insurance; Malpractice claims, insurance against; National health insurance

International Longshoremen's and Warehousemen's Union, 176
Internal Revenue Service, 17
Inter-Society Commission for Heart Disease, 11–12
Isoniazid, 112, 231

Javits, Jacob, 250, 257
Jenkins, Charles C., 148
Johnson, Lyndon B., 50, 182, 190, 197, 228
Johnson, Olive G., 6
Joint Commission on Hospital Accreditation, 17, 63–64, 98–102
Josephs, Deborah, 73
Journal of Nursing Administration, 268
Journal of the American Medical Association, 97

Kaiser-Permanente Health Plan, 7, 150, 162–80; choice of plans in, 169; cost of, 166; patients complaints about, 271; preventive medicine and, 168; waiting times under, 172
Kaitz, Edward, 142–43
Kallet, Arthur, 123
Katz, Leon A., 53
Kavaler, Florence, 53
Kefauver, Estes, 26–30, 111, 233
Kelman, Sander, 139
Kennedy, Edward M., xi, 99, 110–11, 211, 221, 224, 233, 249–50, 257
Kennedy, John F., 181
Kennedy-Mills bill, 211–14, 218–219
Kidney dialysis, 232
Knowles, John H., 15, 17, 79, 82

Larson, Leonard, 169
Lasagna, Louis, 24
Law and Contemporary Problems, 100
Lederle Laboratories, 122
Lembcke, Paul A., 6, 13
Lewis, Charles E., 4

Lewis, Sinclair, 90–91
Librium, 128–29
Licensing laws, 93, 249–50
Lilly, Eli, & Co., 23, 27, 119
Lincoln Hospital, New York, 55
Linkletter, Art, 155
Lloyd, William, 207
Long, Russell, 229
Los Angeles Times, 146–47, 170–71
Loughery, Richard M., 141
Lyford, Joseph, xv

McGill University, 215–17
McGovern, George, 229
McNeil Laboratories, 28
McNerney, Walter J., 159–60
Mail-order health insurance, 154–55
Malpractice claims, 95–109, 234–38; compulsory arbitration of, 236–37; insurance against, 105–109; limit to size of, 236–37; no-fault compensation and, 234–35
Maricopa County Medical Care Foundation, 178
Martens, Vernon E., 17
Martin Luther King, Jr., Health Center, New York, 201, 207, 261
Martin Luther King Hospital, Watts, 195
Massachusetts General Hospital, 79
Mastoidectomy, 102
Meany, George, 210, 225
Medicaid, 181–96; Blue Cross and, 158; cost of, 190; doctors' fees and, 15–16, 53–54, 193; eligibility for, 189–90; exploitation of, 191–92; health centers and, 182, 188; hospital admission and, 62–63; hospital costs and, 135–36; limitations of, 51–52; national health insurance and, 210; quality of care under, 193–94; reimbursement methods of, 240–41; unnecessary surgery and, 6; unwillingness of doctors to take patients on, 53; as welfare medium, 187–88
Medical Care, 205
Medical care, quality of, 34–48; doctor shortage and, 44–48; in emergency rooms, 41–42; in general practice, 43–44; government spending and, 242–45; humanizing to improve, 262–75; infant mortality and, 35–37; nonprofessionals and, 269–73; poor and, 37–38, 193–94; proposals for improving, 231–51; standards of, 39–41
Medical Committee for Human Rights, 204
Medical Economics, 2, 16–18, 71, 90, 147
Medical Letter, The, 123, 126–27
Medical practice, 84–109; commercialism of, 91; group, 89–90; malpractice in, 95–109; responsibility for, 91–94; traditional style of, 84–90
Medical schools, 20–23; AMA and, 21; choosing students for, 263–65; doctor shortage and, 253–55; emotional illness and, 75–76; foreign, 47; nondoctors in, 258; research in, 81–83
Medical Times, 95n
Medical University of South Carolina, 266
Medicare, 51, 181–96; AMA and, 181–82; Blue Cross and, 158; cost of, 184–87; doctors' fees and, 15–16, 18, 183–84; history of, 181–82; nursing-home care and, 186–87; reimbursement methods of, 240–41; unnecessary surgery and, 6
Medicare (Canada), 215–17
Medico Moderno, 127
Medicredit, 209–10, 228
Merck & Co., 23, 112
Messier, Edward A., 146

Messinger, Eli, 204, 206
Metropolitan Life Insurance Company, 30–31, 152
Michigan State Board of Registration in Medicine, 96
Mid-Westside Neighborhood Health Center, 202
Midwives, 37
Mills, Wilbur, 211
Minorities, 50, 56, 188, 192–93, 201
Montefiore Hospital, 89–90, 173
Moore, Francis D., 254
Morehead, Mildred, 193–94
Moser, Robert H., 26
Moss, Frank, 191–92
Motorola Company, 141, 178
Mound Bayou, Mississippi, 198–99
Mueller, Willard, 29
Mumford, Emily, 73, 82–83
Myers, Robert, 190

Nader, Ralph, 4, 99, 142, 220
National Academy of Sciences, 25, 42, 113, 247
National Cancer Foundation, 1
National Center for Clinical Pharmacology, 250
National Council of Senior Citizens, 186
National Farmers Union, 46
National health insurance, 157–61, 209–30; administrating, 224–26; AMA and, 209–10, 217–18, 226–30; areawide plans for, 257–58; in Canada, 214–17, 225; in England, 222; Health Security bill, 211, 219, 221–30; hospital costs and, 238–40; Kennedy-Mills bill, 211–14, 218–19; Medicaid and, 210; Nixon bill, 211–12, 217, 219; payment for, 211, 219, 221–30; regulation of, 219–21. *See also* Group practice plans; Health insurance, private
National Health Service (British), 5, 88, 222, 243; infant mortality and, 36

National Liberty Corporation, 154
National Urban Coalition, 210
Neighborhood Health Services Program, 201, 205
Nelson, Gaylord, 27, 111, 115–16, 233–34, 250
Nesson, Richard, 179
Netherlands, 134
New England Journal of Medicine, 5, 41, 247
New Handbook of Prescription Drugs, 28
New health practitioners (NHPs), 259–61
New Jersey Medical Association, 94
Newman, Harold, 172
New Times, 133n
New York City Health and Hospitals Corporation, 64
New York City Health Department, 53
New York Post, 55
New York Times, 73
Nixon, Richard M., 163, 222, 224
Nixon health insurance bill, 211–12, 217, 219
No-fault compensation, 234–35
Nondoctors, 258–61
Northwestern National, 167n
Nurse practitioners, 258–61
Nursing homes, 186–87

Occupancy rate, hospital, 12–13, 137
Office of Economic Opportunity (OEO), 202–203
Office visits, 43–44
Olson, Culbert L., 151
Ombudsman, patients', 88, 268–69
Open-heart surgery, 11–12
Ortho-Pharmaceutical, 122
Outpatient clinics, 57–61; doctors' attitudes in, 60–61; impersonality of, 59; waiting time in, 58–59

Parke Davis & Co., 115–16
Parrot, Robert H., 147
Participation, community, 206–207, 270–73
Patent laws, 234
Patients' rights, 267–69
Pediatrics, 260
Peer review, 91–95, 101–109; doctors' opposition to, 91–95; government pressure and, 246; health insurance and, 157
Peterson, Osler, 43, 48, 93
Pfizer, 27, 117
Pharmaceutical Manufacturers Association (PMA), 29, 124
Pharmacology. *See* Drug industry
Physician's assistant (PA), 258–61
Physician's Desk Reference, 124
Pillard, Richard, 120
Pills. *See* Prescription drugs
Porterfield, John, 99–102
Poverty. *See* Charity care
Prepaid practice. *See* Group practice plans
Prescription drugs, 23–30, 110–31; advertising of, 117–22; in combinations, 112–13; effectiveness of, 113–15; FDA restrictions on, 125–28; generic vs. brand names for, 28, 128–31; information on, 233–34
President's Commission on Heart Disease, Cancer and Strokes, 12
Preventive medicine, 78–79, 167–68
Professional Liability Newsletter, 107
Professional Standards Review Organizations (PSROs), 104, 185, 226, 228; government pressure on, 245–48; hospitals and, 239–40
Profession of Medicine (Freidson), 92
Providence Hospital, Oakland, 148
Public hospitals, 132; charity care in, 63–66, 79–81
Pure Food and Drug Act, 113, 118

Rapoport, Roger, 133*n*
Real Voice, The (Harris), 28–29
Reinhard, Edward H., 262
Research, biomedical, 81–83, 263
Ribicoff, Abraham, 159, 229
Rights, patients', 267–69
Ritalin, 121–22
Robinson, E. A., xii
Robinson, Janice, 203–204
Robinson, Jerry M., 16
Rockefeller, Nelson, 189
Roemer, Milton I., 34–35, 166–67, 172, 175–76
Rothschild, Edmund O., 64
Roy, William, 255
Rubsamen, David, 107
Rural practice, 45–46, 256–57
Russia, 9–10, 88
Rutstein, David D., 37

St. Luke's Hospital, New York, 145–46, 203
Salber, Eva J., 206
Samuel Merritt Hospital, 148
San Diego Foundation for Medical Care, 18
Sandoz Pharmaceuticals, 120–21
San Francisco General Hospital, 64
San Joaquin (California) Foundation for Medical Care, 176–77
Santa Monica Community Hospital, 265
Schering Corporation, 26–27
Schmidt, Alexander M., 130
Schwartz, Jerome L., 271
Scientific medicine, 67–83; change in doctor-patient relationship in, 71–78; chronic illness and, 78–79; emotional illness and, 75–78; humanizing, 262–75; medical schools and, 81–83; organic disease and, 75; specialists and, 68–71; terminal illness and, 73–75, 78–79; university hospitals and, 79–81
Searle & Co., G. D., 122

Senate Finance Committee, 184
Senate Subcommittee on Antitrust and Monopoly, 26, 29, 115–16, 125
Serentil, 120–21
Serino, Ronald, 122
Shargel, Martin, 26
Shaw, George Bernard, 4
Shortage, doctor, 44–48, 252–61; AMA and, 253; family-practice residencies and, 253–55; foreign medical graduates and, 252–53; Health Security bill and, 255; paramedical personnel and, 258–61; relocating doctors to avoid, 255–58
Sickness and Society (Duff and Hollingshead), 72
Siegel, Barry, 55
Silver, George A., 210
Silver, Laurens H., 100
Simmons, Henry E., 126
Sinequan, 117
Skrbkova, Emile, 89
Slater, Robert E., 154
Smythe, Mrs. Patrick, 32–33
Social Security Administration, 30
Society of Urban Physicians, 64
Space Age Computer Systems, 140
Specialists, 44, 68–71; family-practice physicians as, 70–71; qualifying as, 85–86, 254–55
Squibb & Sons, E. R., 23, 111–12
Standard, Samuel, 205
Standards, performance, 39–41
Steinbeck, John, 11
Stern, Thomas, 266
Stetler, C. Joseph, 29
Stevenson, Robert L., Jr., 41–42, 58
Stolley, Paul D., 24–25
Stone, Joseph, 99
Sudnow, David, 65, 74
Suffolk County Medical Society, 190
Supreme Court of Illinois, 103
Surgeons' fees, 22–23
Surgery, unnecessary, 4–9, 102, 136–37, 232

Sweden, 13–14, 134; infant mortality in, 36–37

Teamsters' Union, 39–40
Terminal illness, 73–75
Tofranil, 120
Tonsillectomies, 5–9, 102
Trademark laws, 128–31
Tranquilizers, 27, 117, 120–21
Truman, Harry S, 181, 209
Tufts University School of Medicine, 198

Undertreatment, 170–71
Union Fidelity Life, 154
United Mine Workers, 7
United Store Workers Union, 7
University hospitals: advantages of, 79–81; charity care in, 62–63; research in, 81–83. *See also* Hospitals
University of Illinois Medical School, 265
University of Pittsburgh, 215–17

Vacek, Milos, 89
Valium, 27
Van Doren, Mark, 71
Venality, 4, 190–92
Verstandig, Charles, 91
Veterans Administration, 182
Vitamin B_{12}, 24, 112
Voluntary hospitals, 132–48; abuses in, 139–43; administration of, 133–36; charity care in, 63; cost of care in, 135–36; denial of funds to, 145–48; health insurance and, 137–46, 154–56; occupancy rate in, 137; unnecessary surgery in, 136–37. *See also* Hospitals

Wallace Laboratories, 119
Warren, James V., 126
Washington, D.C., Hospital Center, 140–41
Washington Post, 12, 17, 140, 147
Weinerman, Richard, 173

Welfare cases. *See* Charity care
Western Voice of Motorola, 141
White, Kerr, 39*n*
Williams, Lawrence P., 9
Winstrol Compound, 127–28
Winthrop Laboratories, 127
Wise, Harold B., 49, 201, 261
Wolfe, Sidney, 4–5
Women's movement, 5

Woodcock, Leonard, 31
Workmen's compensation, 235
Worthington, William, 100

X-rays, 42

Yankee Hospital, 75–78

Zactirin, 114, 123

LIBRARY OF DAVIDSON COLLEGE

Books on regular loan may be checked out for **two weeks**. Books must be presented at the Circulation Desk in order to be renewed.

A fine is charged after date due.

Special books are subject to special regulations at the discretion of library staff.

MAR -9 1976	MAY - 4 1981		
APR. -1 1976			
JAN. 15 1977	DEC 06 1992		
FEB. 13 1977			
FEB. 23 1977			
SEP. 21 1977			
OCT. 29 1977			
MAY -3 1978			
MAR 11 1980			
JAN. -6 1981			
JAN 25 1981			
FEB -9 1981			
FEB 25 1981			
MAR 10 1981			